LOW BACK PAIN
SYNDROME

EDITION 4

LOW BACK PAIN
SYNDROME

RENE CAILLIET, M.D.

Clinical Professor
School of Medicine
Chairman (Retired)
Department of Physical Medicine and Rehabilitation
University of Southern California
Los Angeles, California
Director
Rehabilitation Services
Santa Monica Hospital Medical Center
Santa Monica, California

Illustrations by R. Cailliet, M.D.

 F.A. Davis Company • Philadelphia

Also by Rene Cailliet:

Foot and Ankle Pain
Hand Pain and Impairment
Knee Pain and Disability
Neck and Arm Pain
Scoliosis
The Shoulder in Hemiplegia
Shoulder Pain
Soft Tissue Pain and Disability

Copyright © 1988 by F.A. Davis Company
Fourth printing 1991

All rights reserved. This book is protected by copyright. No part of it may be reproduced, stored in a retrieval system, or transmitted in any form or by any means, electronic, mechanical, photocopying, recording, or otherwise, without written permission from the publisher.

Printed in the United States of America

10 9 8 7 6 5 4

Library of Congress Cataloging-in-Publication Data

Cailliet, Rene.
    Low back pain syndrome.

    Includes bibliographies and index.
    1. Backache.   I. Title.   [DNLM: 1. Backache.
WE 755 C134L]
RD771.B217C35   1988   617'.56   88-11810
ISBN 0-8036-1606-6

Authorization to photocopy items for internal or personal use, or the internal or personal use of specific clients, is granted by F. A. Davis Company for users registered with the Copyright Clearance Center (CCC) Transactional Reporting Service, provided that the fee of $.10 per copy is paid directly to CCC, 27 Congress St., Salem, MA 01970. For those organizations that have been granted a photocopy license by CCC, a separate system of payment has been arranged. The fee code for users of the Transactional Reporting Service is: 8036-1606/88 0 + $.10.

Preface

Ten years have passed since the first volume, and three editions of *Low Back Pain Syndrome* have been presented to the medical public. Every year, new concepts have emerged, new theories have been proffered, new diagnostic terms have emerged, new forms of treatment have been propounded, and much of what was considered verified has been refuted.

So much research and clinical experience has been recorded that a complete rewriting of *Low Back Pain Syndrome* appears needed.

The term "syndrome" appears in the literature and will probably so remain. "Syndrome" is defined by Webster as "in medicine . . . a number of symptoms occurring together and characterizing a specific disease." There is a paradox in retaining the term "syndrome" when viewed in this context, because there are a number of symptoms, but no specific disease can be deduced from them.

With the exception of painful diseases of the bones of the vertebral column—such as metastatic disease, multiple myeloma, Paget's disease—all low back pain and disabilities of the spine can be considered mechanically caused. The term "disease" is therefore in question except in that, to paraphrase Webster, it interrupts or impairs any or all of the natural and regular functions of an organ of a living body and afflicts one with pain or sickness. The "organ," in this case, the lumbosacral spine, must be fully understood in a functional respect. If one assumes that there is a deviation from normal function caused by insult, injury, stress, or trauma, the normal function must be uppermost in the mind of the diagnostician and the therapist in evaluating the patient complaining of and disabled by low back pain.

The magnitude of the low back pain problem is financially formidable and involves many persons. It is a disease that needs a great deal of study and understanding, for low back pain remains an enigma of medical science for the patient, the insurance carrier, attorneys, employers, and family members.

The format of the book has been altered. The sequence of chapters and their contents have changed, and the conclusions have been revised. It is hoped that this new edition will cast light on otherwise unanswered questions and lead to a more rational approach to bringing relief to the afflicted.

RENE CAILLIET, M.D.

Contents

ix

Illustrations

CHAPTER 1

Functional Anatomy

Most pain and disability of the low back (lumbosacral spine) is mechanical in nature. Thus, the **functional** spine must be analyzed, examined, and understood in its normal state before abnormal spine function, causing pain and impairment, can be understood.

The spine, or vertebral column, is an aggregate of superimposed segments that can be termed **functional units** (Fig. 1–1). The functional unit is composed of two adjacent vertebral bodies, one superincumbent on the other, separated by an intervertebral disk. The anterior segment of the functional unit (Fig. 1–2) is essentially a supporting, weight-bearing, shock-absorbing, flexible structure. The posterior segment of the functional unit (see Fig. 1–2) is a non–weight-bearing structure that contains and protects the neural structures of the central nervous system as well as paired joints that function to direct the movement of the unit.

Each functional unit contains all the tissues needed for total function. These tissues may be nociceptive, causing pain. Impairment of any part of the unit may lead to functional impairment of the total system.

Five of these functional units in the lower back constitute the **lumbosacral spine** (Fig. 1–3). The lumbosacral spine, viewed as a functional, mechanical structure, is the basis for clinical evaluation of low back pain.

The spine functions to support two-legged mankind in standing, sitting, walking, bending, and every aspect of the performance of the activities of daily living. It is subservient to the forces of gravity and must conform to these forces with the minimum exertion of energy. It must minimize the ravages of wear and tear and perform repeated tasks without failure.

When the spine "fails," the causative or contributing factors must be analyzed. External forces must be related to the failure, and the tissues that

1

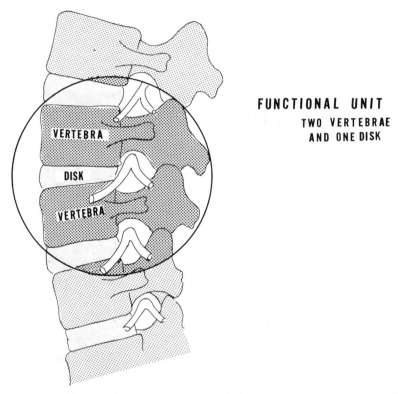

FUNCTIONAL UNIT
TWO VERTEBRAE
AND ONE DISK

Figure 1–1. Functional unit of the spine. The basic structural component of the spine is the functional unit, which consists of two adjacent vertebrae separated by the disk. (Modified from Cailliet, R: Understand Your Backache. FA Davis, Philadelphia, 1984, p 7.)

ultimately fail must be identified. The tissues from which pain originates must also be identified.

Let us analyze the functional unit as a separate structure, then combine the five units of the lumbosacral spine and evaluate the total system.

ANTERIOR WEIGHT-BEARING PORTION OF THE FUNCTIONAL UNIT

The anterior weight-bearing portion of the vertebral functional unit (see Fig. 1–2) is ideally constructed. It is comprised of two adjacent rounded vertebrae flattened at their cephalad and caudal ends.

At birth and throughout maturation, the caudal and cephalic ends of the vertebrae are slightly convex and coated with cartilage. These cartilage endplates gradually undergo ossification from age 15 to 20 and fuse with

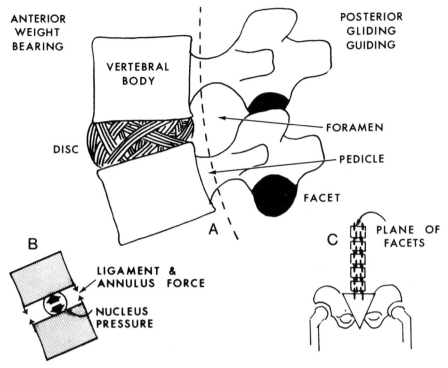

ANTERIOR
WEIGHT
BEARING

VERTEBRAL
BODY

DISC

POSTERIOR
GLIDING
GUIDING

FORAMEN

PEDICLE

FACET

B

A

C

PLANE OF
FACETS

LIGAMENT &
ANNULUS FORCE

NUCLEUS
PRESSURE

Figure 1–2. Functional unit of the spine in cross-section. Anteriorly are two verte-brae separated by the disk and lined by the longitudinal ligaments. Posteriorly is the neural arch containing the facets and forming the spinal canal and the foramina.

the vertebral bodies. There is an ossification layer at each endplate, termed an "epiphysis," that is the growth center of that vertebra (Fig. 1–4). These epiphyseal centers remain active throughout growth and are influenced by Wolff's Law with regard to pressure reaction (Fig. 1–5). The spine main-tains its alignment essentially as the epiphyseal growth progresses symmet-rically.

Within the anterior weight-bearing portion of the functional unit, be-tween each pair of vertebrae, is the intervertebral disk.

THE INTERVERTEBRAL DISK

The **intervertebral disk** is a hydrodynamic elastic structure that is in-terposed between two adjacent vertebrae, separating them and acting as a shock-absorbing mechanism. Its fluid composition permits motion. Struc-turally, it is composed of a central nucleus (pulposus) enclosed within an annulus (fibrosus) (Fig. 1–6).

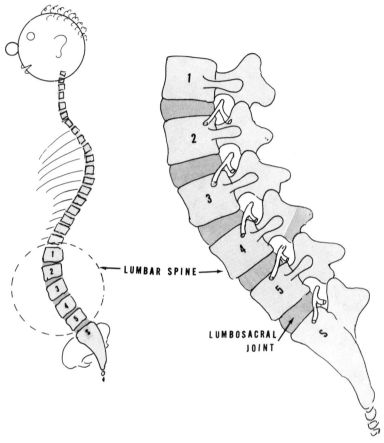

Figure 1–3. The lumbosacral spine. The lumbosacral portion of the spine consists of five functional units in the lower back. (Modified from Cailliet, R: Understand Your Backache. FA Davis, Philadelphia, 1984, p 5.)

The nucleus is a homogeneous, elastic globoid centrally located within a fibrocartilaginous envelope. This nucleus is predominantly a mucopolysaccharide homogeneous matrix containing a rich network of fine banded fibrils layered in a random manner. These fibrils form a sheet with the fibrils interlocking at a 60-degree angle (Fig. 1–7). This orientation imparts tensile strength against deforming forces.

The mucopolysaccharide of the matrix is a soluble protein loosely bound to a complex polysaccharide polymer, which includes hexose sucrose, hyaluronidase, chondroitin sulphate, and many other components. Within the matrix are numerous negative acid radicals that tend to bind water. This combination forms a sponge-like tissue.

The mechanical arrangement of the fibers accounts for its elasticity and

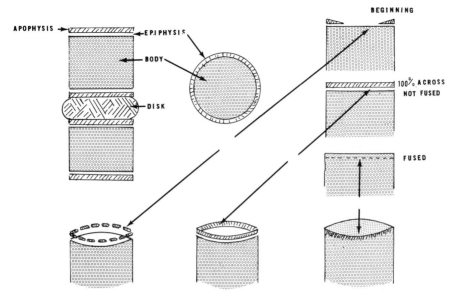

Figure 1–4. Epiphyseal bone growth. As children mature, their vertebral bodies grow from their endplates (epiphyses). By maturity, the endplates "fuse" with the vertebral body and further vertical growth ceases. (From Cailliet, R: Scoliosis: Diagnosis and Management. FA Davis, Philadelphia, 1975 , p 35, with permission.)

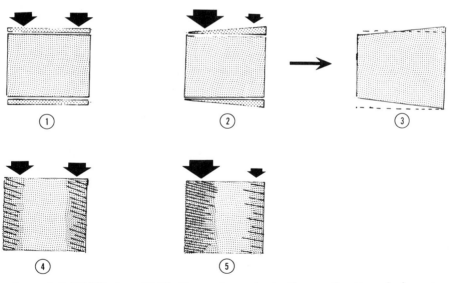

Figure 1–5. Wolff's Law (1868). Every change in the form or function of a bone is followed by certain definite changes in its internal architecture and its external shape. (1) Equal pressure to the epiphyseal plates results in symmetrical growth. (2) Asymmetrical pressure results in (3) asymmetrical growth and vertebral deformity. (4) Internal architecture with equal pressure. (5) Architectural changes from asymmetrical pressure. (Modified from Cailliet, R: Scoliosis: Diagnosis and Management. FA Davis, Philadelphia, 1975, p 46.)

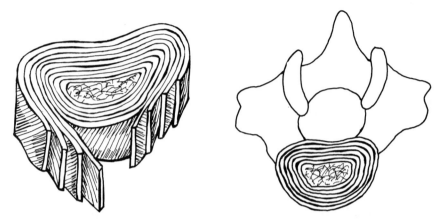

Figure 1–6. Annulus fibrosus. *Left,* Layer concept of annulus fibrosus. *Right,* Circumferential annular fibers around the central, pulpy nucleus (nucleus pulposus).

its tensile strength. The gel status of the matrix is the basis for its hydration pressure.

For years, osmosis was considered the basis for variable hydration of the disk matrix due to its colloidal state and its anion radicals. Further studies (Hendry 1958) have clearly shown that osmosis plays only a small role in the hydration of the matrix. Most disk hydration occurs via imbibition.

The weight-bearing function of the disk based exclusively on hydrodynamic principles is now being questioned (Fanfan et al, 1970). The function of weight bearing is considered to reside within the annular fiber structure. This concept is based on the functional structure of the individual collagen fibers and their unification into sheets with alternating fiber angulation. The central hydrodynamic pressure of the nucleus is related to its action on this annular fiber arrangement.

The disk annulus is composed of layered sheets of collagen fibers. The sheet of collagen fibers reacts to tension elongation as does each individual collagen fiber. Each collagen fiber originates around the circumference of the vertebral endplate passing to the adjacent vertebral endplate at a specific angulation (approximately 30 degrees).

An individual collagen fiber is a trihelix intertwined chain of amino acids connected chemically and electrically (Fig. 1–8). Individual collagen fibers have a physiologic compliance to elongating forces that is their mechanical efficiency and simultaneously their vulnerability to failure from excessive stress.

The collagen fiber, a spiral intertwined structure, elongates by uncurling (i.e., straightening). This uncurling is limited; and when the elongating force is released, the fibril recurls to its original condition (see Fig. 1–8). Excessive tension on the fibril may break the chemical-electrical bond between the constituent amino acids and the collagen fiber will "fail." By frag-

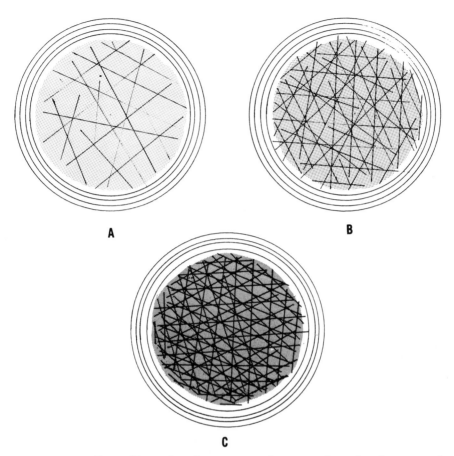

Figure 1–7. Collagen fibers of nucleus matrix. The mucopolysaccharide matrix of the nucleus has sparce, randomly directed collagen fibrils (*A*). As aging or deterioration progresses, the fibrils increase in number and thickness (*B* and *C*).

menting the amino acid chain, the fiber loses its elasticity: it does not recoil, and therefore loses its tensile strength. This physical aspect of the collagen fibril plays an important role in the integrity and the pathology of the annulus of the disk.

It can be summarized that the intervertebral disk functions by virtue of its component parts: mechanically by virtue of the structure and function of the annular collagen fibers, and chemically and hydrodynamically by the dynamics of the mucopolysaccharide matrix.

The natural history of the intervertebral disk evolves with certain contributing factors:

1. The disk in early human development is nourished by direct blood supply. The blood vessels pass through the vertebral endplates directly into

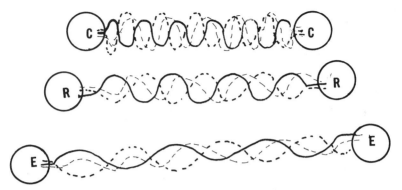

Figure 1–8. Collagen fiber (schematic). A collagen fiber is a coiled trihelix chain of connected amino acids (C). It elongates (E) by uncoiling and has a physiological length when fully uncoiled. Excessive force upon uncoiled fibril fragments the amino acid bonds preventing return to relaxed status (R).

the intervertebral disk. By the age of maturation, when the epiphysis closes with cessation of further physiologic growth, the endplates calcify. The blood vessels are obliterated and the intervertebral disk becomes ischemic. From that point on, nutrition of the disk is by osmosis and by imbibition of a filtrate of adjacent blood supply (Fig. 1–9). If imbibition by the disk is a factor in its nutrition, it is mandatory that there is alternating compression and relaxation of the disk to ensure its "sponge imbibition action." Mechanically, this sponge-like imbibition ensures entry of fluid through the semi-permeable membranes: the endplates of the vertebra and the outer annular envelopes of the disk.

2. There exists an intrinsic internal pressure within the disk that functions to separate the vertebral endplates and maintains pressure on the annular fibers, thus keeping them elongated and under a degree of tension (Fig. 1–10). Mechanically, it is apparent that the annular fibers would become slack if the internal hydrodynamic pressure within the nucleus dropped and did not take up the slack. This becomes a self-monitoring effect.

3. The nucleus undergoes physical chemical changes with aging and from mechanical injuries that impair the function of the annulus. The mucopolysaccharides of the matrix undergo degradation (Naylor 1976) and re-formation into an inferior type of polysaccharide. This degraded and re-constituted mucopolysaccharide absorbs excessive water (hydration) but cannot retain it within the matrix. The reasons for matrix degradation remain unexplained. There are undoubtedly genetic factors that play a part in early and excessive degradation. It is also probable that there are metabolic factors in this chemical process. Endocrine factors also are considered to be involved. These factors will be elucidated later during the discussion of emotional stress. Mechanical "failure" of the annular fibers plays a vital

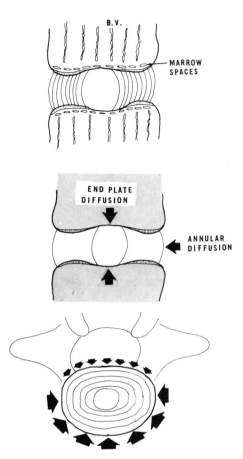

Figure 1–9. Disk nutrition through diffusion. Diffusion of solutes occurs through the central portion of the endplates and through the annulus. Marrow spaces exist between circulation and hyaline cartilage and are more numerous in the annulus than in the nucleus. Glucose and oxygen enter via the endplates. Sulfate to form glucosaminoglycans enters through the annulus. There is less diffusion into the posterior annulus. (B.V. = blood vessels.)

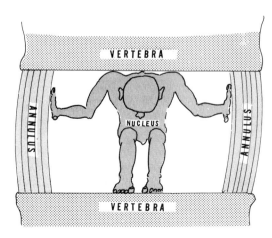

Figure 1–10. Function of nucleus pulposus (schematic). The nucleus pulposus has an intrinsic pressure that keeps the vertical endplates separated and the annular fiber sheets taut. (From Cailliet, R: Understand Your Backache. FA Davis, Philadelphia, 1984, p 17, with permission.)

part in this matrix degradation but the question of which comes first—matrix degradation or annular fiber failure—remains conjectural.

4. The function of the annulus in spinal motion has been re-evaluated (Farfan 1970) in a provocative manner. It has been well documented that a compressive force fractures the vertebral endplates before the force injures the annulus. Flexion and extension of the functional unit are well tolerated by the annular fibers. Excessive flexion is prevented by the posterior elements of erector spinae muscles, the fascia, ligaments, and the longitudinal ligaments. Excessive extension is mechanically, structurally prevented (Fig. 1–11). Rotatory torque is limited by the elongation of the annular collagen fibers of the disk and the mechanical structural limitation posed by the facet alignment. The mechanical limitation plays a major role, as excessive rotational elongation of the annular collagen fibers can disrupt their integrity. It has been postulated that annular fibers "fail" (i.e., disrupt) after exceeding 5 degrees of rotation. The site of failure varies because of the differences in angulation and length of annular fibers in the outer sheets

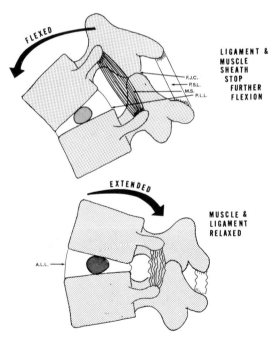

Figure 1–11. Restraints of flexion-extension of the functional unit. Excessive flexion of a functional unit is prevented by the posterior soft tissues: posterior longitudinal ligament (P.L.L.), muscle sheath (M.S.), posterior superficial ligaments (P.S.L.), and facet joint capsules (F.J.C.). Extension is restricted by mechanical impact of the facet joints and by the anterior longitudinal ligament (A.L.L.). (Modified from Cailliet, R: Understand Your Backache. FA Davis, Philadelphia, 1984, p 35.)

compared with the inner sheets (Fig. 1–12). Since the circumference of the annulus is much less in the inner layer than the outer layer, the verticality of the individual collagen fibers differs. The inner fibers are more vertical and thus do not elongate as much as the outer fibers on rotation. This probably accounts for the outer fibers being "torn" (failing) on rotation forces exceeding 5 degrees. With simultaneous compression, bringing the vertical endplates closer together, the fibers further angulate. Failure is thus enhanced by the combination of compression and rotation. These factors are examplified in Fig. 1–12 and Fig. 1–13. With tearing of annular fibers, the remaining fibers of more inner layers cannot maintain "stiffness" (tension of the fiber sheets); thus instability of the functional unit results.

5. The nucleus and annulus mucopolysaccharide, a colloidal gel, is 88 percent water at maturation. As aging occurs the percentage of hydration decreases to 80 percent or less.

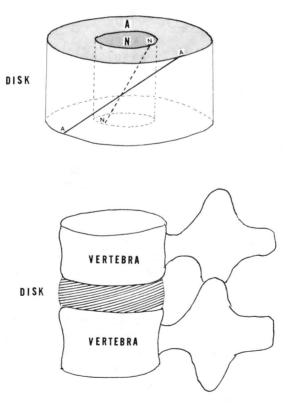

Figure 1–12. Annular fiber. The *upper figure* is a schematic analysis of the intervertebral disk in the functional unit (*lower figure*). A = Annulus. N = Nucleus. There are the same number of collagen fibers in the outer sheath (A _____ A) and in the inner sheath (N_____N). The difference is their angulation and length.

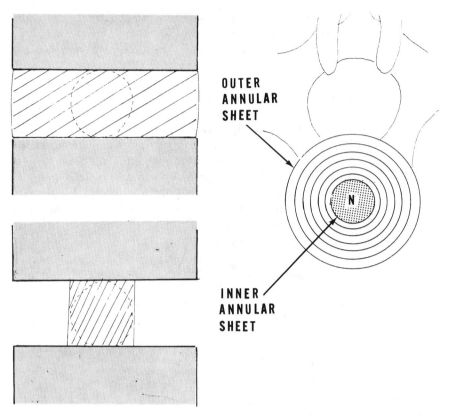

Figure 1–13. Angulation of annular fibers. In the outer sheath, the annular fibers form approximately 30-degree angles. The inner sheath has the same number of fibers as the outer sheath, but a smaller circumference, and thus the fibers have a different angulation. Rotational torque of the disk elongates the outer sheath more than the inner sheath and can cause "failure" of the collagen fibers.

The solutes that nourish the disk diffuse through the central portion of the endplates and through the annulus (see Fig. 1–9). Increased intradiskal pressure probably forces fluid through the minute foramina of the calcified endplates. Upon release of external pressure, which has compressed the disk, the disk reexpands, and fluid is imbibed inward. As the disk ages, be it from age attrition or prematurely from injury to the annulus, the mucopolysaccharide undergoes degradation and loses its normal imbibitory capacity. On degradation the matrix can absorb more water but not retain it. Ions, especially sodium and potassium, migrate through the permeable tissues and act in osmotic action.

The intervertebral disks are reinforced and protected by the longitudinal ligaments. These ligaments run the length of the vertebral column anteriorly and posteriorly. They are adherent to the vertebral body cortex by

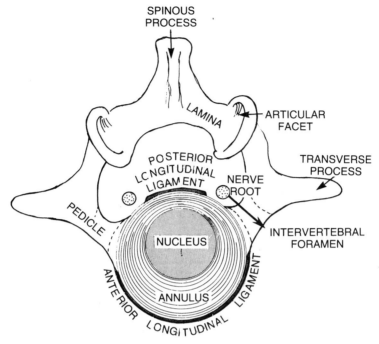

Figure 1–14. Components of the functional unit, viewed from above.

Sharpey fibers and in their passage across the intervertebral spaces are essentially the outer layer of annular fibers (Fig. 1–14). It is of interest that the posterior longitudinal ligament is intact throughout the entire length of the vertebral column until it reaches the lower lumbar region (L3, L4, L5, and S1) where it narrows to approximately half its width (Fig. 1–15).

POSTERIOR PORTION OF THE FUNCTIONAL UNIT

The posterior portion of the functional unit can be considered the neural arch in that it forms the outer walls of the spinal canal (Fig. 1–16, *top view*). The neural arch originates from the posterolateral aspects of the vertebral bodies and extends posteriorly as pedicles to form the lateral transverse processes. It then widens to form the zygapophyseal (facet) joints that reside within the lateral laminae. The laminae continue posteromedially to rejoin centrally and form the posterior superior spine.

The processes of the posterior arch, the transverse processes, the lamina, and the posterior superior processes are the sites of attachment of the extensor musculature. These muscles will receive specific description in discussing the kinetic spine.

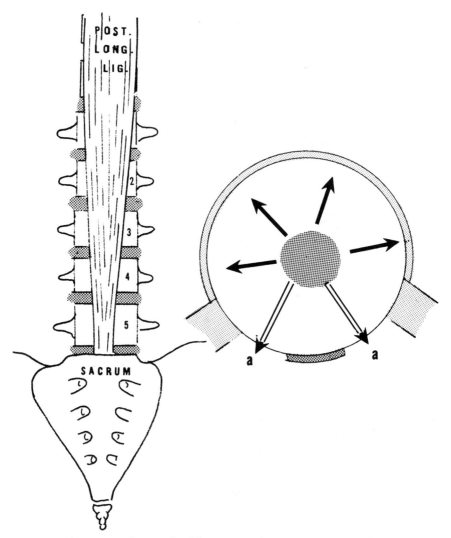

Figure 1–15. Posterior longitudinal ligament. The posterior longitudinal ligament narrows in the lower lumbar region. At L5 it covers less than half of the posterior disk margin (*arrows*). The *double arrows* (a) show where disk herniation may bulge into the spinal canal.

The zygapophyseal joints (facets) lie in a vertical sagittal plane (see Fig. 1–16, *rear view*). The superior facets of an articulation are the inferior facets of the superior vertebrae, and they reside medially to the inferior facets, which are the superior facets of the inferior vertebrae. As stated, the facets, being sagittal (vertical), allow essentially flexion and extension but markedly restrict lateral flexion and especially rotation (Fig. 1–17).

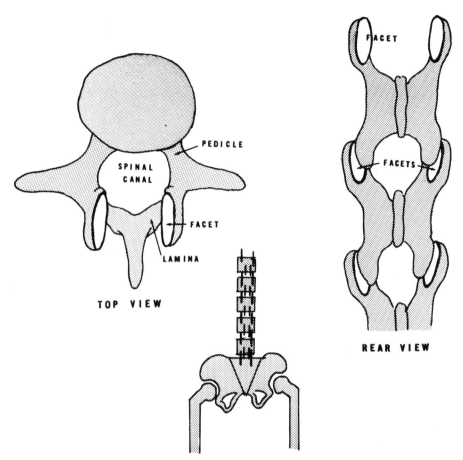

PEDICLE

SPINAL
CANAL

FACET

LAMINA

TOP VIEW

FACET

FACETS

REAR VIEW

Figure 1-16. Facet alignment. The zygapophyseal facets have a vertical alignment and allow flexion-extension but limit lateral and rotational movement.

Rotation of the functional unit causes damage to the annular fibers of the intervertebral disk. As stated during the discussion on the annulus, rotation causes stiffening of the annular fibers with limitation of rotation. The nucleus, being a gel, provides little or no resistance to torsion. Approximately 40 to 50 percent of the torque strength of the whole joint is provided by the disk annulus. The rest is provided by the posterior articulations: the facets, their capsules, and the interspinous ligaments.

With flexion of the lumbosacral spine and simultaneous rotation and lateral flexion, there occurs some separation of the facets on the convex side of the curvature. The facets on the concave side become approximated and act as a fulcrum around which the functional unit rotates. Rotation about this facet approachment causes lateral shear of the anterior aspect of the

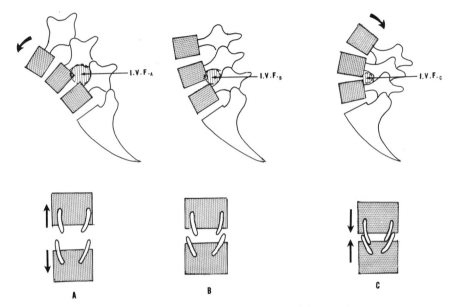

Figure 1–17. Facet movement in flexion and hyperextension.

functional unit, the disk; thus, further damage can occur to the outer annular fibers (Fig. 1–18).

As the lumbar spine laterally flexes, there is mandatory simultaneous rotation toward the side that the spine bends (Lovette 1907). In this motion the following occurs within the functional unit (see Fig. 1–18).

1. The facets on the concave side (toward which the spine is bending) approximate.

2. The facets on the side from which the spine is bending separate. This separation is physiologically permitted due to the flexibility of the joint capsule. Excessive flexion and rotation can sublux the joint with stretching or tearing the capsule.

3. The intervertebral disk is sheared laterally with a degree of rotation. Normal movement of limited flexion and rotation of the annular fibers permits this degree of extensibility. Excessive rotatory movement results in tearing of the annular fibers. The tearing of the annular sheets is usually and initially of the outer sheet of collagen fibers.

4. Normal movement does not change the width or the content of the foraminae to an abnormal unphysiologic degree. The spinal canal and the intervertebral foraminae remain patent. Abnormal movement can alter these spaces and compress or injure their contents.

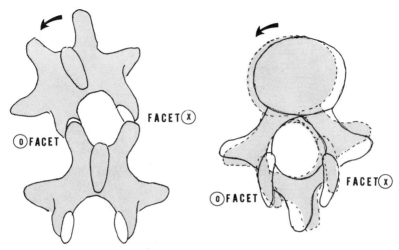

FACET (X)

(O) FACET

FACET (X)

(O) FACET

Figure 1–18. Lateral flexion-rotational torque. When a person bends to the side, the facets on the concave side (O) approximate and can become the axis of rotation. The opposite facets (X) open and cause the vertebral bodies to shear (*arrow*) toward the concave side. If this movement is excessive, the concave facets (O) can "jam," the convex facets (X) can sublux, and the disk annular fibers can tear.

MUSCLES OF THE FUNCTIONAL UNIT

The erector spinae (sacrospinalis) muscles originate from the last two thoracic vertebrae, the lumbar vertebrae, the sacral spine, the sacrum, the sacroiliac ligament, and the medial aspect of the iliac crest. Below the twelfth rib, the muscle splits into three columns (Fig. 1–19):

1. Iliocostal—lateral band
2. Longissimus—intermediate band
3. Spinalis—medial band

The iliocostal (lateral band) muscle inserts into the angle of the rib cage and ultimately extends to C4 to Th6. The muscle extends over six rib segments in the thoracic spine.

The longissimus (intermediate band) inserts into the transverse processes cephalad to T1. It is the only erector spinae muscle to reach the skull.

The spinalis (medial band) is essentially a flat aponeurosis muscle. Its medial border attaches to the posterior spines of the thoracic vertebrae. The lateral margin of this muscle is free of bony attachment.

Under the erector spinae muscles is located the transverse spinae muscle, which is comprised of three layers:

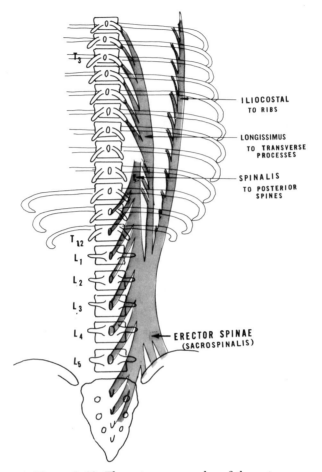

Figure 1–19. The extensor muscles of the spine.

1. Semispinalis
2. Multifidus
3. Rotatores

The semispinalis (superficial layer) arises from the tips of the transverse processes of the vertebrae and inserts into the tips of the posterior spinous processes. It spans three to five segments.

The multifidus arises as a thick, fleshy mass on the dorsum of the sacrum, between the spinous and transversus crest, from the overlying erector spinae aponeurosis, and from all the transverse processes up to C4 vertebrae. This muscle spans three vertebral segments to attach to the inferior border of the next transverse process above it.

The rotatores (rotator) span only one segment: from the transverse process of one vertebra to the spinous process of the adjacent vertebra (Fig. 1–20).

In the lumbar spine there are other small muscles (see Fig. 1–20):

1. Interspinalis (interspinal), which unite adjacent lumbar spinous processes.

2. Intertransversarii (intertransverse), which unite transverse processes of adjacent vertebrae.

The erector spinae muscles are considered extensors in that they cause the spine to return to the erect position after the person has bent over. They are powerful extensors, but they also act eccentrically in that they elongate to allow the spine to forward flex.

The speed and degree of muscle elongation or contraction, depending on whether spine flexion or reextension is occurring, is a neuromuscular activity that is dependent on proprioceptive sensory stimuli that are transmitted via intrinsic unmyelinated and myelinated nerves within the muscles and their muscle sheaths. These impulses are then transmitted and coordinated by a complex neurologic reflex pattern within the spinal cord. This will be further discussed, to the degree it is currently understood, in discussion of the kinetic spine.

The erector spinae muscles, as are all muscles of the musculoskeletal system, are contained within myofascial sheaths. These fascial sheaths play a mechanical activity in musculoskeletal function. They are involved in proprioceptive as well as nociceptive sites of stimuli. They become involved pathologically after injury.

The thoracolumbar fascia plays a major role in spine function and merits special consideration. There is controversy as to whether and to what degree the fascia plays a role in the re-extension of the bent over spine and

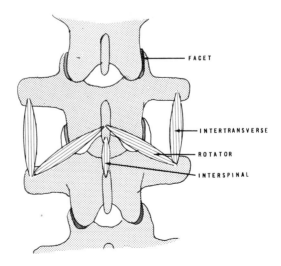

Figure 1–20. Deep extensor spinal muscles.

in lifting activities. There is also consideration as to whether and how the fascia plays a role in the maintenance of the erect static spine. These controversies will be considered in subsequent chapters. At this point it is pertinent to merely evaluate the structural aspect of the spinal erector muscles and their fascia.

The thoracolumbar fascia consists of three layers: deep, middle, and superficial. The **deep** layer covers the quadratus lumborum. It attaches to the transverse processes of the vertebrae (Fig. 1–21). This deep layer forms bands that attach to the posterior-superior aspect of the transverse process. The fibers radiate posterocaudally as shown in Fig. 1–22.

The **middle** layer arises from the ends of the transverse processes of the vertebae. This layer is thick and at the lumbar levels 1 to 3 has two

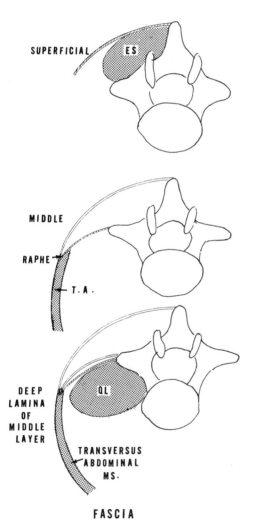

FASCIA

Figure 1–21. Thoracolumbar fascial layers. There are three layers of the thoracolumbar fascia. The superficial covers all the erector spinae muscles but does not attach to the transverse abdominal muscles. The middle fascial layer is divided into two layers that attach primarily to the lateral tips of the transverse processes and to the laminae. The deep muscle groups and their fascia (as depicted in Fig. 1–22) emit a downward lateral pull on the spine.

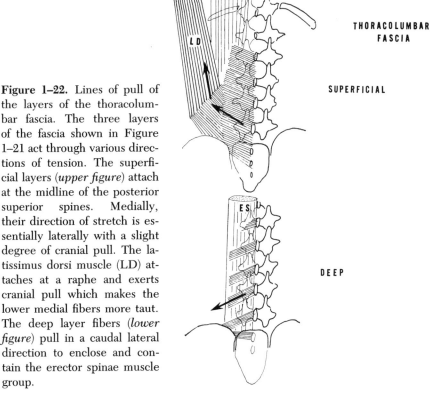

Figure 1–22. Lines of pull of the layers of the thoracolumbar fascia. The three layers of the fascia shown in Figure 1–21 act through various directions of tension. The superficial layers (*upper figure*) attach at the midline of the posterior superior spines. Medially, their direction of stretch is essentially laterally with a slight degree of cranial pull. The latissimus dorsi muscle (LD) attaches at a raphe and exerts cranial pull which makes the lower medial fibers more taut. The deep layer fibers (*lower figure*) pull in a caudal lateral direction to enclose and contain the erector spinae muscle group.

THORACOLUMBAR FASCIA

SUPERFICIAL

DEEP

laminae, at levels L3 to L5 has three laminae, and at levels L4 to S1 has five laminae. Laterally the middle fibers fuse with the superficial layers of the thoracolumbar fascia forming a raphe that forms the lumbosacral ligament. The middle fibers, the tendinous termination of the oblique, and the transversus abdominal muscles do not attach to the superficial fibers.

The **superficial** fascial layer covers all the low back muscles. It attaches to the contralateral superficial fascia at the midline, to the supraspinatus ligament and the posterior-superior (see Fig. 1–21) spinous process. The supraspinous ligament does not extend below the L3 spinous process onto the sacrum. At its caudal extension it blends with the distal end of the erector spinae muscle group where it also attaches to the sacrum and into the fascia of the gluteus maximus.

At the rostral end the superficial fascia blends with the fascia of the splenius, rhomboids, and trapezius muscles and also has a firm contact with the latissimus dorsi muscle.

Laterally the superficial fascia attaches at several levels. At the lowest level it attaches to the posterior-superior crest of the ilium. At midlumbar area it attaches to the lateral margin of the erector spinae muscles.

The reason for such a detailed discussion of this fascia is that the fascia of the erector spinae muscle and its attachment to the abdominal wall muscles are considered to play a significant role in spinal function. The adage that a "back is as strong as is a strong abdominal wall" is a truism. The need is to confirm, justify, and explain this statement and concept.

LIGAMENTS OF THE FUNCTIONAL UNIT

There are interspinous ligaments other than the anterior and posterior longitudinal ligaments that were discussed in relation to the intervertebral disks. There are ligaments connecting the vertebral arches. These are the interspinous and intertransversus ligaments. They connect the opposing transverse processes and the opposing posterior-superior spinous processes and laminae.

THE NERVES OF THE FUNCTIONAL UNIT

The nerves within the functional unit are involved both in normal spinous function as well as in abnormal function and in the production of pain. They transmit impulses of a nociceptive nature to tissues within the functional unit or are referred into the lower extremity.

The major nerve supply to tissues within the functional unit is the posterior and anterior primary divisions of the nerve root and the recurrent nerve of von Luschka (recurrent meningeal nerve).

The nerve root is a sensory-motor nerve (Fig. 1–23). The anterior pri-

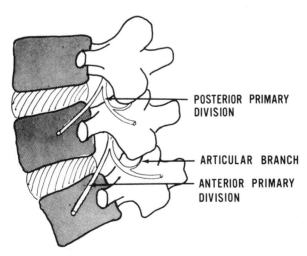

POSTERIOR PRIMARY DIVISION

ARTICULAR BRANCH

ANTERIOR PRIMARY DIVISION

Figure 1–23. Division of nerve root. The nerve root divides into the anterior primary division and the posterior primary division. A small articular branch is sensory to the facets.

mary division contains sensory and motor fibers descending into the lower extremities to form the lumbosacral plexus. The posterior primary division branches posteriorly to divide into the cutaneous branch, the muscular branch, and the articular branch (to the facets).

The recurrent meningeal nerve (the recurrent nerve of Luschka, Fig. 1–24), is a sensory nerve that enters the gray matter of the spinal cord, into the dorsal horn (Lissauer's tract), and into the substantia gelatinosum. The recurrent meningeal nerve contains fibers from the sympathetic ganglia. The nerve reenters the foraminae to innervate the posterior and anterior longitudinal ligaments, the dural sac of the nerve roots, and possibly the very outer layer (annular sheet) of the intervertebral disk.

There are sensory nerve unmyelinated endings in the human lumbar tissues within the lumbar fascia, the supraspinous and interspinous liga-

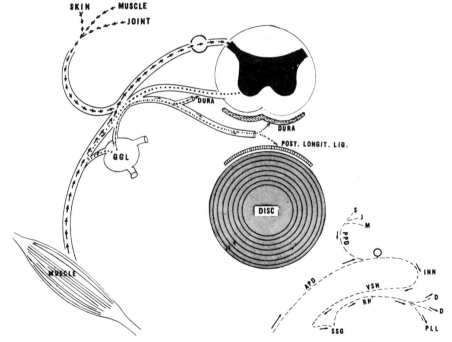

Figure 1–24. Innervation of the recurrent nerve of Luschka.
PPD—posterior primary division
APD—anterior primary division
GGL—sympathetic ganglion
INN—internuncial neurons
VSN—ventral sensory nerve
SSG—sensory sympathetic ganglion
RN—recurrent nerve of Luschka
D—to dura
PLL—posterior longitudinal ligament

ments, the capsules of the facets, the erector spinae muscles, and the long longitudinal ligaments. All these tissues are potential sites of nociception in the production of pain. They are also potential sites of proprioception in the moderation and coordination of neuromusculoskeletal function of the lumbar spine. Their role in controlling the kinetic spine function will receive full evaluation.

REFERENCES

Bogduk, N and Long, DM: The anatomy of the so-called "articular nerves" and their relationship to facet denervation in the treatment of low back pain. J Neurosurg 51:172, 1979.

Bogduk, N and MacIntosh, JE: The applied anatomy of the thoracolumbar fascia. Spine 9:164, 1984.

Epstein JA, et al: Lumbar nerve root compression at the intervertebral foramina caused by arthritis of the posterior facets. J Neurosurg 39:362, 1973.

Farfan, HF, et al: The effects of torsion on the lumbar intervertebral joints: The role of torsion in the production of disk degeneration. J Bone Joint Surg 52A:468, 1970.

Gordon, EE: Natural history of the intervertebral disk. Arch Phys Med Rehabil Nov: 750, 1961.

Gracovetsky, S and Farfan, HF: The optimum spine. Spine 11:543, 1986.

Hendry, NGC: The hydration of the nucleus pulposus and its relation to intervertebral disk derangement. J Bone Joint Surg 40B:132, 1958.

Hirsch, C and Miller, M: The anatomical basis for low back pain. Acta Orthop Scand 32:1, 1963.

Hirsch, C and Schajowicz, F: Studies on structural changes in the lumbar annulus fibrosus. Acta Orthop Scand 22:184, 1953.

Inman, VT and deC. M. Saunders, JB: The clinico-anatomical aspects of the lumbosacral region. Radiology 38:669, 1942.

Kellgren JH: The anatomical source of back pain. Rheumatol and Rehabil 16:3, 1977.

Lovett, RW: Lateral Curvature of the Spine and Round Shoulders. P. Blakiston's Son & Co., Philadelphia, 1907.

Maroudas, A: Biophysical chemistry of cartilaginous tissues with special reference to solutes and fluid transport. Biorheology 12:233, 1975.

Nachemson, A, Lewin, T, and Freeman, MAR: In vitro diffusion of dye through the endplates and the annulus fibrosus of human lumbar inter-vertebral disks. Acta Orthop Scand 41:589, 1970.

Naylor, A: Intervertebral disk prolapse and degeneration: The biochemical and biophysical approach. Spine 1:108, 1976.

Pedersen, HE, Blunck, CFJ, and Gardner, E: The anatomy of lumbosacral posterior rami and meningeal branches of spinal nerves (sinu-vertebral nerves). J Bone Joint Surg 38:377, 1956.

Selby, DK and Paris, SV: Anatomy of facet joints and its clinical correlation with low back pain. Contemp Orthop 3:1097, 1981.

Stilwell, DL: Nerve supply of the vertebral column. Anat Rec 125:139, 1956.

Stilwell, DL: Regional variations in the innervation of deep fasciae and aponeuroses. Anat Rec 127:635, 1957.

Wyke, B: The neurological basis of thoracic spinal pain. Rheumatol Phys Med 10:356, 1967.

Wyke, B. The neurology of joints. Ann R Coll Surg Engl 41:25, 1967.

CHAPTER 2

Total Spine

The **total spine,** the vertebral column, can be visualized as an aggregate of all superimposed functional units balanced against gravity and capable of functional flexibility. The vertebral column can be evaluated as a static and a kinetic structure.

STATIC SPINE

As seen from the side the spine has four physiologic curves: two lordotic and two kyphotic. The cervical and lumbar lordotic curves have flexibility and the dorsal kyphotic curve has limited flexibility, but the sacral kyphotic curve is a "fixed" inflexible curve (Fig. 2–1).

The entire spine is balanced on the sacral base. The lumbar curve, a lordosis, is immediately cephalad to the sacrum. This curve is convex anteriorly and concave posteriorly. It comprises, as a generality, six functional units termed L1, L2, L3, L4, L5, and S1. As this text considers essentially **low back pain syndrome,** it is the lumbosacral spine that will receive major consideration.

The next curve cephalad is the thoracic spine comprising 12 vertebrae. The curve is a kyphosis with convexity dorsally and concavity anteriorly. The vertebral bodies of the thoracic spine and the intervertebral disk are smaller than those of the lumbar spine. There is essentially no forward flexion or extension flexibility of the thoracic spine after maturity, and the thoracic spine has limited rotation due to the muscular attachment of the ribs.

The ribs attaching to the transverse processes of the vertebral bodies and connected to each other by intercostal muscles and ligaments allow lit-

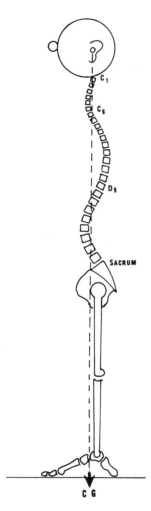

Figure 2–1. Posture. The physiologic curves of the erect vertebral column transect the center of gravity (CG) at the regions shown.

tle individual movement. The thoracic spine moves on the thoracolumbar articulation within a transitional functional unit.

The cervical spine has eight vertebrae forming a lordosis and is divided into an upper cervical segment: the occipital-atlanto-axis upper segment including C3 and a lower segment including C3 to C7. The curve is convex anteriorly and concave posteriorly. Within the total segments of the cervical spine, movement is permitted in flexion, extension, lateral flexion, and rotation. (The cervical spine is discussed in detail in Cailliet, R: Neck and Arm Pain, ed 2. FA Davis, Philadelphia, 1981.)

The facet joints of the functional units of the lumbar, thoracic, and cervical regions differ in their angulation which, in part, determines the direction of motion permitted and the motion prevented or restricted (Fig. 2–2).

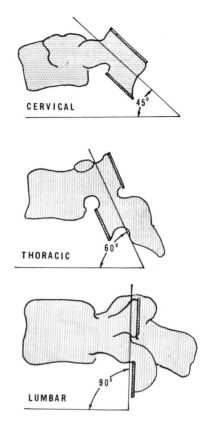

Figure 2–2. Angulation of planes of vertebral facets. The angulation that determines the direction of movement at various vertebral levels is depicted.

All three curves, the cervical, thoracic, and lumbar, bisect the center of gravity and balance each other. These three curves viewed in an erect position can be considered human **posture**.

The sacrum is the foundation platform on which the superincumbent vertebral column is balanced. The sacrum is firmly attached to both ilia via the sacroiliac joints. These three bones move en masse as one unit, forming the pelvis. The pelvis is centrally balanced on a transverse axis between two ballbearing joints of the femoral heads, which articulate within the acetabulae. This articulation permits rotatory motion in a sagittal anterior-posterior plane. Any rotation of the pelvis within this sagittal plane changes the angulation of the sacral base.

The upper surface of the sacrum, on which is balanced the lumbar spine, is known as the lumbosacral angle (Fig. 2–3). The articulation of the lumbar vertebra to the sacrum is termed the lumbosacral spinal joint.

As the pelvis rotates, proper terms used for clinical description relate to its effect on the lumbosacral angle. Upward movement of the anterior aspect of the pelvis is termed "upward rotation," which lowers the sacral aspect and **decreases** the lumbosacral angle. Downward movement of the

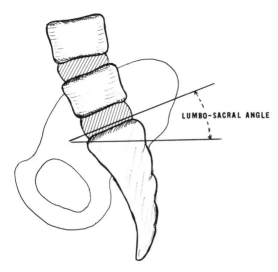

LUMBO-SACRAL ANGLE

Figure 2–3. Physiologic lumbosacral angle. The lumbosacral angle is computed as the angle from a base parallel to horizontal and the hypotenuse drawn parallel to superior level of the sacral bone. The optimum physiologic lumbosacral is in the vicinity of 30 degrees.

anterior portion of the pelvis accomplishes the exact motion and elevates the sacral position, **increasing** the lumbosacral angle. These pelvic motions are termed **pelvic tilting**.

The lumbosacral angle is determined by drawing a line parallel to the superior level of the sacrum and angled to a true horizontal level (Fig. 2–4).

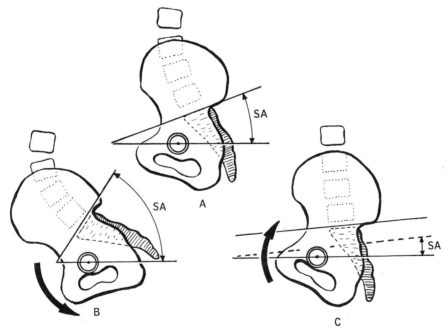

Figure 2–4. The lumbosacral angle is determined by drawing a line parallel to the superior level of the sacrum and angled to a true horizontal level.

28

As the lumbosacral angle changes so does the superincumbent lumbar lordotic curve. An **increase** in the lumbosacral angle results in an **increase** in the lordosis as does a **decrease** result in a **decrease** of the lordotic curve (Fig. 2–5).

The lordotic curve changes but the cephalad thoracic curve remains balanced as a **fixed** curvature so the total spinal curvature relies on the lumbosacral angle and the thoracolumbar angulations. As has been earlier stated there is *no* significant flexibility of the thoracic spine after spinal maturity. There is also an effect on the lumbosacral angulation and the resultant lumbar lordosis exerted by the cervical lordosis. This will be discussed in the section on **posture**.

The lumbar lordotic curve also is determined by the angular shape of the intervertebral disks. The disks are wider anteriorly and narrower posteriorly (Fig. 2–6). Because the lower lumbar vertebrae, predominantly L5, L4, and L3, are angled, as is the lumbosacral articulation, there is a **shearing** force component to these functional units. As was noted earlier, there are ligamentous structures that unite the posterior bony element of the functional units. These are the posterior superior spinous ligament, the intertransversus ligaments, and the posterior longitudinal ligaments. These act to minimize the shear effect of the angulation of the lower lumbar vertebrae (Fig. 2–7).

As will be noted in the section on **posture** the posterior ligaments remain slack in the erect posture, but they still exert static support. In the erect posture, however, there is opposition of the facet joints, and the ligaments also exert action to minimize anterior shear (Fig. 2–8).

The three physiologic curves that comprise the static spine and designate erect posture are unequivocally influenced by the sacral angle and the shape of the intervertebral disks.

As one quarter of the adult spine comprises disk material, and the endplates of the vertebral bodies are essentially parallel, if all the disk material were removed and the vertebrae placed one on the other, there would be no significant curvature as viewed from the lateral aspect. This is the spine of the newborn.

The spine of the newborn has no physiologic curves as noted later in the erect adult. The infant **in utero** is curled in total flexion. All curves— cervical, thoracic, and lumbar—are kyphotic.

During the first 6 to 8 weeks of life the child raises his or her head and by this antigravity maneuver initiates action of the erector spinae muscles. This gradually forms the cervical lordosis. As crawling and sitting gradually evolve, the lower lumbar curve is formed.

The thoracic curve does not significantly change, but as the total spine gains the erect position, the iliopsoas muscle does not fully elongate and mechanically causes the lumbar spine to assume a lordosis (Fig. 2–9). When the hips and knees are flexed against the abdomen, the curled posi-

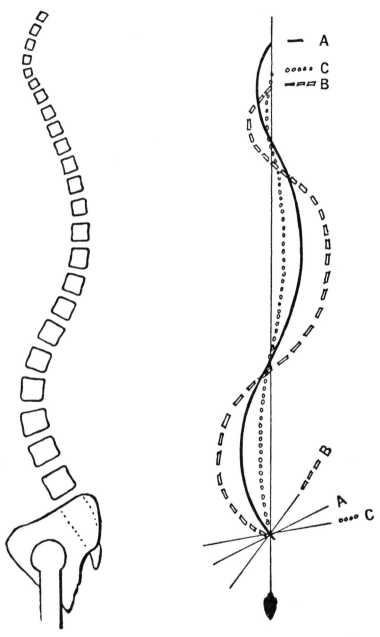

Figure 2–5. Static spine considered erect posture (relationship of physiologic curves to plumb line of gravity). *Left:* Lateral view of the upright spine with its static physiologic curves depicting posture. *Right:* The change in all superincumbent curves as influenced by change in the sacral base angle. All curves must be transected by the plumb line to remain gravity balanced. *A* is physiologic; *B,* increased angle; and *C,* decreased sacral angle with flattened lumbar lordosis.

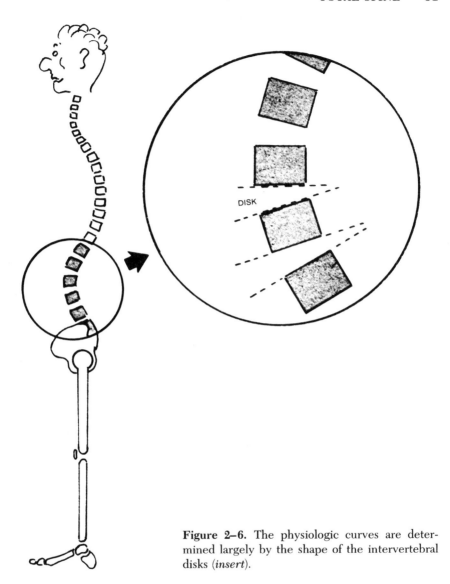

DISK

Figure 2–6. The physiologic curves are determined largely by the shape of the intervertebral disks (*insert*).

tion is known as the **fetal position**. The iliacus muscle acting on the femora keeps the hips flexed. The psoas portion of that muscle originates from the anterior portion of the lumbar spine and attaches to the anterior aspect of the femur. As the femora extend, they gradually pull on the lumbar spine to affect a lordosis.

The erect spinal configuration constitutes **posture,** the basis for the next chapter.

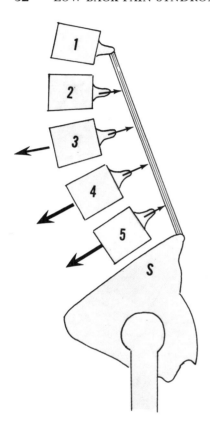

Figure 2–7. Shear stress. The lordosis of the lumbar spine causes the vertebrae to have an incline plane shear force (*large arrows*). The ligaments (*small arrows*) attach to the posterior spinous ligaments which minimize shearing.

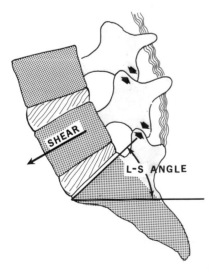

Figure 2–8. Shear stress on facets. Forward and downward shear of the fifth lumbar vertebra upon the sacrum is borne by the facet (*arrows*) when the longitudinal ligaments are lax.

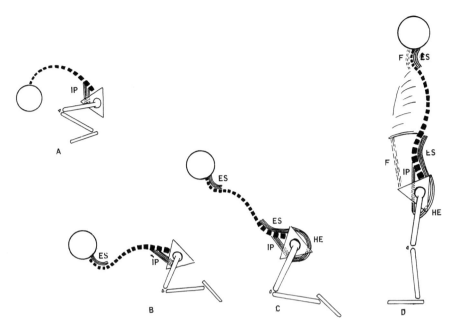

Figure 2–9. Chronologic development of posture. *A*. The total curve of the fetal spine *in utero*. *B*. Formation of the cervical lordosis when the head overcomes gravity. *C*. Formation of the second lordotic (lumbar) curve due to the antigravity force of the lumbar erector spinae (ES) muscles and the restriction of the iliopsoas muscles (IP). *D*. Erect adult posture showing the strong antigravity erector muscles (ES and HE hip extensors) and the weak flexor (F) muscles of the neck and abdomen.

CHAPTER 3

Posture

The erect static spine constitutes posture. Mankind stands erect on a sacral base with all the superincumbent vertebral functional units forming four physiologic curves.

Balance must be maintained against gravity. The body must be balanced using the minimum of energy; it must be energized economically and with minimal wear and tear. This concept must not be altered or violated. In its normal status of structure and function, this concept is not significantly modified.

The spine remains erect by virtue of its soft tissue components: ligaments, capsular tissues, and muscles. The muscles play a lesser role in maintaining erect posture to minimize the energy expenditure that sustained muscular action would evoke.

Only ligamentous restraint is possible without energy expenditure. When ligamentous strain exceeds the physiologic limit, muscular action intervenes and spares further ligamentous stress. This neurologic reflex mechanism remains to be confirmed, but it stands to reason that sensory nerve endings of a mechanoreceptor nature would be used with prolonged ligamentous and capsular stretch. This reflex invokes an isometric muscular response-dispelling further ligamentous and capsular elongation.

Good posture, meaning an energy-economical cosmetically acceptable stance, requires balance between ligamentous and muscular tone. Whereas proper posture mandates balance between ligamentous support and muscular tone, improper posture means an imbalance with resultant fatigue, skeletal symmetry, and creation of pain producing nociceptive impulses.

Proper posture, which means maintaining an erect spinal column, requires the spine be supported on the sacrum, which assumes a physiologic angle.

The pelvis is supported by ligamentous control on the hip joints. These congruous joints cannot be extended past neutral, as they are restricted by a thickening of the anterior capsular tissues that form the "Y" ligament (iliopectineal) of Bigelow. In the standing position mankind "leans" on this ligament in the hip joint capsule (Fig. 3–1).

The knee joint also can be "locked" when the leg is placed in full extension. The posterior knee capsule, in this position, becomes taut and prevents any further extension. At this stage there is no need for quadriceps

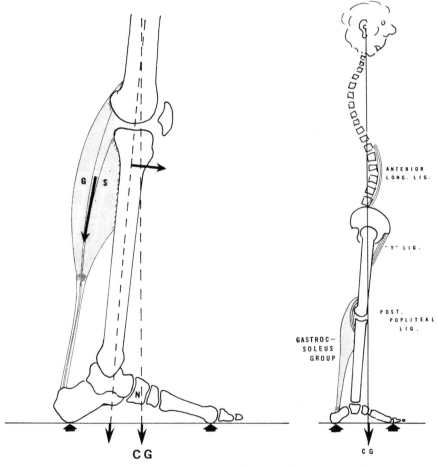

Figure 3–1. Static spine support. The relaxed person leans on his ligaments: the iliofemoral ligament, ("Y" ligament of Bigelow), the anterior longitudinal ligament, and the posterior knee ligaments. The ankle cannot be "locked," but by leaning forward only a few degrees the gastrocnemius must contract to support the entire body. Relaxed erect posture is principally ligamentous with only the gastrocnemius-soleus muscle group active.

contraction to sustain the erect leg and body position. All the support is ligamentous.

The ankle joint cannot be "locked" by ligamentous capsular tissue as there is free dorsi and plantar flexion motion at the tibiotalar joint. To stand vertical, the lower leg leans forward, ahead of the center of gravity, causing proprioceptive stimulation on the gastrocnemius-soleus muscle, which then contracts isometrically and prevents the tibia from moving further forward. This minimal isometric sustained contraction of the gastrocnemius-soleus expends minimal energy; the remaining action of erect posture is essentially ligamentous.

The pelvis is additionally supported by the tensor fascia lata. This fascia courses from the iliac crest downward and backward to insert into the iliotibial band at the knee. It reinforces the hip support and prevents knee hyperextension.

The lumbosacral angle, which is dependent on the rotation of the pelvis, maintains the base on which the spine is supported. This too depends on ligamentous support. When this support is upset, muscular effort is required to support the spine, which impairs the energy efficiency of primarily ligamentous erect posture.

Viewed from behind, the spine must also, in this view, be erect and properly aligned to the center of gravity. There must be no or minimal deviation to either side of the center. From this view the spine also is supported on the sacrum, which is contained between both ilia and hip joints.

To be horizontal, the pelvis, thus the sacrum, must be supported on two legs of equal length (Fig. 3–2).

The erect spine, balanced on the oscillating sacrum, can rotate only in the sagittal plane. As the pelvis rotates, so does the superincumbent spinal curves: the lumbar, the thoracic, and the cervical. Ultimately the head is held directly above the spine and supported on the total spine. The head, therefore, is held efficiently, requiring minimal energy expenditure of the cervical spine and the capital muscles, based on the integrity of the total spine alignment.

Viewed anteroposteriorly, the bilateral leg lengths determine the horizontality of the pelvis and the sacrum. A discrepancy in leg length or a deformation of the pelvis will result in an imbalance of the superincumbent spine. Shortness of one leg, for any reason, will depress the height of the pelvis on that side, and the sacrum will also be slanted. The lower lumbar vertebra will "take off" at an angle and result in a segmental scoliosis (Fig. 3–3).

There are numerous reasons for one leg being shorter in length than the other. These include congenital hypoplasia, previous poliomyelitis, postfracture, severe genu varum and valgum, hip dysplasia, or degenerative arthritis, to mention a few. The result on the spine is a relative "functional" scoliosis.

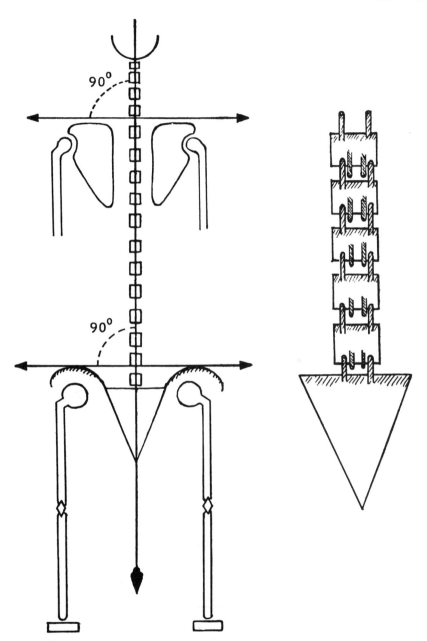

Figure 3–2. Spinal alignment from anterior-posterior aspect. Anterior-posterior view of the erect human spine. With both legs equal in length, the spine supports the pelvis in a level horizontal plane and the spine, taking off at a right (90-degree) angle, ascends in a straight line. The facets shown in the enlarged drawing on the right show their parallel alignment and proper symmetry in this erect position.

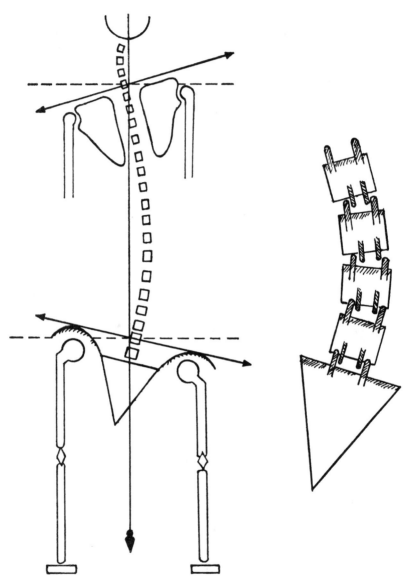

Figure 3–3. Pelvic obliquity and its relationship to spinal alignment. Anterior view of an oblique pelvis due to a leg-length discrepancy. Owing to pelvic slant in a lateral plane, the spinal take-off is at a lateral angle. The flexible spine will curve in an attempt to compensate, and the facets of the curving spine will become asymmetrical in relationship to each other.

POSTURE

Posture generally implies evaluation of the spine as viewed from the side—a lateral view. The physiologic curves, which comprise posture, are the lumbar lordosis, the dorsal kyphosis, the cervical lordosis, and the sacral kyphosis—the last being essentially the lumbosacral angulation.

As initially stated, erect posture must conform to the balance within the center of gravity and be maintained with minimal energy expenditure.

From an engineering viewpoint, the body can be considered to be poorly designed insofar as, during erect stance, the heavy parts are on top of a narrow base (Fig. 3–4) at all three major levels: the head, the thorax, and the pelvis.

This apparent paradox is explained by the fact that all three triangles have their base at the center of gravity, and the upper widths of the triangles are well balanced. Little energy is needed to balance this structure because none of the parts are far from the vertical axis.

Ligamentous support has been discussed. Studies have revealed that the erector spinae muscles are essentially inactive in the erect spinal posture. Some activity of the lumbar erector spinae muscles occurs when merely the head moves ahead of the center of gravity; otherwise *no* muscular activity has been revealed by electromyographic (EMG) studies. This is the basis of effortless erect stance.

There are spurts of neuromuscular activity demonstrated as the body sways to one side or the other from the center of gravity. These are undoubtedly "righting reflexes."

These EMG studies were done in the laboratory with clinical electromyographic equipment that measures 100 μV of neuromuscular activity. At this microvolt level any EMG activity measured requires isotonic muscular activity. Laboratory studies performed with special equipment that can measure 1.0 μV reveal that there is a continuous sustained muscular activity. This EMG microvoltage essentially measures muscle "tone": a sustained isometric contraction of low amplitude requiring little energy expenditure.

It appears that effortless erect postural stance is accomplished by:

1. Intradiskal pressure separating the adjacent vertebral endplates, which in turn impose

2. Tension on the annular fibers: both the deep and the superficial layers and

3. Create tension on the anterior and posterior longitudinal ligaments.

4. The pelvis is supported by the ligamentous support of the iliopectineal ligaments of the hips, the posterior popliteal ligaments of the knee, and the sustained muscular contractions of the gastrocnemius-soleus muscles.

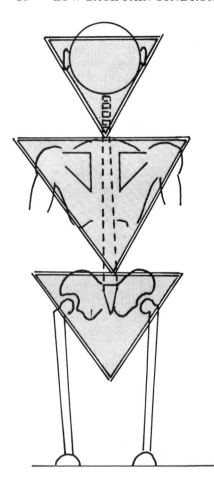

Figure 3–4. Body engineering of stance performed with broad, heavier parts at the top, situated upon a narrow base.

It can be summarized that posture, the erect static stance, exhibits balanced physiologic curves, is effortless, thus nonfatiguing, and is pain free. An acceptable posture must also present an aesthetically acceptable appearance.

Standard posture is defined by the Posture Committee of the American Academy of Orthopedic Surgery (1947) as "Skeletal alignment refined as a relative arrangement of the parts of the body in a state of balance that protects the supporting structures of the body against injury or progressive deformity." These criteria remain pertinent in regard to the lumbosacral spine.

There are many factors that influence adult posture, but there are three that are predominant in their influence and frequency:

1. Familial or hereditary postures such as marked dorsal kyphosis or excessive lumbar lordosis.

2. Structural anomalies, either congenital or acquired: neurologic; muscular; skeletal; or ligamentous, static or progressive.

3. Postures of habit or training during the developmental years.

Postural deviations attributable to familial or hereditary origins or diseases can be identified by a correct, thorough history and a complete physical examination, and can be confirmed by appropriate laboratory studies.

The effects of habit and training during the formative years are more difficult to recognize. Postural training in childhood is indoctrinated by school procedures and by parental influence. These postural "habits" gradually become deeply ingrained and subconsciously become accepted as "normal." These acquired postural habits may be deeply embedded in the psyche and the neuromuscular proprioception, but they can be modified and corrected.

CULTURAL ASPECTS OF POSTURE

The customary upright posture with the arms dangling at the sides or clasped in front of or behind the body is and has been an accepted universal standard. Sitting in a chair has not been a daily occurrence nor universally implemented. In fact, sitting in a chair is actually of recent origin.

One quarter of the human race habitually take the weight off their feet, legs, and backs by crouching in a deep squat both at rest and at work (Fig. 3–5).

Chairs, stools, and benches were used in Egypt and Mesopotamia 5000 years ago, but the Chinese used chairs only as recently as 2000 years ago. Before that time the Chinese sat on the ground as did the Japanese and the Koreans. The Islamic cultures of the Middle East and North Africa have returned to sitting on the floor or the ground for "cultural and religious prestige and ritual."

The deep squat position for working and resting is currently used by millions of people in Asia, Africa, and some countries of Latin America. The Turkish or "tailor" crossed-legged squat position is used in the Middle East and India as much as it is used in much of Asia.

The crossing of one's legs or folding them under the body while sitting was originally thought to be assumed by women because of their narrow skirts, but it is now recognized that this sitting posture is also assumed in cultures where no clothing is worn.

Standing posture is influenced by the use of footwear as well as by physiologic, psychologic, social, sexual, occupational, and environmental factors too numerous to elucidate.

Posture has also been influenced by religious rituals that instituted kneeling, standing with bowed head, or lying prone or in a posture of "meditation-Yoga."

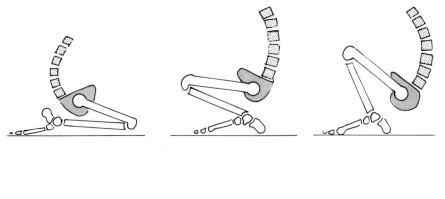

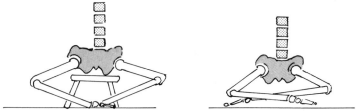

Figure 3–5. Sitting postures common to Eastern cultures.

Western social postural codes have become relaxed in the course of the past century with the availability of soft cushioned chairs and sofas replacing the hard seat with erect chair backs. Regardless of changes in cultural precepts, our children are still admonished to assume a posture assumed to be "normal and desirable" whether it is physiologic or musculoskeletally proper.

Posture also must be viewed from the cultural influences of parental training, school, and peer pressures. Parental example, as well as intended teaching, plays a formative part of posture as does competition from siblings and classmates.

The psyche contributes formidably to posture. Posture can be considered as a somatization of the psyche. We stand and move as we feel. Our postural stance and our movement clearly mirror, to the astute observer, our psychologic inner drives or their absence. Consciously, but usually unconsciously, we assume a pose that portrays our inner feelings. We move in a manner that clearly depicts our attitude toward ourselves, our fellow man, and our environment. Our posture is **body language** in all its studied aspects.

The depressed, dejected person stands in a "drooped" postural manner with the upper back, the thoracic spine, rounded and the shoulders rounded forward and depressed. This is the expressed "carrying the weight of the world on our shoulders." This is the postural expression of "being too tired to **stand** any more of this burden."

This posture is an expression of fatigue and ultimately becomes a fatiguing posture to assume and maintain. By placing the head and upper body ahead of the center of gravity, abnormal postural spinal ligamentous strain with resultant nociceptive reaction occurs, and the extensor muscles must assume a burden of bodily support that adds to the acquired fatigue.

On the opposite side of the coin from the lethargic depressed person is the hyperkinetic aggressive individual who portrays his or her inner feelings in posture and abruptness of actions. This posture depicts the combative attitude with either an attack or aggressive posture or crouch. This posture also places the person ahead of the center of gravity and all the muscles in a constant state of sustained contraction.

The self-conscious tall girl may decrease her apparent height by bending over. Her counterpart, the short girl or boy, may stand erect in an abnormal, arched back posture to appear taller. The full-bosomed girl, self-conscious in her early formative years, may wish to decrease the apparent buxom appearance by slumping forward.

All patterns of assumed posture in early childhood may result in deep-seated patterns that persist into adolescence and adulthood. The tissues become structurally the engram of the assumed psychologic posture even when mature thought belying the need for this posture occurs.

Feldenkrais stated that improper head balance is rare in children except in those with structural skeletal abnormalities. He postulated that repeated emotional upheavals cause the child to adapt attitudes (postures) that ensured safety. He claimed that these emotional upheavals evoked contraction of the flexor muscles of the neck and trunk with resultant inhibition of the extensor musculature. His analogy to animals showed that when frightened, they react with violent contraction of all the flexor muscles and an inhibition of the extensor muscles, preventing walking or running.

The attitude of a child with repeated emotional stresses is that of "curling within": resuming the fetal position—a contraction of the flexor muscles and an inhibition of the extensor tone. This posture, when maintained, becomes habitual and "normal."

The abnormal postures described are well known to play a role in the causation of pain and functional impairment leading to disability. This is the basis of further chapters.

REFERENCES

Feldenkrais, M: Body & Mature Behavior: A Study of Anxiety, Gravitation & Learning. International Universities Press, New York, 1949.
Inman, VT, Ralston, HJ, and Todd, F: Human Walking. Williams & Wilkins, Baltimore, 1981.

Joseph, J: Man's Posture: Electromyographic Studies. Charles C Thomas, Springfield, 1960.

Lovett, RW: Lateral Curvature of the Spine and Round Shoulders. P. Blakiston & Son, Philadelphia, 1907.

Lowman, CL: Postural Fitness: Significance and Variances. Lea & Febiger, Philadelphia, 1960.

Roaf, R: Posture. Academic Press, New York, 1977.

CHAPTER 4

The Kinetic Lumbosacral Spine

The total erect spine that has been described in its static postural state is endowed with the capability of controlled movement. The total spine moves as an aggregate of movement of each functional unit, so each specific isolated functional unit merits detailed evaluation.

Movement is initiated by implementing the forces of gravity and by the kinetic action of the musculature on the structural system. All these actions are well coordinated and controlled by biofeedback from the proprioceptive nervous system. All actions are subservient to the forces of gravity with an attempt at retaining balance with the center of gravity.

Movement of each functional unit occurs within the anterior weight-bearing portion involving the disk and within the guidance of the posterior neural arch tissues, including the facet joints. Limitations of movement are exerted by the constraints of the ligaments, joint capsules, and the muscular fascial tissues.

The following can be recapitulated:

1. The intervertebral disks permit compression allowing flexion, extension, lateral flexion, and rotation. The latter two motions, lateral flexion and rotation, occur simultaneously, being limited in their range of motion by the elasticity of the annular collagen fibers.

2. The nucleus of the disk deforms to allow these motions but remains within the container of the inner annular fiber sheets.

3. The facet (zygapophyseal) joints glide on each other in a sagittal plane permitting flexion and extension but markedly limiting lateral and rotatory motion. They contribute to the weight bearing of the erect vertebral column but only to an estimated 15 to 24 percent of weight borne.

4. Extension of each functional unit is limited by mechanical approximation of the rear zygapophyseal joint structures with flexion being limited

by the extensibility of the posterior longitudinal ligaments, intervertebral ligaments, and the erector spinae muscle fascial sheaths.

Extension causing an excessive lordosis is greater in young children but remains possible throughout life as long as all intervertebral disk spaces are adequate.

Flexion of the total lumbosacral spine is that of reversal of the lumbar lordosis to achieve a kyphosis. Each functional unit flexes approximately 8 to 10 degrees of flexion with the total lumbar spine, comprised of five functional units, for a total of 45 degrees (Fig. 4–1).

Flexion occurs at a different degree at each functional unit (Fig. 4–2) with 75 percent of flexion occurring at the L5-S1 and L4-5 interspaces. Motion occurs primarily at the lumbosacral joint, within the functional units of the lumbar spine, and to a limited degree at the thoracolumbar junction. No significant flexion occurs within the thoracic spine.

LUMBAR PELVIC RHYTHM

As a person attempts to bend forward, as in trying to touch the floor ahead, the total spine flexes in a very specific manner termed the **lumbar pelvic rhythm**.

It has been stated that the lumbar spine, the five lumbar functional units, flex forward to approximately 45 degrees of flexion. This is a reversal of the lumbar lordosis into a lumbar kyphosis. Each functional unit flexes approximately 9 degrees; five units equal 45 degrees. This allows the person to bend over forward only a portion of the amount of flexion required to allow touching the floor ahead.

For additional forward flexion a simultaneous rotation of the pelvis must occur. Once both have occurred, the reversal of the lumbar lordosis and the full rotation of the pelvis, the person has bent over forward to the full degree allowed by the soft tissues of the spine and pelvis.

The neuromuscular mechanism by which the **lumbar pelvic rhythm** (Fig. 4–3) occurs currently presents unanswered questions about the specific extent of muscular and ligamentous-fascial tissue involvement. Enough, however, has been confirmed and accepted that a concept can be postulated (Fig. 4–4).

FLEXION

As the person bends over forward to attempt to reach the floor with the hands, the following sequence of activities occurs within the functional units that comprise the lumbosacral spine.

1. In the erect static posture the extensor muscles are relaxed and the three physiologic curves transect the center of gravity.

2. On the decision of attempting forward flexion the head moves

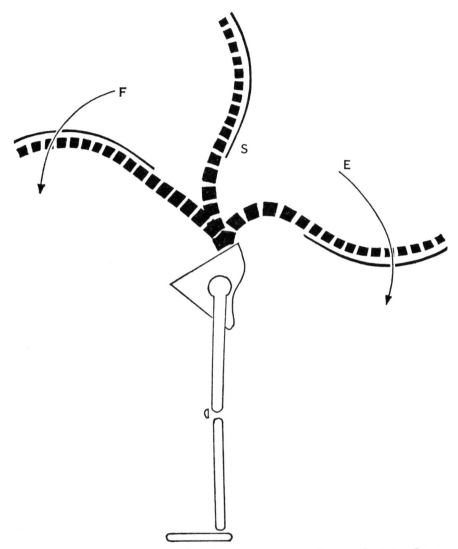

Figure 4–1. Flexion-extension of total spine. Composite diagram depicting flexion and extension of total spine. Flexion of the lumbar spine occurs to the extent of reversing slightly past the lordosis, whereas extension is moderate. In all movements of flexion, extension, or static erect position, the thoracic spine does not alter its curve. (F = flexion; S = static spine; E = extension.)

ahead of the center of gravity, initiating contraction of the erector spinae muscles. Floyd and Silver (1955) showed electromyographically that the lumbar erector spinae muscles at the full erect relaxed posture were inactive but immediately became activated by flexing the head ahead of the center of gravity.

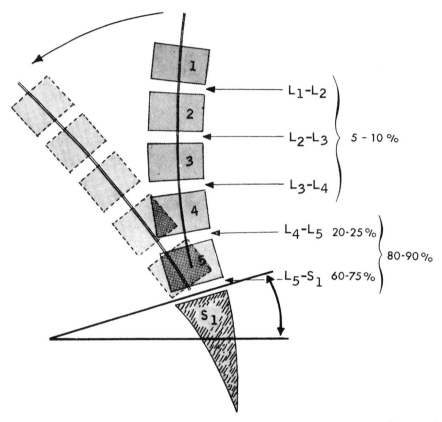

Figure 4–2. Segmental site and degree of lumbar spine flexion. The degree of flexion noted in the lumbar spine as a percentage of total spine flexion is indicated. The major portion of flexion (75 percent) occurs at the lumbosacral joint; 15 to 20 percent of flexion occurs at the L4–5 interspace; and the remaining 5 to 10 percent is distributed between L1 and L4. The forward-flexed diagram indicates the mere reversal past lordosis of total flexion of the lumbar curve.

3. With further forward flexion the lumbosacral spine begins the reversal of the lordosis into kyphosis. The spindle system of the extensor back muscles becomes elongated and reflexly initiates an impulse via the gamma fibers to the grey matter of the cord, reflexly initiating excitation via the alpha fibers to the extrafusal fibers with resultant contraction of the extensor muscles. The extent of tonus is determined by excitation of appropriate impulses and a "resetting" of the spindle system via motor fibers to the spindle system.

4. The extensor muscles gradually elongate to smoothly and gradually allow the lumbosacral spine to assume a kyphosis. The speed and extent of this neuromuscular action depend on the intended and desired action.

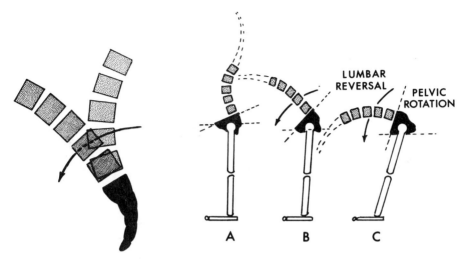

Figure 4–3. Lumbar pelvic rhythm. With pelvis fixed, flexion-extension of the lumbar spine occurs mostly in the lower segments L4–5 and L5–S1.

5. The erector spinae muscles accordingly act to decelerate, an eccentric contraction. Each functional unit flexes about 9 degrees during this action.

6. The pelvis through this lumbar phase of the flexion moves very little, if at all, with the extensor muscles of the pelvis (the glutei) maintaining an isometric contraction.

7. The lumbar spine flexes until it becomes restrained by the erector spinae muscle fascia, the posterior superior ligaments, the intertransversus ligaments, the posterior longitudinal ligaments, and the facet capsules. When the muscles are fully elongated and the ligaments become taut, further flexion of the lumbar spine is prevented; muscular activity ceases. Full lumbar kyphosis has been reached.

8. During the last portion of lumbar flexion the pelvis begins forward rotation by elongation and deceleration of the hip extensor (glutei) and the hamstring muscles. The ratio of lumbar flexion and pelvic rotation is not a fixed degree of one with the other; both occur simultaneously. The lumbar flexion occurs first and completes its range often before any significant degree of pelvis rotation has occurred.

9. On full flexion the pelvis is restricted by the ligamentous and fascial tissues of the posterior thigh and pelvis—the gluteal and hamstring muscles.

10. Now fully flexed there is **no** muscular activity. Only fascia and ligaments are operative (Fig. 4–5).

The proprioceptive stimuli that control, by feedback, the degree, rate, and force of flexion have not been confirmed but undoubtedly reside in the

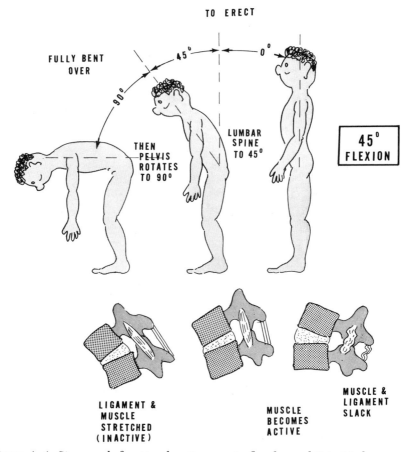

Figure 4–4. Since each functional unit opens to flex forward 8 to 10 degrees and there are five lumbar units, the lumbar spine bends forward about 45 degrees. (Modified from Cailliet, R: Understand Your Backache. FA Davis, Philadelphia, 1984, p 36.)

spindle systems of the muscles (Fig. 4–6), the Golgi system of the ligaments, and the mechanoreceptors of the facet joints and their capsules.

For normal pain-free flexion it is apparent that:

1. The soft tissues of the functional units, the facet capsules, the ligaments, and the fascia must have normal flexibility.

2. The neuromuscular control coordination must be established by proper training and habit formation.

3. The intended task must be an expected physiologic action.

4. There must be no interference of neuromuscular activity such as fatigue, anxiety, anger, etc.

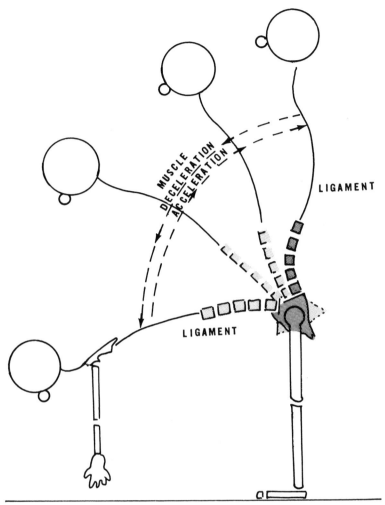

Figure 4–5. Muscular deceleration and acceleration of the forward-flexing spine from the erect ligamentous support to the fully flexed ligamentous restriction. Muscle eccentric and concentric contraction permits forward flexion and re-extension.

RE-EXTENSION TO THE ERECT POSITION

Once forward flexed until the lumbar spine is fully flexed and residing upon ligamentous restraint with no muscular activity and the pelvis is fully rotated to the point of posterior thigh ligamentous restraint, the person must now return to the erect position (Fig. 4–7).

The spinal tissues involved in this re-extension maneuver remain con-

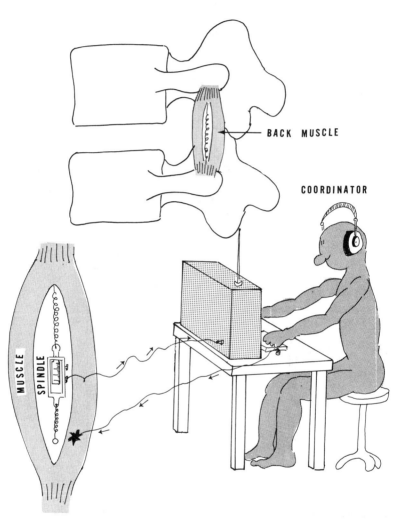

BACK MUSCLE

COORDINATOR

MUSCLE SPINDLE

Figure 4–6. Proprioceptive autonomic control of neuromuscular function (schematic). Of the neuromuscular proprioceptors controlling muscular function, the spindle system is the best documented. The tension invoked on the spindle system transmits an impulse via gamma fibers to the cord. The cord then relays via alpha fibers to the extrafusal fibers causing muscular contraction of a specific intensity. Simultaneously, the neurological circuit "resets" the spindle system to react at a different level of tension. All these are instantaneous and well coordinated to ensure the proper tension within the extrafusal fibers to accomplish the intended muscular action. (Modified from Cailliet, R: Understand Your Backache. FA Davis, Philadelphia, 1984, p 31.)

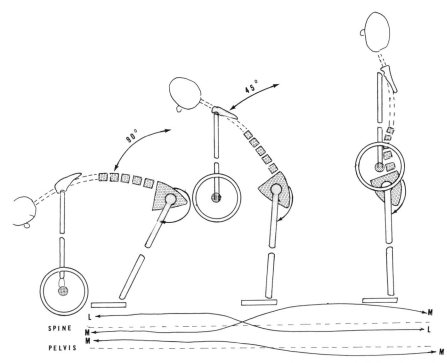

Figure 4–7. Muscle-ligamentous control in lifting. In lifting from full flexed (90 degrees) to half erect (45 degrees), the lumbar spine is supported by its ligaments (L) with posterior pelvic muscles (M) bearing the stress effort. From 45 degrees of flexion to full erect, the spine extensor muscles contract and complete the full extension.

troversial and vary according to whether the spine returns to the erect position unresisted or is lifting a heavy object.

As the spine returns to the erect position from the bent-over stance the following physiologic aspects of spinal function that are accepted are:

1. The pelvis should rerotate first before the lumbar spine resumes its lordosis (Fig. 4–8).

2. The hips and knees should be slightly flexed.

3. Any object being lifted should be close to the body.

4. The spine must resume the erect posture without excessive rotation and derotation.

The mechanism of derotation of the pelvis is unquestioned. The gluteal and hamstring muscles are the rotators of the pelvis and to do so they must initiate and sustain a smooth gradual shortening (contraction).

The pelvis should derotate from the fully bent over position until the

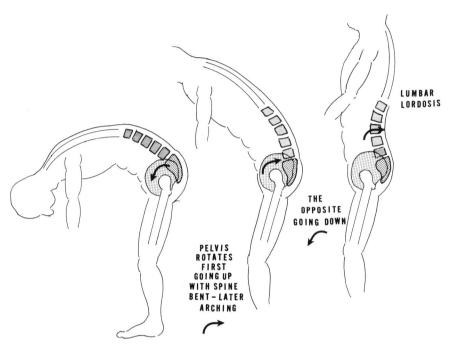

LUMBAR LORDOSIS

THE OPPOSITE GOING DOWN

PELVIS ROTATES FIRST GOING UP WITH SPINE BENT-LATER ARCHING

Figure 4–8. Lumbar pelvic rhythm in re-extension. The lordosis reverses in forward flexion with simultaneous synchronous pelvic rotation. In returning to the erect position, the pelvis should "derotate" first, with the lordosis being regained when the person still flexes forward to approximately 45 degrees.

lumbar spine is flexed to 45 degrees ahead of the center of gravity. Then, and only then, should the lumbar spine resume its lordosis.

On reaching a point 45 degrees of forward flexion (lumbar kyphosis) the lumbar lordosis should then be gradually and smoothly regained.

All these motions must be gradual and smoothly coordinated. They must never be performed in an erratic or excessive manner. It is apparent that the rapidity and the force required, as well as the direction, must be appropriate to accomplish the intended task. This implies that the "computer" of the central nervous system must be set to accommodate:

1. The size of the object being lifted.
2. The weight of the object being lifted.
3. The position of beginning and ending the task to be accomplished.
4. The rapidity of the lift.
5. The repetitive nature expected.
6. The position of the body during the lifting activity.

Even in the absence of an object being lifted, the body must flex and re-extend **as if a heavy object were being lifted.** By instilling this concept and this pattern into a person's mind, the normal manner of bending over and lifting or merely returning to the erect position will be done correctly. Repeatedly doing the activity in the proper manner will ensure the establishment of an appropriate **habit** pattern even when the mind is otherwise preoccupied.

LIFTING A HEAVY OBJECT

There is unresolved controversy regarding which of the spine tissues are involved in the act of lifting a heavy object from a level below the waist line. There are also questions as to when and to what degree these tissues become involved in the lifting act.

Whether the low back extensor muscles "lift" the body and the heavy object being lifted or whether the myofascial-ligamentous tissues bear the brunt remains unresolved.

It has been postulated that the erector spinae muscles, in their attachments from the vertebral bodies to the transverse processes, act through a fulcrum too small to accomplish the act without failure. The weight of the forward flexed body, ahead of the center of gravity, places a load upon the spine considered to be overwhelming to the erector spinae muscles. Such a weight acting at a distance from the center of gravity is considered to create a stress that results in the muscle fibers "failing."

The exponents of this "muscle failure" concept allege that the spine, in the forward flexed position, returns to the erect position via the thoracolumbar fascia and that the muscles essentially remain quiescent or at "best" partially isometrically active to moderate the ligamentous function.

The thoracolumbar fascia is considered to mechanically be able to sustain the stress forces of the magnitude imposed on them from the forward fully flexed spine position to the erect upright position in the act of lifting.

In the fully flexed position the fascia and the ligaments of the lumbosacral spine are fully taut (fully in the state of tension). The muscles are essentially inactive. All the forces at this point are borne by the fascia and ligaments.

The concept of "physiologic" lifting is that the lumbosacral spine remains fully flexed during the first stage of lifting until 45 degrees of forward flexed position (Fig. 4–9) is reached. Then, it is assumed, the erector spinae muscles contract (isometrically shorten) and "take over" from the fascia and ligaments.

This concept justifies the need of lifting an object close to the body by "derotating" the pelvis first (Fig. 4–10), which places the stress of the lift on the pelvic muscles and the taut fascia and ligaments of the low back (Fig. 4–11).

The role of the thoracolumbar fascia in lifting heavy objects has been

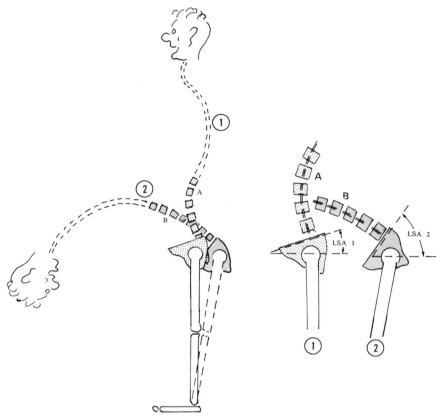

Figure 4–9. The concept of "physiologic" lifting.

recently refuted by McGill and Norman (1986). In their studies they claimed that the lumbodorsal fascia was not observed to be used until the end of the lift and **not** at the period of high loading. These authors claim that the extensor muscles do most of the lifting and, because of their alignment, unload the compression upon the disks and decrease the shear stress on the disk.

These findings also refute the original findings of the classic work of Floyd and Silver (1955) who claimed "in full flexion of the trunk, all layers of the exertor spinae are relaxed, thus, suggesting that the intervertebral ligaments are the structures most likely to sustain the gravitational moment."

Floyd and Silver also had claimed that the erector spinae muscles in trunk flexion do not undergo a lengthening reaction. They found that instead of the muscles elongating they change their angulation on the points of attachment and develop intrinsic "tension." This reaction, along with the

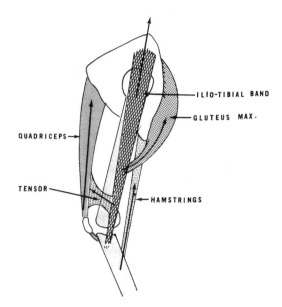

Figure 4–10. Pelvic extensor mechanism. By flexing the knees, the quadriceps tense the iliotibial band to which is attached the glutei. This combination strengthens the pelvic rotation which extends the back in lifting.

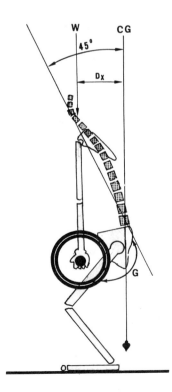

Figure 4–11. Mechanical advantage in lifting an object close to the body from 45 degrees to erect. The erector spinae muscles extend the spine upon the pelvis and "do the lifting." The shorter the distance of the weight (D_x) to the center of gravity (CG), the more efficient is the lever arm. The pelvis is rotated by the glutei (G), which are aided by the quadriceps and tensor band.

increased tension within the ligaments, invokes mechanical "negative" work.

Both of these schools of thought undoubtedly have some validity and both theories need to be associated. A recently published (Tesh, Dunn, and Evans, 1987) study partially attempts to clarify the problem.

Lifting an object from the fully flexed position is primarily ligamentous and fascial but the erector spinae muscles concurrently also contract. This is demonstrated by the electromyographic studies of the above reports. Muscular contraction during lifting presumably prevents compression and shear of the vertebrae by creating pressure within the fascial compartment (Fig. 4–12), causing a hydrodynamic effect on the fascia compartment.

Paraspinal muscular activity gives rise to intercompartmental pressure. This, in turn, increases the cross section of the compartment, which causes an increase in the caudiocervical tissue tension. This tension within the intercompartment places tension on the thoracolumbar fascia without requiring simultaneous abdominal muscular tension.

These facts may explain why lifting throughout the entire phase from fully bent over forward to the full erect position occurs in the following stages, with the specific muscular, ligamentous, and fascial components.

1. In the fully flexed position the erector spinae muscles are quiescent.

2. The thoracolumbar fascia is taut.

3. As recovery to the erect position is commenced, the thoracolumbar fascia bears the brunt of the stress.

4. The erector spinae muscles contract sufficiently to increase intercompartmental pressure, which increases the tension of the fascia and ligaments.

5. Contraction of the abdominal muscles increases the tension within the abdominal "air bag" to further "unload" the spine.

6. Contraction of the abdominal oblique muscles adds to the tension of the thoracolumbar fascia which is bearing the brunt of the lifting forces.

7. On reaching 45 degrees of forward flexion the "proprioceptive" neurologic receptors, via the central nervous system network, indicate a decrease in tension and thus initiate contraction of the erector spinae muscles.

8. The extensor muscles now assume the role of further lifting by contracting and restoring the lumbar spine to a lordosis. After 45 degrees the fascia and the extensor ligament have been relaxed.

In the process of lifting a "heavy" object, as evident by professional athletic weight lifters, the lumbar spine has been shown to assume a slight kyphosis during the initial lift. This could be construed to indicate that the fascia does not initiate the lift but rather that the erector muscles do. The probability is that the central nervous "computer," realizing that the load

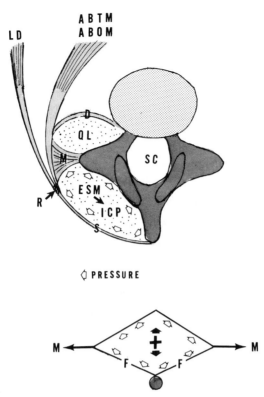

Figure 4–12. Schematic concept of intracompartmental pressure. The intracompartmental pressure (ICP) (*small arrows*) that distends the thoracolumbar fascia is initiated by contraction of the erecto-spinae muscles (ESM). The outer superficial layer of the fascia (S) is made taut by the latissimus dorsi muscle (LD) and the oblique abdominal muscles, ABTM (abdominal transversus muscle) and ABOM (abdominal oblique muscles). The front part of the compartment is the lamina, transverse process, and posterior superior spine of the vertebrae. The transversus ligament that connects two adjacent vertebrae is not shown. The middle (M) layer of the fascia completes the anterior wall of the compartment. The deep layers of the thoracolumbar fascia (D) forms a compartment with the middle (M) layers that contains the quadratus lumborum (QL). The spinal canal (SC) is noted. The abdominal muscles tense the middle layer of the fascia. The superficial fascia is made tense by the latissimus dorsi muscle. Both tendinous insertions fuse at a raphe (R). The lower drawing depicts the forces (M—muscles) upon the fascia (F) causing an increase in compartment pressure which in turn increases caudal-cranial tension (*large plus sign with black arrows*).

is excessive, calls into play more muscular activity to moderate ligamentous and fascial stress. The erector spinae muscles spare the ligaments and simultaneously increase the intercompartmental pressure. This is aided also by a greater increase in intra-abdominal pressure with an increase in the air bag pressure.

59

The pelvis is undoubtedly a forceful component of the lifting effort. Its rotation changes the base on which the spine is supported. It derotates as the spine extends. The pelvis derotates about the bilateral hip joints activated by the gluteus maximus muscles (see Fig. 4–10).

The admonition "that all lifting must be done with the knees and hips bent" has a physiologic basis. As the rotation is accomplished by the gluteus maximus, when the hips are slightly flexed this muscle is placed under tension, causing it to be more effective in its contracture.

Fifty percent of the gluteus attaches to the femur and 50 percent to the tensor fascia lata. By flexing the hips the tensor is made more taut and becomes more efficient because of this altered site of muscular (gluteus) attachment. By flexing the knees in a weight-bearing stance, the lateral ligaments of the quadriceps mechanism are attached to the tensor, making it more taut.

All these factors—hips flexed, knees flexed, and lengthening the gluteal attachment—make the pelvic derotation more powerful in aiding the person lift a heavy object from the bent-over position.

FLEXION-ROTATION AND EXTENSION-DEROTATION DURING LIFTS

To this juncture, the spine has been discussed in regard to flexing and re-extending in the **sagittal** plane. Most lifting episodes are done with some degree of rotation. A person bends over and to one side and returns from that point to the erect position in the midline.

The alignment of the facets (zygapophyseal) joints has been stated to permit flexion and extension but to **limit if not restrict lateral flexion and rotation**. This is true but not to the degree implied of limiting *all* lateral and rotatory movement. Some rotation and lateral flexion (along the ideas of Lovette) is physiologically permitted without injury or impairment.

In the erect position some degree of lateral flexion and rotation is possible in the lumbosacral spine. In the hyperextended position the facets are approximated to essentially become **locked in**. In this position *no* lateral flexion or rotation is possible.

As the spine flexes—goes from lordosis to kyphosis—the posterior structures separate. The facets literally "unlock." The facets separate. Their capsules elongate. Movement at this point is permitted laterally and rotatorily.

The anterior weight-bearing aspect of the functional unit restricts movement in all directions by the resistance and inflexibility of the annular fibers and the longitudinal ligaments. The disk annular fibers have been deducted to permit 5 degrees of rotation before they "fail" (disrupt).

The degree and safe range of rotation are thus determined by the posterior degree of separation and rotation and must not exceed 5 degrees.

In flexion and simultaneous rotation the facets on the concave side approximate and those on the convex side separate. There is also simultaneous rotation of the disk within the limits of annular elongation (collagen fiber elongation, i.e., uncoiling). The posterior tissues, the erector spinae muscles, and the ligaments also have elongated similarly (Fig. 4–13).

Return to the erect position must conform to the same **tract** of motion, in reverse, as was done in flexion. Derotation must follow the same pathways, which implies symmetrical derotation with gradual re-extension. In doing so properly the facets disengage and the torque of the tissues is not abused or misused.

Improper re-extension (i.e., failure to derotate sufficiently or appropriately during the course of re-extension) causes failure with the facet (on the concave or approximated) side remaining approximated and the disk annular fibers exceeding their torque limits.

This is a mechanical exposé of proper (and improper) flexion and extension. This will be discussed relating to the resultant symptoms later in the text.

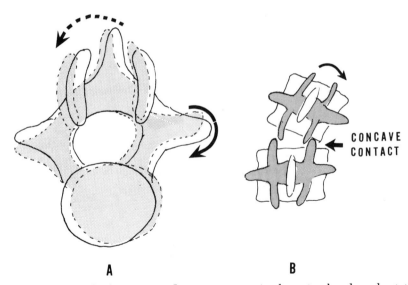

A   **B**

CONCAVE
CONTACT

Figure 4–13. Vertebral torque on flexion-rotation. As the spine bends and rotates, the vertebrae of each functional unit laterally flex and rotate one upon the other. The facets on the concave side approximate (*arrow in figure B*). Viewed from above (A), the facets glide as does the intervertebral disk (*the dotted outline upon the solid*). The degree of rotation can physiologically rotate and shear 5 degrees before "failing."

THORACOLUMBAR JUNCTION

This is the junction of the caudal aspect of the thoracic spine to the upper aspect of the lumbar spine. This is the transitional functional unit T12-L1.

It is a "transitional" unit as the superior facets and the lower facets within that unit differ in their planes to allow rotation and flexion, whereas the thoracic (above) allow only rotation and those below (lumbar) only flexion extension.

The emerging nerves from this thoracolumbar unit have a particular distribution that will be discussed in the clinical situations later in the text.

REFERENCES

Asmussen, E: The weight-carrying function of the spine. Acta Orthop Scand 1:276, 1960.

Bogbuk, N and Macintosh, JE: The applied anatomy of the thoracolumbar fascia. Spine 9:164, 1984.

Edgar, MA and Nundy, S: Innervation of the spinal dura mater. J Neurol Neurosurg Psychiatry 29:530, 1966.

Floyd, WF and Silver, PHS: The function of the erectores spinae muscles in certain movements and postures in man. J Physiol 129:184, 1955.

Froning, EC and Froning, B: Motion of the lumbosacral spine after laminectomy and spine fusion. J Bone Joint Surg 50A:897, 1968.

Gracovetsky, S and Farfan, H: The optimum spine. Spine 2:543, 1986.

Hendry, NGC: The hydration of the nucleus pulposus and its relation to intervertebral disc dehydration. J Bone Joint Surg 40B:132, 1958.

Hirsch, C and Lewin, T: Lumbosacral synovial joints in flexion-extension. Acta Orthop Scand 39:303, 1968.

Kaplan, EB: Recurrent meningeal branch of the spinal nerves. Bull Hosp Joint Diseases 8:108, 1947.

McGill, SM and Norman, RW: Partitioning of the L4-L5 dynamic moment into disk, ligamentous, and muscular components during lifting. Spine 11:666, 1986.

Morris, JM, Benner, G and Lucas, DB: An electromyographic study of the intrinsic muscles of the back in man. J Anat (London) 96:509, 1962.

Portnoy, H and Morin, F: Electromyographic study of postural muscles in various positions and movements. Am J Physiol 186:122, 1956.

Splithoff, CA: Lumbosacral junction. JAMA 152:1610

Steindler, A: Kinesiology of the Human Body. Charles C Thomas, Springfield, IL, 1955.

Tesh, KM, Dunn, JS and Evans, JH: The abdominal muscles and vertebral stability. Spine 12:501, 1987.

Wyke, B: The neurology of joints. Ann R Coll Surg Engl 41:25, 1967.

Wyke, B: The neurological basis of thoracic spine pain. Rheumatol Phys Med 10:356, 1967.

CHAPTER 5

Tissue Sites of Low Back Pain

Pain considered to occur within the low back or from the low back implies that tissue(s) within a functional unit has become the site of nociception. There has been insult or injury to this (these) tissue(s) from an abnormal stress that results in transmission of impulses through the sensory neurologic pathways to the cord then to the cerebral cortex where the symptom of **pain** becomes apparent to the patient.

The tissue site capable of becoming a site of nociceptive stimulus must be innervated by nerve endings and fibers that can transmit impulses which, in time, convey "pain." The mechanism of pain sensation transmission via the central nervous system and the factors influencing the interpretation of pain will be fully discussed in a subsequent chapter, but an analysis of the specific tissue site within the functional unit appropriately innervated must be clarified.

The major sensory nerve of the functional unit has been well documented as being the recurrent nerve of von Luschka (Fig. 5–1). There undoubtedly also is transmission of sensation via the somatic nerves within the anterior and posterior primary branches through the dorsal ganglion (Fig. 5–2).

Within the functional unit each specific tissue will be mentioned that is capable of being a site or source of nociceptive stimuli. The end organs of nerve fibers that are functionally mechanoreceptors will not be mentioned here.

1. The intervertebral disk mentioned so prominently as "the" site and source of low back pain is essentially an aneural tissue. No unmyelinated nerves or end organs of nerves have been found in the nucleus or in the middle and inner annular fiber sheets of normal intact disks.

Recent studies have claimed that microscopic end organs of unmyelin-

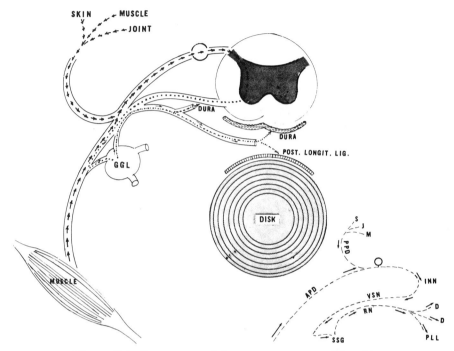

Figure 5–1. Innervation of the recurrent nerve of Luschka.
  PPD—posterior primary division
  APD—anterior primary division
  GGL—sympathetic ganglion
  INN—internuncial neurons
  VSN—ventral sensory nerve
  SSG—sensory sympathetic ganglion
  RN—recurrent nerve of Luschka
    D—to dura
PLL—posterior longitudinal ligament

ated nerves have been identified in the extreme outer layers of the annulus. Whether these end organs belong to nerves penetrating into the annulus or are extensions of nerve endings from the longitudinal ligaments has not been clarified. It is currently accepted that, at most, only the very outer layer of the annulus is innervated and may possibly be a site of nociceptive stimuli.

The nerve that supplies this outer annular layer, which is possibly a sensitive tissue site, is the recurrent nerve of von Luschka at each root segment.

2. The vertebral body is an insensitive tissue unless it is invaded by metabolic or metastatic disease. Multiple myeloma, Paget disease, osteitis, fracture, etc., are acceptably pain-producing, but otherwise the "normal"

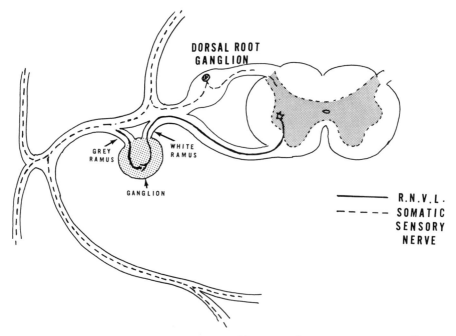

Figure 5–2. Somatic sensory nerve. In addition to the recurrent nerve of von Luschka (R.N.V.L.), sensory transmission of nociceptive stimuli ascend via the somatic sensory nerve through the dorsal root ganglion into the dorsal gray matter of the cord (the S.G.).

vertebral body is insensitive. Its periosteum is innervated and thus is capable of being the site of pain. Tissue site as a source of pain is difficult to ascertain clinically or by laboratory confirmation.

3. The anterior longitudinal ligament is a proven pain-sensitive tissue. This ligament is innervated by the recurrent meningeal nerve and has clinically been confirmed as a painful tissue site. Surgical experiments on the awake patient, in which the longitudinal ligament has been irritated chemically, mechanically, or electrically, have caused local pain or referred pain in sclerotomal distribution areas.

4. The posterior longitudinal ligament has also been confirmed as being innervated by unmyelinated somatic and sympathetic sensory nerves. When this ligament is irritated, a sensation of pain can be elicited.

5. The nerve root, per se, is not sensitive (Fig. 5–3). Irritation of the nerve root (axones) from traction, pressure, or trauma does not cause pain. As in a peripheral nerve, pressure or mechanical trauma may cause paresthesia, dysesthesia, analgesia, or motor paresis but rarely "pain." If trauma to a peripheral nerve does not cause pain, why does mechanical irritation of a nerve root that is basically a peripheral nerve—containing sensory and motor fibers—cause pain? It does not!

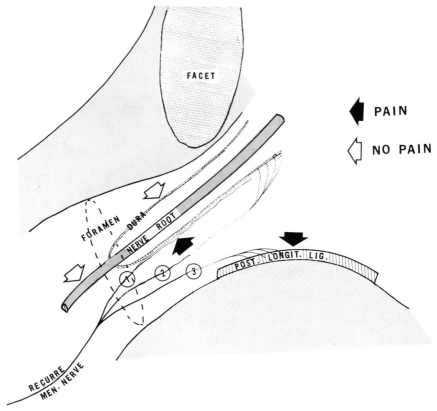

Figure 5–3. Dura accompanying nerve root through intervertebral foramen with its innervation by the recurrent meningeal nerve. *1* and *2* proceed to the anterior dural sheath, illustrating the sensitivity of that portion of the dura. The posterior dural sheath with no innervation is insensitive. *3*. Innervation which is capable of pain supplies the posterolongitudinal ligament.

The tissue of the nerve root within the intervertebral foraminae that is irritable and supplied by sensory nerve fibers capable of transmitting pain is the recurrent nerve. Within the dural sheath is contained spinal fluid, venules, arterioles, lymphatics and nervosus nervosum (Fig. 5–4).

The mechanism of irritating this nerve and relating it clinically will be fully discussed in the chapter relating to low back and radicular pain. It is enough here to merely state that the nerve roots (the axones) are not sensitive, but their dural sheath is. Trauma to a peripheral nerve can cause hypalgesia, hypesthesia, and motor paresis because the sensory and motor fibers within the nerve root are located in a position close to the intervertebral disk and the facet joints (Fig. 5–5). Irritation from either of these structures, the disk or the facet joints, can irritate the nerve root and,

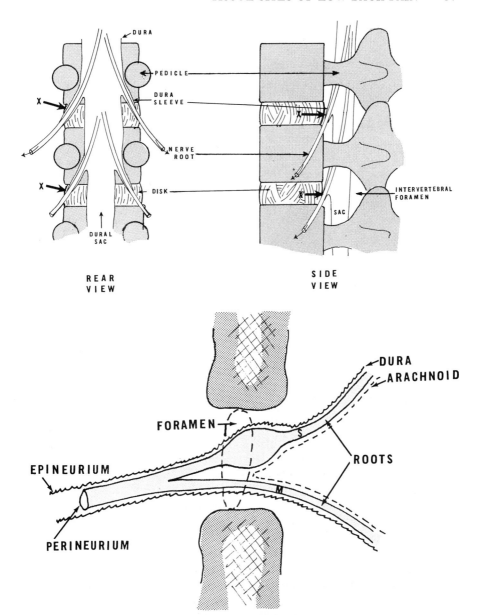

Figure 5–4. Dural and arachnoid sheaths of the nerve root complex. The arachnoid follows the sensory and motor nerve roots to the beginning of the intervertebral foramen and follows the sensory root to the beginning of the ganglion. The dura follows the nerve roots until they become the combined sensory and motor nerve outside the foramen and continues as the perineurium and epineurium. Neither the dura nor the arachnoid attaches to the intervertebral foramen.

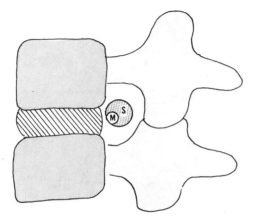

Figure 5–5. Sensorimotor aspect of nerve root. Within the intervertebral foramen, the motor roots are smaller than the sensory and are inferior and posterior near the disk.

depending on which irritant, the sensory or the motor nerve fibers affected will cause appropriate symptoms.

The dorsal root ganglion was implicated as the source of low back pain by Lindblom and Rexed in 1948, with pressure on the ganglion from the disk or facet joints being the primary basis. Newer studies of neurotransmitters have evoked some clarification and contradiction in this alleged simplistic pain mechanism.

Chemical transmitters were originally few, but many neuropeptides are now relegated to the role of neurotransmitters and neuromodulators within the central nervous system.

The cells within the dorsal root ganglion were originally divided into large cells giving rise to large myelinated fibers and small cells giving rise to thin unmyelinated fibers. The latter fibers are now considered to terminate within the substantia gelatinosum (lamina II of Rexed) in the dorsal column of the spinal cord. Stimulation of these fibers and cells apparently liberates substance P and calcitonin gene-related peptides, which are considered to mediate the sensation of pain.

The conflict that has arisen is whether mere pressure of the disk on the nerve root, as claimed by Mixter and Barr (1957), could cause radicular pain. Howe (1977) demonstrated that long periods of repetitive firing of the nerve resulted following minimal acute compression of the **normal** dorsal root ganglion. Chronic injury to the dorsal root, however, increased the sensitivity to mechanical irritation and markedly increased firing. Thus, pressure on a **normal** dorsal ganglion nerve does not produce pain, but pressure on the irritated nerve root ganglion fibers can cause pain. The conclusion is that formation of neuropepetides at the site of nerve damage predisposes that nerve to increased sensitivity and may result in transmission of pain on mere pressure.

The nerve root and the dorsal root ganglia of the lumbosacral plexus (sciatic and femoral nerves) emerge from the spinal canal through the inter-vertebral foraminae. This foramen has been discussed as being between two contiguous vertebrae, bounded anteriorly by the posterior annular lam-inae of the intervertebral disk and the posterior margins of the vertebral bodies (Fig. 5–6). It is bounded posteriorly by the facet joints, their cap-sules, and the ligamentum flavum.

As the nerve roots of the cauda equina proceed caudally within the spinal canal, they cross the disks immediately above the foramen. The roots

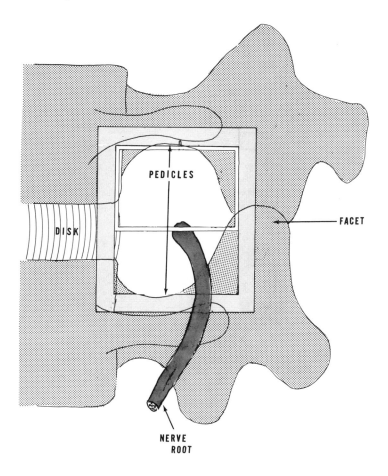

FORAMEN

Figure 5–6. The intervertebral foramen. The "window" through which the nerve root emerges is bordered in front by the disk, above and below by the pedicles of two adjacent vertebrae, and behind by the facets. (Modified from Cailliet, R: Un-derstand Your Backache. FA Davis, Philadelphia, 1984, p 50.)

then enter the foraminae beneath the pedicle. As they leave the foramen, they proceed downward, outward, and forward (Fig. 5–7). In the lower disk level the nerve enters the origin of the psoas muscle. By virtue of their ventral site of entry into the foramen they are located in the superior aspect of that foramen. This is shown in the upper half of Fig. 5–4.

At their site of entry into the foramina toward their extraspinal course,

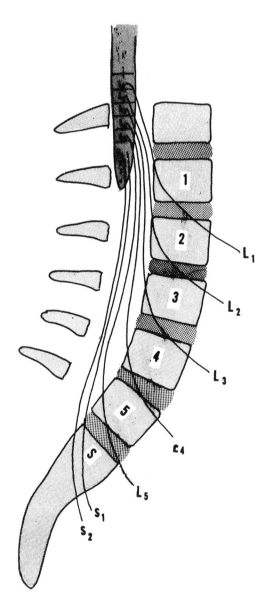

Figure 5–7. Relationship of nerve roots to vertebral levels.

the nerve roots invaginate the dura and the arachnoid carrying the dural sheath into the foramen. The arachnoid continues along the nerve root as far as the sensory ganglion (see Fig. 5–4). The dura continues along the combined (sensory and motor) nerve until it fuses with the arachnoid forming the distal end of the sleeve. The dura continues along the distal nerve forming the outer, fibrous, sheath of the peripheral nerve, the perineurium. Only the dural sheath, within the foramen, is innervated and thus is sensitive.

On emerging from the foramen each nerve root divides into an anterior and a posterior primary division (see Fig. 5–1).

Chronic pain has been attributed to fibrosis of the nerve root and dorsal ganglion within the foramen. This fibrosis has been equated with "inflammation" as a cause of neuritic pain from disk herniation, foraminal stenosis, or arachnoiditis. The exact cause and evolution of this fibrosis have not, to date, been clarified.

Fibrin deposit blended within the connective tissue as a result of irritation has been noted. Recently impaired or defective fibrinolytic activity has been identified in patients with chronic low back pain and radicular symptoms (Pountain, Keegan, and Jayson, 1987). This discovery may cast significant light on the reason certain patients undergo chronic radicular symptoms while others fail to do so.

The basis and cause of fibrinolytic activity remain unclear, but if a fibrinolytic drug or activator is found, the answer to arachnoiditis and even chronic nerve root pain may evolve.

6. The ligamentum flavum is a yellow ligamentous tissue composed essentially of elastin fibers with minimal collagen or fibrous fibers. By being very elastic and having rapid recoil capabilities its major function is to prevent the capsule of the facet from becoming entrapped within the facet joints when they open and close during motion of the lumbosacral spine. No nerve supply to the ligamentum flavum has been identified; thus this tissue is aneural and insensitive.

7. The erector spinae muscles, as all skeletal muscles, are highly innervated by nociceptive sensory nerves situated within the muscles' masses, their fascial sheaths, the intramuscular septa, the tendinous insertions into bone periosteum and within the intramuscular blood vessels. These nerves are somatic, sensory, recurrent meningeal nerves with various end organs. They subserve proprioception as well as nociception.

Where pain sensation originates in the muscle is not fully documented. Ischemia has been implemented as a cause of muscular pain. The accumulation of metabolites such as substance P, kinins, prostaglandins, histamine, lactate, and numerous others has been considered a cause of muscle nociception. Accumulation of tissue metabolites has been attributed to a sustained muscular contraction ("tension") or to mechanical trauma to the muscle.

The fascia of muscle tissue is also well innervated by sensory fibers and is considered to play a role in the production of pain in the low back. A good example of such a painful condition is the so-called myofascial pain.

Low back pain, with pain referred into the lower extremities and concurrent "spasm" of the back and the hamstring muscles, has always been attributed to a "disk origin." These symptoms of low back pain with leg pain radiation and concurrent back spasm have been induced in a normal person by chemically or mechanically irritating specific tissues of the low back. These tissues that can be irritated to produce back and leg pain must be tissues innervated by the lumbar dorsal rami.

To differentiate symptoms occurring from a cause other than pain being mediated by disk pathology causing "nerve root pain," a diagnostic label of **lumbar dorsal ramus syndrome** (LDRS) has been postulated by Bogduk (1980). The symptoms of this syndrome are created by irritation of the dorsal ramus nerve rather than by irritation or compression of the nerve root.

The symptoms of LDRS are those of a pain that is deep, dull, and aching rather than sharp and precisely located. The pain is felt in the back and in the posterior lateral aspect of the leg. LDRS is not a sensation related to a specific site or resulting from a distinctive motion. These symptoms are not mediated by irritation of a nerve root and have no segmental distribution.

The neurologic basis for these symptoms has not been clearly described or accepted. The acceptance of pain as a result of this "syndrome" is based on the fact that similar symptoms have been reproduced in "asymptomatic" people by the irritation of a soft tissue of the low back. These "soft tissues" include the interspinous ligaments, the multifidus muscle, and the zygapophyseal joints (facets). Irritation of these tissues of the low back is invariably accompanied by radiation of a pain into the lower extremities.

As will be mentioned in the differential diagnosis of "sciatic pain," pain considered to be a radicular pain, occurring from pressure or traction on a nerve root by a bulging disk within the intervertebral foramen of the L4-5 S1 root, radiates below the knee (Fig. 5–8).

A referred pain that radiates down the leg below the knee is usually considered to result from a nerve entrapment from a bulging disk at the L4-5 or L5-S1 levels. Pain from a nerve entrapment by disk pressure at disk levels of L3-4 or higher does not radiate below the knee.

The conclusion is that a radiating pain below the knee must be from nerve pressure at the lower two disk levels.

The pain that resulted from experimental chemical or electrical irritation of tissues other than the disk or nerves contiguous to the disk **was** felt in the low back **and** radiated below the knee. In these experimental studies causing low back and radiating pain, it was demonstrated that it was the strength of the irritating stimulus to the soft tissue—not irritation of

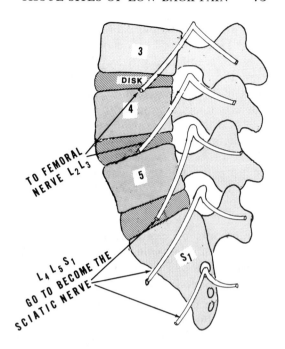

Figure 5–8. Sciatic nerve roots. The fourth and fifth lumbar nerves and the sacral nerve form the sciatic nerve. This nerve goes down the back of the leg to the foot and toes. The second and third lumbar nerves do *not* go into the sciatic nerve. They merge to form the femoral nerve, which goes down the *front* of the thigh to the thigh muscles. (Modified from Cailliet, R: Understand Your Backache. FA Davis, Philadelphia, 1984, p 81.)

the nerve root—that was responsible for causing radiation distally into the lower extremity.

Pain from soft tissue irritation was originally created by injecting hypertonic saline into the tissues being studied. Relief from the pain resulting from the chemical irritant injection was afforded by injecting an anesthetic agent into the same site. As there was a diffusion of the injected irritating solution within the tissues of this injected chemical irritant, the exact tissue site of irritation could not be confirmed. Electrical stimulation of a **precise isolated** tissue site replaced the chemical injection as the irritant used to produce the pain. This confirmed a more precise tissue site as being a ligament, facet joint, or specific muscle.

"Spasm" of the low back muscles and the hamstring muscles resulted from the injection into intervertebral ligaments and facet joints. Electromyographic studies of these muscles confirmed that a "reflex" neurologic pattern occurred when a ligament, facet joint, or the multifidus muscle was injected or electrically irritated. Besides the low back erector spinae muscles and the hamstring muscles going "into spasm" so also did the gluteus maximus and the tensor fascia lata. The "protective muscles reflex pattern" was established by these experiments, and the painful low back situation, so often seen clinically, was considered as occurring from irritation of the soft tissues of the low back that are innervated by the lumbar dorsal (posterior) ramus.

All these findings have led to clinically accepting the premise that low back and leg radiating pain could result from irritation of the tissues inner-vated by the dorsal ramus of the posterior primary division (Fig. 5–9).

Interruption of the dorsal ramus thus was considered as needed to re-lieve the pain when other modalities failed. Interruption of the primary ra-mus of the nerve root chemically, electrically, or surgically has been postulated and attempted to alleviate the pain of the low back patient.

8. Ligamentous pain from trauma to the posterior superior ligaments and the intertransversus ligaments. These ligaments are supplied by the ar-ticular branches (somatic and sympathetic) of the posterior primary division of the nerve roots. Ligamentous trauma such as overstretching or direct blunt trauma has been accepted as being responsible for the production of pain.

9. The zygapophyseal joints are nociceptive sites of pain production. These joints are typical synovial joints containing cartilage, synovium, and synovial capsules, which are copiously supplied by somatic and sympathetic nerves contained within the articular branch of the posterior primary divi-sion of a typical segmental nerve root.

There is voluminous literature as to the presence of, mechanism of, and distribution of pain originating from facet joints and its role in common low back pain. The ultimate basis and the prevalence of low back pain origi-nating from the zygapophyseal joints remain controversial but are currently acceptable.

Having dwelt on the tissues within the functional unit capable of being

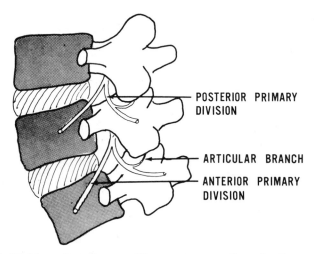

Figure 5–9. Division of nerve roots. Upon emergence from the foramen, the roots divide into the anterior primary division and the posterior primary division. A small articular branch is sensory to the facets.

the site of nociceptive pain we now can turn to the mechanisms by which these tissues can be traumatized and from which pain in and from the low back can occur.

REFERENCES

Barbut, D, Polak, JM and Wall, PD: Substance P in spinal cord dorsal horn decreases following peripheral nerve injury. Brain Res 205:289, 1981.

Bogduk, N: Clinical review: Lumbar dorsal ramus syndrome. Med J Aust 2:537, 1950.

Bogduk, N and Long, DM: The anatomy of the so-called "articular nerves" and their relationship to facet denervation in the treatment of low-back pain. Neurosurg 51:172, 1979.

Dodd, J, Jahr, CE and Jessell, TM: Neurotransmitters and neuronal markers at sensory synapses in the dorsal horn. In Kruger, JC (ed): Advances in Pain Research and Therapy, Chap 6. Liebeskind. Raven Press, New York, 1984, p 105.

Gunn, CC and Milbrandt, WE: Tenderness at motor points. J Bone Joint Surg 58A:815, 1986.

Hakelius, A and Hindmarsh, J: The significance of neurological signs and myelographic findings in the diagnosis of lumbar root compression. Acta Orthop Scand 43:239, 1972.

Hirsch, C, Ingelmark, B-E, and Miller, M: The anatomical basis for low back pain. Acta Orthop Scand 33:19, 1963.

Howe, JF, Loeser, JD and Calvin, WH: Mechanosensitivity of dorsal root ganglia and chronically injured axons: A physiological basis for radicular pain of nerve root compression. Pain 3:25, 1977.

Kellgren, JH: The anatomical source of back pain. Rheumatol Rehabil 16:3, 1977.

Lindahgl, O: Hyperalgesia of the lumbar nerve roots in sciatica. Acta Orthop Scand 37:367, 1966.

Mixter, WJ and Barr, JS: Rupture of intervertebral disk with involvement of the spinal canal. N Engl J Med 211:120, 1957.

Pedersen, HE, Blunck, CF and Gardner, E: The anatomy of lumbosacral posterior rami and meningeal branches of spinal nerves (sinu-vertebral nerves). J Bone Joint Surg 38:377, 1956.

Pountain, GD, Keegan, AL, and Jayson, MIV: Impaired fibrinolytic activity in defined chronic back pain syndrome. Spine 12:83, 1987.

Selby, DK and Paris, SV: Anatomy of facet joints and its clinical correlation with low back pain. Contemp Orthop 3:1097, 1981.

Smyth, MJ and Wright, V: Sciatica and the intervertebral disk. J Bone Joint Surg 40A:1401, 1958.

Stilwell, DL: Regional variations in the innervation of deep fasciae and aponeuroses. Anat Rec 127:635, 1957.

CHAPTER 6

Abnormal Functional Deviation of Spinal Function Resulting in Pain and Impairment

The protocol for pertinent and meaningful clinical examination of the patient with **low back pain** is the same as that for the patient with any musculoskeletal complaint: **to know the normal function and to recognize the deviation from normal; to establish the exact mechanism that initiated the pain and be able to reproduce the pain by reproducing the abnormal position or motion that elicits the pain.**

The history must elicit the precise position or movement that initiated or can reproduce *the* pain. The history must specifically describe the pain: where and when it is. It must reveal the exact mental and emotional status of the person at the time of causation of the pain as well as describe the exact physical position that was assumed by the injured person at the time of onset or recurrence of the pain. All these factors, and many more, will constitute the following discussion of the **abnormal deviation of spinal function causing low back pain and impairment.**

The normal spine must by definition be pain-free, both in the static and in the kinetic status. A person should stand, sit, bend, lift, twist, turn, and lie in a perfectly balanced situation and be pain-free. The presence of pain indicates that one of the component structural tissues has been abused, misused, or injured. Pain is nature's warning sign of tissue insult.

It behooves the examiner to establish what injury has occurred and which tissue has been infracted. In the situation where the low back is implicated, the spinal function must be divided into the static or the kinetic aspect.

76

THE STATIC SPINAL FUNCTIONAL
DEVIATION

The static spine can be viewed as the erect, nonmoving spine. When pain occurs from assuming or implementing this posture, the basis for the production of the pain must be sought.

A person should be able to stand effortlessly and painlessly with cosmetic acceptance if the erect position—the posture—is "normal." When pain intervenes, "normalcy" is questioned.

For many centuries an excessive lordosis—a marked "sway back"— has been considered abnormal and a frequent cause of static low back pain. This diagnosis has been based on the assumption that the sway back noted in numerous conditions, such as pregnancy, was symptomatic and that by decreasing the lordosis, pain decreased or disappeared. This assumption led to the frequently prescribed "Williams exercises," which are intended to decrease lordosis. A corset, allegedly decreasing the lordosis, also affords comfort to many patients by "decreasing the lordosis."

It is a safe assumption that the vast majority of patients with static low back pain suffer from an excessive lordosis, but recent postulations have refuted this concept.

Let us review what is accepted as influencing lumbar lordosis.

The lumbosacral angle is measured by the angulation of the surface level of the sacrum as compared with the true horizontal level (Fig. 6–1). As the lumbar spine ascends on this base, the base changes its angle or "tilts" away from the horizontal level, and the curve of the lumbar spine changes appropriately.

The fifth lumbar vertebra lies on the sacrum and thus resides on an inclined plane (Fig. 6–2). The fifth vertebra is prevented from sliding downward on this inclined base by certain mechanical factors:

1. The opposition of the facets joints—mechanically the opposing surfaces of the facets are in direct relationship and are held immobile by muscular and ligamentous action. Significant shear is minimized.

2. When the lordosis is increased, approximately 16 percent (Fig. 6–3) of the compressive forces on the spine are transmitted through the tips of the facet surfaces (Fig. 6–4). On decreasing the lordosis the shear force is no longer resisted by the facets but now falls on the tensile forces (Fig.6–5) of the disk annulus.

The concept, therefore, that excessive lordosis results in low back pain must relate to the fact that pain originates within the posterior elements and not in the disk.

A model presentation of the causation of lordotic low back pain is offered in Fig. 6–6. In excessive lordosis three things can occur: (1) The facets approximate with compression and can become a site of nociceptive

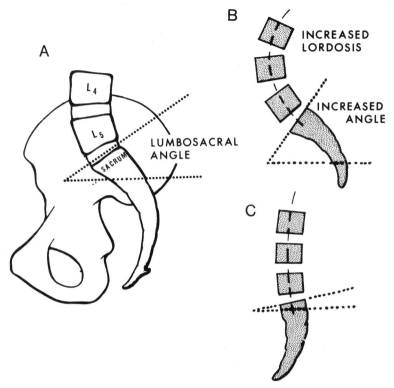

Figure 6–1. Lumbosacral angle. *A*. Erect posture angle. *B*. With increased angle, the lumbar lordosis is increased. *C*. The lordosis decreases with decrease of lumbosacral angle.

impulses; (2) the intervertebral foramen closes and encroaches on the nerve root dura and all its contents; and (3) the disk can bulge posteriorly, putting pressure on the posterior (Fig. 6–7) longitudinal ligament. Myelographic studies have revealed a posterior "bulge" in the low back extended (excessive lordotic) position.

Initiating an exercise program that decreases the lordosis is beneficial to many patients complaining of static low back pain. The benefit derived from wearing a corset that decreases the lordosis also enforces the frequency of low back pain attributed to excessive lordosis.

In recent years MacKenzie, a New Zealand physical therapist, presented a contrary concept that has proved to have some validity. He postulated that lordosis is "physiological" and that the nucleus of the intervertebral disk is "forced" anteriorly, away from the contents of the spinal canal, during lordosis. He advocated extension exercises and claimed benefit.

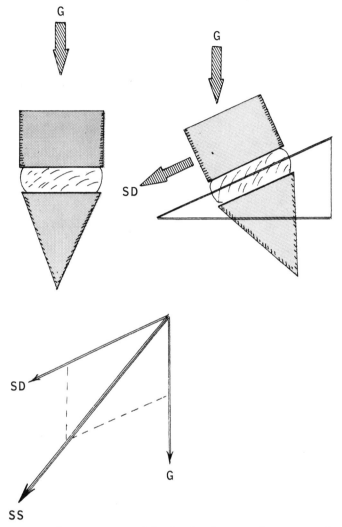

Figure 6–2. Static shearing stress of the last lumbar vertebra in its inclined plane relationship to the sacral vertebra. G implies the gravity stress of the entire body upon the weight-bearing hydraulic system of the intervertebral disk. SD is the force of a body sliding down an inclined plane. SS represents the resultant force and its direction of G and SD and is the shearing stress exerted on the elastic fibers of the annulus.

MacKenzie also claimed that most people today personally and professionally spend many daily hours in the flexed position. In this flexed position the posterior element tissues—the posterior superior spinous ligaments, the facet capsules, the posterior longitudinal ligaments, and the

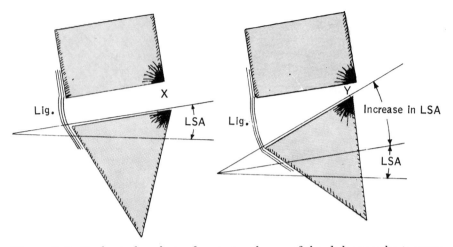

Figure 6–3. Mechanical analysis of posterior closure of the disk space by increase of the lumbosacral angle (LSA), anterior restriction of the anterior longitudinal ligament (Lig.). Narrowing of space X to space Y also portends approximation of the facets in their posterior relationship of the functional unit.

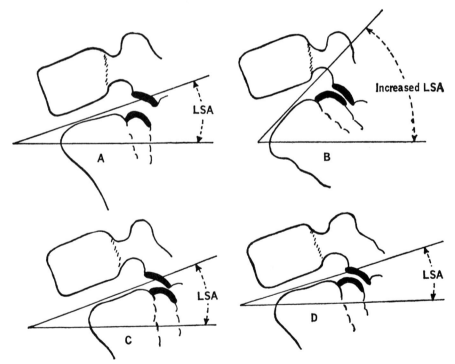

Figure 6–4. Variations in posterior articular relationships. *A*. Normal lumbosacral angle with intact disk: normal relationship of articular facets. *B*. Increase in lumbosacral angle (LSA) with posterior closure of the facets. *C*. Spondylolisthesis with a normal LSA exerting traction on the posterior longitudinal ligament and disruption of facet alignment. *D*. Disk degeneration with narrowing of intervertebral space and approximation of facets.

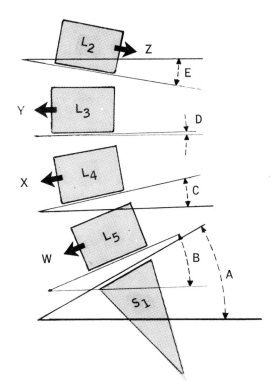

Figure 6–5. Differential shearing stress of lumbar vertebrae. The shearing stress of the last lumbar vertebra upon the first sacral differs from the shearing stresses of each successive cephalad vertebra. At each intervertebral level the inclined plane angle decreases and thus the shearing stress and its direction decrease.

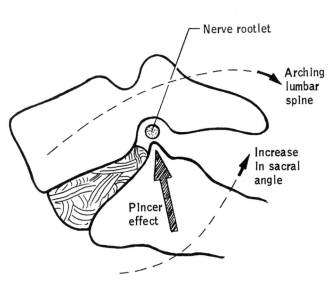

Figure 6–6. Nerve root impingement due to hyperextension of the lumbosacral spine. Greater extent of impingement can be expected with a degenerated disk.

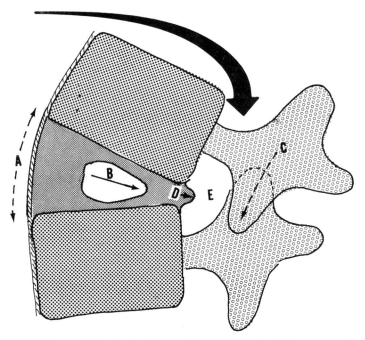

Figure 6–7. Disk protrusion in lumbosacral hyperextension. The anterior longitudinal ligament restricts further extension (A). The nucleus has deformed to the maximum, cannot migrate further anteriorly, and thus moves posteriorly (B). This causes a "bulge" (D) with encroachment into the intervertebral foramen (E). The facets overlap (C), which also narrows the foramen as well as causing painful weight-bearing.

posterior annular fibers of the disk—become excessively elongated. This position, he claims, forces the nucleus posteriorly against the posterior longitudinal ligament and against the posterior annular fibers of the disk causing "bulging" and possibly some herniation (Fig. 6–8).

These factors "result in low back pain that extension exercises and daily positions diminish or eliminate." The clinical results are promising, whereas the proposed anatomic basis remains unsettled. It behooves the clinician to determine whether the symptoms claimed by the patient are the result of flexion or extension. The original adage in the first paragraph of this chapter, **"to reproduce 'the' pain by reproducing the abnormal position . . . that elicits 'the' pain"** applies in this instance. In essence, if "the" pain is reproduced by hyperextension, the cause, and thus the remedy, is apparent. If the history and examination indicate that flexion is the culprit, the causation then becomes evident.

Radicular pain symptoms, as well as low back pain in discogenic dis-

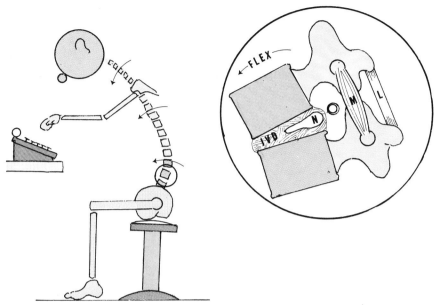

Figure 6–8. Disk "bulging" from prolonged flexed posture: MacKenzie Concept. MacKenzie postulated that man spends much time in the flexed position: standing at work, sitting, etc., which overstretches the posterior tissues (muscles, ligaments, capsules) but especially pushes the nucleus posteriorly and thus is responsible for disk bulging. The remedy (MacKenzie) is to institute extension (recreate the lordosis). (From Cailliet, R: Soft Tissue Pain and Disability, ed 2. FA Davis, Philadelphia, 1988, with permission.)

ease and from spinal or foraminal stenosis, as related to extension or flexion diagnosis and treatment, will receive further evaluation in subsequent chapters.

KINETIC LOW BACK PAIN

Pain in or from the low back caused by improper functional use of the lumbosacral spine is termed **kinetic** low back pain. It behooves us to briefly review how the spine **normally** flexes and re-extends to the erect posture in simple bending over or in the act of lifting. Then, we need to evaluate how the spine bends over and returns to the erect posture **improperly**.

As a person bends forward, the lumbosacral spine functions in a precise, coordinated manner. The act of bending is initiated by bringing the head forward **ahead** of the center of gravity. This initiates a gravity neurologic reflex throughout the entire spine.

The erect **static** spine has been balanced without active muscular contraction other than a slight sustained isometric (tone) contraction (Fig. 6–9). By bringing the head ahead of the center of gravity the erector spinae muscles are slightly elongated. This initiates an elongation of the spindle system and Golgi fibers of the erector spinae muscles (Fig. 6–10).

The reflex action via the Ia fibers to the cord initiates an extrafusal contraction via the alpha fibers of the exact amount of contraction for the intended act. The muscles then elongate. They essentially contract eccentrically and slowly decelerate the flexing spine. The rapidity of this deceleration is monitored within a complex neurologic system pattern so that elongation decelerates the spine flexion at the "pre-set," desired, and intended speed.

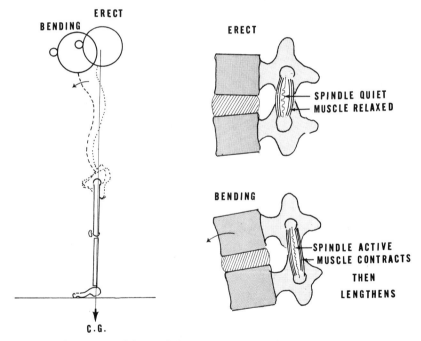

Figure 6–9. Initiation of forward flexion. Once the decision of "bending over" is entertained, the head goes ahead of the center of gravity (C.G.). The intrafusal fibers of the erector spinae muscles (in each functional unit) which have been dormant in erect posture are activated by elongation of the spindle system. A reflex mechanism ensues in which the spindle system now activates the extrafusal fibers (that have also been dormant in the erect stance posture) that gradually progressively elongate to "open" the functional units allowing the lumbar spine to flex. (From Cailliet, R: Soft Tissue Pain and Disability, ed 2. FA Davis, Philadelphia, 1988, with permission.)

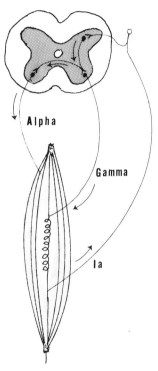

Figure 6–10. Spindle system. The spindle system of the muscle controls and moderates the tone of the extrafusal fibers. It transmits the "information" to the cord via Ia fibers where it (at the cord level) modifies the tone of the extrafusal muscle fibers (innervated by somatic alpha fibers). Via the gamma fibers, the spindle system is "reset" to the appropriate tone needed. (From Cailliet, R: Soft Tissue Pain and Disability, ed 2. FA Davis, Philadelphia, 1988, with permission.)

SPINDLE SYSTEM

The proprioceptive fibers within the muscles, fascia, joint capsules, and ligaments feed back the accomplished action to the central nervous system, which in turn "resets" the spindle system at the repeated new degrees of flexion, new speeds, and the changing mandated efforts. This is a complex pattern that is inbred but has been learned and can be modified.

Each functional unit flexes as the erector spinae (extensor muscles) slowly decelerate flexion initiated by gravity and maintained by gravitational forces. Only gravity is implicated when there is no weight being held, lifted, or supported other than the upper body.

Each functional unit flexes to approximately 9 degrees. By this degree of flexion the erector spinae muscles have elongated to their fullest as restricted by the fascia (Fig. 6–11). At this point of flexion the posterior superior spinous ligaments have also gone from relaxation to full extension. The functional unit can flex no further (see Fig. 6–11).

The proper function of the mechanoceptors of the low back tissues is as yet not fully understood. These nerve endings have been studied by B.D. Wyke and are currently classified as to morphology, physiology, and

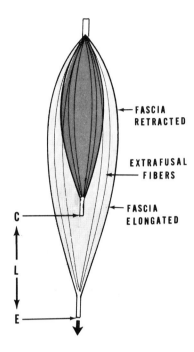

FASCIA
RETRACTED

EXTRAFUSAL
FIBERS

FASCIA
ELONGATED

C

L

E

Figure 6–11. Fascial limits to muscular elongation. Any muscle bundle will elongate to the extent that its fascial sheath will permit. The extrafusal fibers elongate fully, but the fascia must passively be elongated. It is fascial contracture that restricts muscular elongation and joint range of motion. (From Cailliet, R: Soft Tissue Pain and Disability, ed 2. FA Davis, Philadelphia, 1988, with permission.)

pathology but are not yet fully equated into the total low back kinesiologic function.

The nerve endings within the tissues (here of the lumbosacral spine) that subserve proprioception are classified as **types** 1 to 4. It behooves us to pause and evaluate these mechanoreceptors.

Types 1, 2, and 3 have a corpuscular end organ and are situated within a precise type of tissue. Once these end organs are activated, they discharge via the nerves into the central nervous system. Their response reflects the direction, velocity, and amplitude of movement. These nerve endings are not motor nerves, but they influence the intensity, velocity, and direction of the motor action by proprioceptive feedback. In an inadvertent action, where there is excessive muscular action for the intended action, their reaction is too late or too intense to have a remedial effect.

Types 1 and 2 are embedded in the joint capsule, with type 1 in the superficial layers of the joint capsule and type 2 in the deeper layers. Type 3 endings are located within the ligaments. All three are exclusively mechanoreceptors and do not transmit nociceptive sensations. Type 4 end organs and their nerves subserve nociceptive sensation transmission but no proprioception.

Nerve adaptation relates to the duration of time that the nerve continues to discharge impulses when it is exposed to a mechanical stimulus. Type 1 adapts slowly. Type 2 adapts rapidly. Type 1 receptors fire constantly whereas type 2s do not. Both have a low threshold in that they fire with very little stimulus intensity. Type 3s are ligament mechanoreceptors with a thin capsule; thus they are slow reactors and have a high threshold.

It becomes obvious that each type is affected by the direction, the rapidity, and the intensity of the stimulus acting on the ending. Each reacts, therefore, by the stretch imposed on the capsule, given the force, rapidity, and specific duration and direction of the stretch.

Type 4 receptors are not encapsulated. They have free endings and are found within capsules and ligaments. They are quiet at rest, firing only when irritated or stimulated. Their nerve endings are stimulated by mechanical and chemical substances such as prostaglandin E, lactic acid, potassium ions, polypeptides, and histamine substances. They subserve nociceptive impulses resulting in the sensation of pain.

Type 4 nerve impulses enter the cord via the anterior ramus. The other types (1, 2, and 3) enter via the posterior ramus into the tracts to the basal ganglia and subserve proprioception. Through internuncial neuronal connections they influence motor strength, contraction rapidity, and duration. They also, obviously, can initiate the sensation of pain.

KINETIC LOW BACK PAIN

Kinetic low back pain implies irritation of pain-sensitive tissues by **movement** of the lumbosacral spine. Pain can originate in one of three basic manners:

1. Normal stress on unprepared normal back.
2. Abnormal stress on a normal low back.
3. Normal stress on an abnormal low back.

The term **normal** can be assumed to imply a stress of reasonable magnitude that should be efficiently and comfortably handled under average conditions. It can be added to the definition **normal:** "a stress that under normal conditions will not cause **failure** of any of the tissues of the low back involved in that particular function."

A **normal** low back refers to a structural integrity with no inborn or acquired abnormal deviations. The term **normal** understandably has relative interpretation in which the "norms" have not yet all been clearly established, delineated, and totally accepted.

A low back that has normal anatomic structures but has been allowed to deteriorate by failure to maintain normal flexibility and normal strength should not be considered to be "normal"; yet according to acceptable nomenclature, inadequate conditioning is rarely used in describing a low back as being **abnormal**. Structurally, the anatomic aspects of the lumbosacral spine may be normal but functionally the low back is not.

The low back in which function has not been well indoctrinated to perform proper neurophysiologic function by training in and by repetitive proper use of normal habit patterns should not be considered **normal** either. This aspect that ultimately is termed abnormal is, unfortunately, so labeled by retrospective reasoning.

NORMAL STRESS ON AN UNPREPARED NORMAL LOW BACK

A **normal** stress imposed on a **normal** low back that is **unprepared** exposes all these nerve endings within the involved tissues to a stimulation that can result only in an inappropriate reaction. A similar adverse reaction can result when there is an abnormal (excessive) stress on the **normal** back that is prepared. In this instance, the **normal low back** is anticipating the stress, but is overwhelmed by being subjected to excessive stress.

The stress on the unprepared low back initiates a neurophysiologic tissue reaction to that stress as a result of the proprioceptive endings (types 1, 2, and 3) getting inappropriate, inaccurate stimuli. These stimuli, in turn, send improper messages to the nervous system and an inappropriate reflex action occurs.

Simplistically, this neurologic reaction implies that pain will be initiated by irritation of the type 4 fibers within the capsules of the involved joints. As stated, these fibers transmit pain sensation. The stimuli transmitted via fibers 1, 2, and 3 initiate reflex action that not only does not appropriately protect the musculoskeletal system from the imposed stress but creates a secondary source of difficulty by causing an overreaction of the reflex muscles intended to "protect" the functional unit. "Spasm" results.

Low back pain can result from insult to any of the tissues innervated with nerves that subserve nocioceptive impulses. These have been discussed as being innervated by the lumbar-dorsal posterior nerves and include ligaments, facet joints, and deep muscles of the low back.

Spasm, an acute isometric muscular contraction that was intended to be a reflex muscular reaction to immobilize the functional unit from incurring further injury, now becomes a site of nociceptive stimuli. The muscle itself, undergoing sustained violent contraction as it does in spasm, becomes a site of pain. The force of the muscular contraction also compresses the injured tissues of the functional unit, further adding insult to the original inciting accident.

The term "unprepared" merits consideration. The input into the "computer" of the central nervous system that calibrates the size, speed, distance, frequency, duration, and so on, of the intended action is inaccurate.

The weight or the size of the object being lifted may be underestimated or overestimated. The mind sets the resultant neurophysiologic, neuromuscular action for "that" precise action only to have an excess or a deficient reaction. The "light" box is actually heavier than the neuromuscular reaction intends to lift.

The opposite may occur. The "heavy" box for which a powerful neuromuscular action is contemplated is actually empty. There is neuromuscular "overreaction." Failure of the reacting tissues occurs in spite of the fact that "normal" stress on a "normal" low back has been present.

The person lifting or merely bending and resuming the erect position may be distracted, ill-trained, fatigued, angry, impatient, depressed, or unconditioned. The result is the same.

The erector spinae muscles that should gradually synchronously elongate during flexion and smoothly synchronously shorten during re-extension do so erratically and inappropriately.

Low back pain is the usual symptom. Radiating pain into the leg related to the low back symptoms also presents a frequent clinical picture. The exact mechanism of these symptoms—low back pain with or without leg radiation—will be discussed in subsequent sections. It is enough at this juncture to discuss the mechanism of a **normal stress on an unprepared low back**.

Clinically we may revert to whether the injury is a normal stress on a normal back or whether either the stress or the low back is abnormal. The tissue site of nociceptive stimuli is, in most cases, within the posterior soft tissues of the low back supplied by the LDRN. It may also be related to the intervertebral disk and all the contiguous tissues in the vicinity of the disk.

NORMAL STRESS ON A DECONDITIONED "NORMAL" LOW BACK

The "unprepared" low back has been discussed, but another aspect of this painful condition needs to be elucidated. This is the condition in which the low back can be considered **normal,** yet the low back tissues not prepared for the flexion movement by not being limber. In this condition the flexibility of the soft tissues has not been prepared for the activity that is contemplated.

It has been previously stated that the lumbar spine flexes approximately 9 degrees at each functional unit. This is a total of 45 degrees for the five functional units comprising the lumbosacral spine. Adequate flexion is possible if the erector spinae muscles, their fascia (Fig. 6–12), and the posterior longitudinal ligaments are flexible. Flexibility of these tissues can be acquired only by their being passively elongated by exercise.

If a flexion activity is imposed on the low back that is not, at that mo-

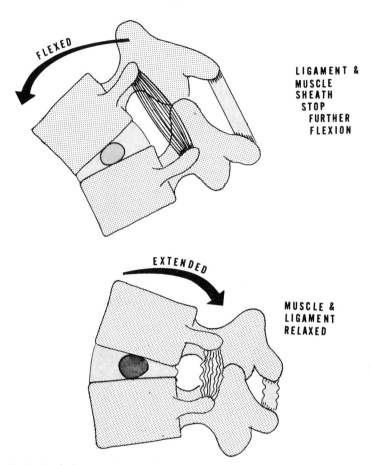

Figure 6–12. Each functional unit flexes (bends forward) as the back muscles elongate. Muscles elongate as far as their sheaths (skin) allow. Once fully stretched, the posterior ligament stops further movement. As the back arches backward, the muscles and the ligaments relax. (Modified from Cailliet, R: Understand Your Backache. FA Davis, Philadelphia, 1984, p 35.)

ment, flexible, the tissues will be injured. An attempt to flex the lumbosacral spine 45 degrees when the tissues have only enough flexibility to allow 35 degrees of flexion can only result in injury to the ungiving soft tissues.

After 45 degrees of lumbosacral spine derotation from lordosis to kyphosis has been achieved, the remaining forward flexion of the body occurs at the pelvis. The pelvis rotates about the hip joints to the degree allowed by the elongation of the hamstring muscles. If the hamstring muscles are inflexible, they will elongate just so far until further pelvic rotation is stopped. Any further forward bending then must occur within the lumbar spine, which has already flexed its maximum. As the fascia of the hamstring muscles is less resilient than the fascia and ligaments of the low back, it does not "give" and stops any further pelvic motion. The low back bears the burden in this flexion against unyielding hamstring muscles (Fig. 6–13).

Normally the pelvis will rotate about the hip joints symmetrically if both hip joints are adequate and if both pairs of hamstrings are symmetric in their flexibility. If one of the hip joints is limited by degenerative arthritic changes, full motion of that hip joint will be limited and thus the pelvis will not rotate evenly. Limited movement about the damaged hip will cause excessive movement about the other hip joint and the pelvis will rotate as well as flex in an abnormal manner. The superincumbent low back will also move in an abnormal manner.

Unilateral inflexibility of a hamstring muscle group will also cause the pelvis to derotate asymmetrically. As the pelvis attempts to rotate about the hip joints, each pair of hamstrings must elongate sufficiently and evenly. If one of the hamstring muscle groups is limited, the pelvis will be limited in flexion on that side. In a low back patient with evidence of kinetic low back abnormality it behooves the examiner to ascertain the hip joint range of motion and evaluate hamstring symmetric flexibility.

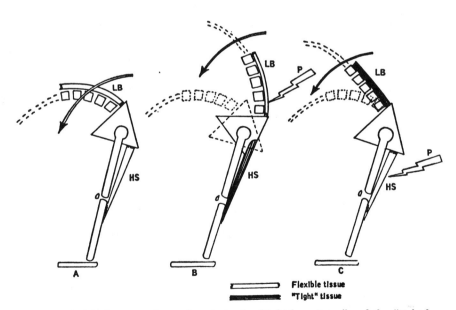

Figure 6–13. Mechanism of stretch pain in the "tight hamstring" and the "tight low back" syndromes. *A*. Normal flexibility with unrestricted lumbar-pelvic rhythm. *B*. Tight hamstrings (HS) restricting pelvic rotation and thereby causing excessive stretch of low back (LB) resulting in pain (P). *C*. Tight low back (LB) performing an incomplete lumbar reversal and thus, by placing excessive stretch on the hamstrings (HS), causes pain (P) in both the hamstrings and the low back as well as a disrupted lumbar-pelvic rhythm.

In summary:

1. A low back that is not flexible (limber) at the time it is subjected to a flexion activity may result in overstretching the extensor soft tissues of the spine.

2. A low back that is flexible but has limited pelvic rotation due to hamstring inflexibility may cause the low back to be overstretched if flexion persists after the pelvis has rotated its maximum.

3. A low back that is flexible but flexes improperly due to pelvic asymmetric rotation as the pelvis derotates abnormally about a limited hip joint.

4. Asymmetric low back flexion is caused by asymmetric hamstring elongation causing abnormal pelvic rerotation.

All the above are examples of low back pain and impairment occurring with a **normal** stress on a **normal** low back with the exceptions noted.

THE NORMAL LOW BACK USED IMPROPERLY IN LIFTING

In resuming the erect posture from being bent over, such as in lifting, it has been generally accepted that the lumbar lordosis is not regained within the first degrees of straightening until 45 degrees of forward flexion, ahead of the center of gravity, has been reached.

This is postulated because during this range of movement, regaining full erect position, with the lumbar spine flexed, the thoracolumbar fascia assumes most of the stress. It is accepted that the fascia is structurally

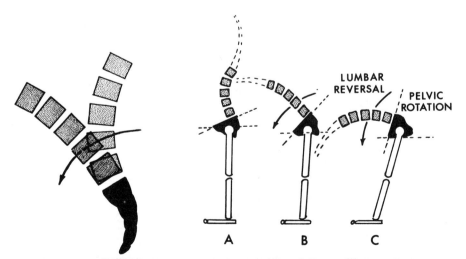

Figure 6–14. Lumbar pelvic rhythm. With pelvis fixed, flexion-extension of the lumbar spine occurs mostly in the lower segments L4–5 and L5–S1.

strong enough to sustain these stresses, whereas the contracting erector spinae muscles are not. This is the basis for "lifting with a straight or forward flexed lumbar spine."

If a person, during the act of lifting or merely resuming the erect position assumes the lordosis prematurely, the stresses on the lumbosacral region are the same as were discussed in the erect **static** spine, namely:

1. Gravity forces on the facet joints.
2. Closure of the intervertebral foramen.
3. Forward migration of the nucleus but a posterior protrusion of the posterior annular fibers against the posterior longitudinal ligament.
4. Increased shear stresses on the unit.

These forces, assumed in the erect static posture, are markedly increased when the body is held forward ahead of the center of gravity. This is so because the weight of the upper body and the weight of the arms and material being lifted are added. The erector spinae muscles forcefully contracting to lift also acts to compress the tissues within the lower functional units. Fig. 6–14 shows the normal lumbar reversal in the act of flexing with re-extension being initially derotation of the pelvis. Fig. 6–15 depicts the wrong way of lifting.

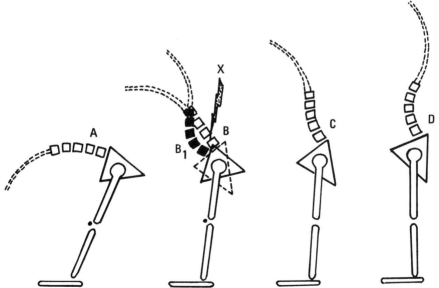

Figure 6–15. Mechanism of acute facet impingement. A, B, C, and D depict the proper physiologic resumption of the erect position from total flexion with reverse lumbar-pelvic rhythm. B_1 shows improper premature lordotic curve which cantilevers the lumbar spine anterior to the center of gravity. This position approximates the facets at X and, coupled with the eccentric leading of the spine, requires greater muscular contraction of the erector spinae group. Facet impingement can occur.

FAULTY ROTATION-DEROTATION IN THE ACT OF LIFTING

The act of properly bending over and lifting or merely resuming the erect position **in the sagittal plane** has been discussed. This act, with some rotation, merits discussion, as this is the general manner in which a person bends over and returns to the erect position. To avoid pain and impairment, it must be done physiologically.

It has also been amply stated that the facet (zygapophyseal) joints, by their alignment in a sagittal plane (Fig. 6–16), permit essentially flexion-extension and markedly limit lateral flexion and rotation.

There is a deviation from that concept as, in the act of forward flexion, with the assumption of beginning lumbar kyphosis, the **posterior facet joints do separate slightly**. They separate sufficiently to allow a slight degree of lateral flexion **and rotation**.

As the spine flexes, there is a degree of rotation. This is consistent with the concept postulated by Lovett (1907) that "with flexion of a flexible rod there is a simultaneous degree of rotation."

The degree of rotation is limited posteriorly by the facet joint capsules and the fascia and erector spinae muscles. Anteriorly, rotation is limited by the anterior and posterior longitudinal ligaments and the annular fibers of the intervertebral disks.

It has been stated that the annular fibers permit only 5 degrees of rotation torque stresses before failure; therefore, it is within these limitations of degrees of rotation that the facets protect the annular disk fibers in the act of bending over and simultaneously "twisting" to one side.

It is only when rotation exceeds these limits that damage to the spine tissues occurs. Excessive rotation can overstretch the ligaments, the muscle fascia, and the facet capsules but, more seriously, injure the annular fibers of the disk. More of this last point constitutes a later chapter on disk disease.

Excessive rotation during the act of flexion can overstretch and even tear the posterior tissues of the spine. These are the tissues enumerated as being subserved by the posterior dorsal lumbar ramus of the spinal nerve with all the symptoms of the sustained insult.

Once flexed forward to the point of the lumbosacral spine being fully flexed, albeit also fully rotated to one side, the person must return to the erect position. The **spine must derotate as it rotated during forward flexion: it must return along the exact path delineated by the plane of the facets. Derotation must occur to the precise degree of the extent of re-extension along the path of movement.**

From the above it is apparent that during re-extension there must be a proportional synchronous derotation. The alignment of the vertebral components of the functional unit must, at each point of the path, be in proper

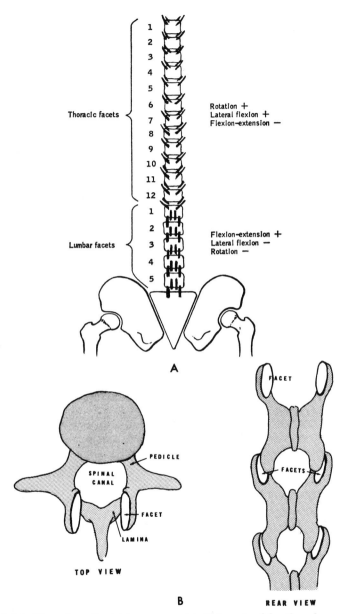

Figure 6–16. Direction of spinal movement is determined by the planes of the articular facets. *A*. The planes are vertical in the lumbar region, thus only anterior-posterior motion (flexion-extension) is possible in this region. Lateral bending and rotation are prevented. The plane of the thoracic facets permits rotation and lateral flexion but denies flexion and extension. The direction of movement permitted and prevented is indicated for the individual sections. Plus signs indicate possible motion; minus signs mean motion prevented. *B*. Details showing facets.

relationship. We must return to the upright along the same path as we bent over.

For proper flexion, rotation, and re-extension the following must exist:

1. The tissues of the spine, the fascia, the ligaments, the joint capsules, and the muscles must be sufficiently flexible to allow full, physiologic range of motion.

2. The spinal segments (the adjacent functional units) must be properly aligned throughout the intended motion:

a. The facets must be parallel.

b. The pelvis must be horizontal.

c. The hip joints must be symmetrically fully flexible (i.e., with the hamstring muscles flexible).

3. The neuromuscular pattern that initiates this motion must be well programmed and be properly implemented. **The person must bend over and return to the erect position, albeit with simultaneous rotation, correctly.**

Faulty re-extension is a frequent cause of pain and impairment of the low back. As we normally return to the erect position from the bent-over and laterally flexed-rotated position, the facets engage and disengage their approximation (Fig. 6–17).

In flexion and rotation to the right the facets **on the right** approximate; they engage. Those on the left **separate** (see Fig. 1–18). Excessive flexion **and rotation,** theoretically, can sublux the open facet joints, on the convex side, by overstretching the interspinous ligaments and joint capsules. This excessive motion can also excessively compress the facets on the concave side.

Assuming that there has been **no excessive flexion,** re-extension to the erect posture must accept this facet relationship. The approximated facets on the concave side must open smoothly and those on the convex (open) side reapproximate equally smoothly **and synchronously.**

If the person resumes the lordosis with **inadequate appropriate derotation,** the approximated facets on the concave side do not separate. They become the axis of rotation by their contact about which the functional unit rotates. There is excessive shear of the anterior portion of the functional unit, which is borne by the annular fibers.

Injury obviously occurs wherein these possibilities result:

1. The approximated facets compact with synovial insult.

2. The excessively separated facets undergo stretch or tear of their capsules.

3. The annular disk fibers are exposed to excessive rotation and torque shear and may "fail."

4. Excessive erector spinae muscle spasm results, causing lateral functional scoliosis, antalgic spine, and added disk-facet compression.

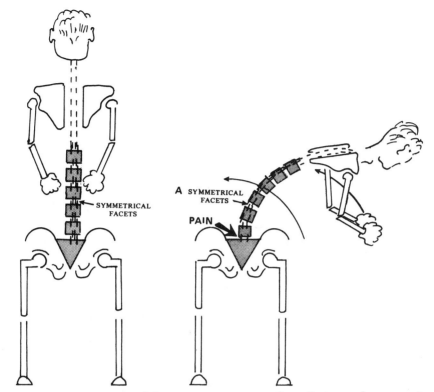

Figure 6–17. Asymmetrical facets. Pain can occur from flexion and re-extension when the facets are anatomically asymmetrical or when there is faulty derotation.

Nociceptive impulses are generated from these tissue insults within the nerves that supply them. These are the LDRN fibers that have been discussed. They react to the reflexly contracted muscles comprising the "spasm" and can become the focal site of further nociceptive stimuli.

The "why" of faulty re-extension from the flexed position justifies clarification. During normal development a child returns to the erect position from numerous bent-over positions without effort or thought. The child is small and usually flexible. Bending over is through a small range of motion and is done frequently.

As we age, besides growing taller and thus having to bend over through a greater range of motion, the tissues of the body—the muscles, their fascia, and the ligaments—tend to lose their flexibility unless exercised daily. The "normal pattern" of bending over and returning to the erect position is stressed repeatedly by being exposed to different positions, actions, and demands in everyday activities and in various vocations.

Fatigue occurs. Distraction is rampant. Deconditioning exists. Poor habit becomes accepted as normal. Work conditions impose hazards to permit faulty actions.

ABNORMAL STRESS ON A NORMAL
LOW BACK

An excessive weight-bearing stress on a person who must stand or sit flexed for long periods of time may pose an abnormal stress on a normal back. Unfortunately, such a situation occurs frequently in today's society—professionally, recreationally, and in many activities of daily living.

This stressful situation can be considered a cause of **static low back pain**. Prolonged standing in a forward flexed posture imposes excessive loading on the posterior spinal tissues as well as on the intervertebral disks. If only the weight of the arms or if a weight is held in the arms ahead of the body, the weight stress is increased.

Nachemson, in his intra-diskal pressure studies, demonstrated that this posture of leaning forward ahead of the center of gravity, in either standing or sitting positions, greatly increases the intradiskal pressure. MacKenzie (1980) claims that this flexed posture has an adverse effect on the posterior ligamentous, muscular, and fascial tissue. He actually postulates that this prolonged flexed posture adversely affects the disk nucleus by causing the nucleus to migrate posteriorly.

Prolonged flexed postures can initiate a sustained isometric muscular tonus of the erector spinae muscles. This sustained isometric muscular contraction causes a vascular compression with resultant ischemia and an accumulation of muscle metabolites. These metabolites are nociceptive tissue irritants that further intensify the muscle contraction. Pain results that prolongs the sustained isometric muscular contraction.

When the muscles become "overwhelmed," they fatigue and no longer maintain their antigravity function. The ligaments now bear the brunt of the posture and become another site of nociception.

Emotional anxiety places a similar stress on the tissue of the low back by causing the erector spinae muscles to assume a sustained isometric contraction. The term **tension myositis syndrome** (TMS) has been applied to this emotionally induced low back pain by Sarno (1984) and others.

Tension myositis syndrome indicates the production of low back pain predominantly caused by sustained muscle contraction of the low back extensor muscles from deep-seated anxiety. This condition undoubtedly occurs frequently and must be accepted as a diagnosis and never as an accusation. Kraus (1905) also has been a strong advocate of tension as causing low back pain and dysfunction.

TMS is an example of an abnormal stress on a normal spine, which affects the static low back but also may affect the kinetic spine, resulting in pain and impairment. In movement such as bending forward or the process of lifting, the erector spinae muscles must elongate eccentrically in a slow and gradual manner. Muscles that are "tense," albeit from an emotional cause, fail to relax adequately, or, if they do relax, do so in an erratic manner. Tissue irritation and inflammation result.

A weight being lifted, which normally can be considered acceptable to a normal back, if lifted repeatedly to an excessive degree can result in fatigue. Fatigue, per se, can cause undesirable muscular reaction with accumulation of metabolites or can lead to failure to perform the needed function. "Strain" and "sprain" result.

NORMAL STRESS ON AN ABNORMAL LOW BACK

It must be candidly stated that a low back that is "abnormal" can fail on being exposed to an otherwise "normal" everyday activity. The term "abnormal," as applied to the low back, requires further evaluation.

Structural abnormalities have been enumerated in medical literature. Spondylolysis and spondylolisthesis will be considered in a subsequent chapter. Spondylosis is a term applied to a spine with multiple diskogenic spaces having undergone significant degenerative changes. "Degenerative arthritis" is also often used as a diagnostic label with little comprehension or consistency. Let us evaluate these conditions and others that are considered to constitute an **abnormal** spine.

STRUCTURAL SCOLIOSIS

It has been stated that a person with a structural rotoscoliosis is more prone to backache than a person with a straight spine. Statistics bear this contention out, but many people with severe rotoscoliosis do not suffer from low back pain. It is also evident that many people without scoliosis have low back pain, so what is the relationship of scoliosis to symptomatic low back pain?

Rotoscoliosis, of a significant degree, evolves causing each functional unit, within the curve, to undergo structural changes. Each vertebra within the curve deforms structurally. The vertebral bodies and the laminae change over the years. The facets within the laminae also become deformed (Fig. 6–18). This structural malalignment of two adjacent deformed vertebrae has been termed spinal "tropism."

The facets, which gradually become structurally deformed, no longer permit proper normal "tracting" of the spine during flexion-extension.

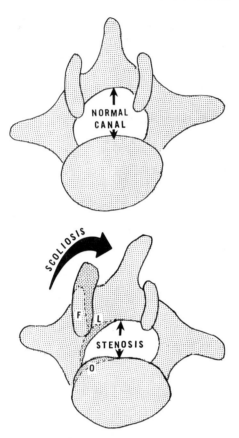

Figure 6–18. Spinal canal stenosis in scoliosis. The deformity that occurs from lateral and rotational forces causes spinal canal stenosis as a result of thickening of the lamina (L), osteophytosis of the vertebral bodies (O), and thickening of the facets (F). (From Cailliet, R: Scoliosis: Diagnosis and Management. FA Davis, Philadelphia, 1975, p 103, with permission.)

Movement of adjacent vertebrae is no longer symmetric. The lumbar-pelvic rhythm thus becomes impaired by the abnormal segment of the spine not moving appropriately. The proper sequence of spine pelvic motion, previously discussed, is altered, and pain results.

The relationship of the fifth lumbar vertebra to the sacrum may become "tilted." The "tilt" implies that the fifth lumbar vertebra does not "seat" symmetrically on the sacrum. The three-point weight bearing of this functional unit—the anterior intervertebral disk and the two posterior facet joints—as in a three-legged stool, become altered and asymmetric. Rotation about its normal axis in movement is changed.

SEGMENTAL SCOLIOSIS

Tropism of the lower functional unit of the lumbosacral spine can exist without the remainder of the spine being scoliotic. An asymmetry of the lumbosacral unit, in which the last vertebra is laterally "tilted" on the sacrum, often exists but is ignored in the radiologic report or in the evaluation of the roentgenogram by the clinician. This asymmetry, a "tropism," is a common cause of static low back pain and kinetic malfunction.

SHORT LEG SYNDROME

A "short leg" may cause a pelvic obliquity with a resultant segmental scoliosis of the superincumbent vertebrae. This segmental "scoliosis," due to a short leg pelvic obliquity, has been considered to cause low back pain. Retrospective studies of a short leg causing a pelvic obliquity in patients with low back pain have revealed that a leg length discrepancy of less than ½ inch is of no clinical significance. A leg length discrepancy of ½ inch apparently compensates of its own, but any degree above ½ inch should be corrected with an appropriate shoe-heel lift.

SPONDYLOSIS

As a spine undergoes disk degeneration, each disk space narrows and each pair of facet joints therefore also approximates. The facet joint surfaces no longer function adequately and the intervening articular cartilages undergo degenerative changes. There results degenerative changes that are termed "osteoarthrosis." This subject will be more fully discussed in the chapter of that title but a word about spondylosis is justified in the current discussion of the **abnormal** low back.

With one or more disks degenerating, there is excessive stress on the contiguous functional units. As the greatest degree of degeneration usually occurs at the L5-S1 and the L4-5 disk spaces, the illustration is focused best here.

In normal spinal movement it has been stated that each functional unit flexes approximately 9 degrees, for a total of 45 degrees for the entire lumbosacral spine. If one (L5-S1) is limited by disk degeneration, the remainder of the lumbosacral spine must compensate. Excessive motion must therefore be imposed on the cephalad functional units. These units have their own limitations and total movement is restricted. If the force of flexion or bending and lifting is excessive, the tissues of the limited units will be injured. The cephalad units will also be overstressed. This is the reason that a person who suffers a localized disk injury may in the future be limited in performing activities the "recovered" patient would otherwise consider to be normal.

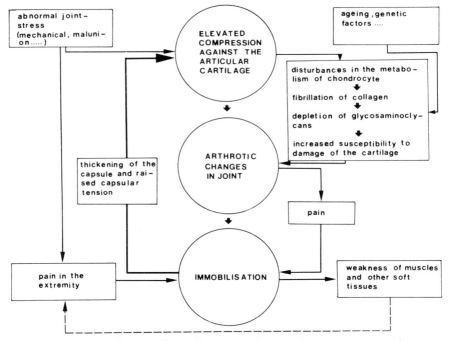

Figure 6–19. Hypothesis of the pathogenetic chain in degenerative joint diseases.

FACET ARTHRITIS

The cartilage of the facet joints, like cartilage of any joint, will undergo degeneration from abnormal use. Excessive lordosis, asymmetry of facets, from whatever cause, or faulty re-extension from prolonged improper body function will inevitably result in facet cartilage degeneration or "arthritis" (Fig. 6–19).

BONE PATHOLOGY

Low back pain, both static or kinetic, can occur in the presence of bone pathology. These conditions are numerous and include Paget's disease, multiple myeloma, metastatic disease, and other metabolic diseases. Diskitis, an infection of a disk, also causes severe pain.

Any pain that cannot be related to a position or movement, that does not respond to appropriate treatment within a reasonable time, that awakens a patient from sleep without movement, or that is "constant" and unrelieved by medication and appropriate modalities should raise a warning signal that some significant organic structural tissue change is responsible and lead to appropriate studies.

SUMMARY

Low back pain symptoms should be clinically evaluated and categorized as to being **static** or **kinetic**. The history, carefully elicited, can give the exact mechanism that led to the symptoms.

Static low back pain is pain that occurs during a stationary position, be it sitting or standing. The tissues that elicit the nociceptive transmission are discernible. The symptoms can be reproduced by placing and holding the patient in **that position** that causes **that pain**.

The **kinetic** low back pain is caused by a specific movement occurring from an assumed position to accomplish a specific result. The history reveals **the movement** and the specific pain resulting from **that movement**.

Where the pain is felt specifies **the tissue** that has been injured and is transmitting the nociceptive impulses. The pain may be felt in the low back, the leg, or both. **Where** exactly the pain radiates into the leg clarifies whether a nerve root is involved, which nerve root, or whether the tissue site is a tissue innervated by the posterior ramus of a nerve root.

When the pain occurred is valuable in the history, and **how** it can be reproduced during the examination clarifies the mechanism and the tissue involved.

The results of the history and physical examination, supplemented by appropriate laboratory findings, clarify whether (1) the stress has been abnormal; (2) the low back has been structurally abnormal; (3) the low back was deconditioned; or (4) the low back was unprepared for the activity that initiated the pain.

Having a complete knowledge of the **functional anatomy** of the tissue site of nociceptive stimuli and the ability to reproduce the symptoms complained of by the patient assure that a meaningful diagnosis can now be elicited by clinical diagnostic procedures.

REFERENCES

Adams and Hutton. J Bone Joint Surg 62B:358, 1980.

Altschule, MD: Emotion and skeletal muscle function. Med. Sci. 2:163, 1962.

Behan, RC and Hirschfeld, AH: The accident process. II. Toward more rational treatment of industrial injuries. JAMA 186:300, 1963.

Bogduk, N: Lumbar dorsal ramus syndrome, Med J Aust Nov. 1980, 537.

Bogduk, N and Long, DM: J Neurosurg 51:172, 1979.

Cyron and Hutton. Spine 5:168, 1980.

Hirschfeld, AH and Behan, RC: The accident process. JAMA 186:193, 1963.

Hirschfeld, AH and Behan, RC: The accident process. III. Disability: Acceptable and unacceptable. JAMA 197:125, 1966.

Hockaday, JM and Whitty, CWM: Brain 90:481, 1967.

Jacobson, E: Electrical measurements of neuromuscular states during mental activities: Imagination of movement involving skeletal muscles. Am J Physiol 91:567, 1930.

Jainsbury, P and Gibson, JG: Symptoms of anxiety and tension and the accompanying physiological changes in the muscular system. J Neurol Neurosurg Psychiatry 17:216, 1954.

Kraus, H: Backache, Stress and Tension: Cause, Prevention and Treatment: A Fireside Book. Simon and Schuster, New York, 1905.

Kellgran, JH: Clin Sci 3:175, 1938.

Lovett, RW: Lateral Curvature of the Spine and Round Shoulders. P. Blakiston & Son, Philadelphia, 1907.

Lundervold, A: Electromyographic investigation during sedentary work—especially typewriting. Br J Phys Med 14:32, 1951.

Lundervold, A: Electromyographic investigation of position and manner of working on typewriting. Acta Physiol Scand 24(Suppl 84), 1951.

MacKenzie, RA: The Lumbar Spine: Mechanical Diagnosis and Therapy. Waikanae, New Zealand, 1981.

Mooney, V and Robertson, J: J Clin Orthop 114:149, 1976.

Nachemson, A and Morris, J: In vivo measurements of intradiscal pressure. J Bone & Joint Surgery 46A,1077–1092, 1964.

Sarno, J: Mind Over Back Pain. William Morrow & Co, New York, 1984.

Shealy, CN: Technique for Percutaneous Spinal Rhizotomy. Radionics, Burlington, 1974.

Weinstein, MR: The illness process. JAMA 204:209, 1968.

Wyke, BD: Neurology of the cervical spine joints. Physiotherapy 65:72, 1979.

CHAPTER 7

Clinical Diagnosis of Low Back Pain Syndromes

The history and physical examination of the patient complaining of low back pain must have as its basis a **functional diagnosis**. A diagnosis must be based on ascertaining the deviation from normal of the static or kinetic function of the spine. The tissue site of symptoms must also be ascertained and the mechanism by which functional anatomy has been jeopardized must be determined.

LOCALIZATION OF PAIN SITE BY HISTORY

The complaint by a patient of "pain in the low back" must be clarified. The exact site alluded to by the patient as being the "low back" must be delineated. The symptom site claimed to be the low back may be stated by the patient as being the "kidney" area, the hip, or the sacrum. The exact site of the pain must be identified precisely.

The site may be pointed to by the patient's finger, by a verbal description, or by the patient pinpointing a specific area such as "my disk," "my sacroiliac joints," "my buttocks," or "my tail bone." These words must be anatomically substantiated by the examiner.

The characteristics of the pain, as described by the patient, have great value. Much has been written about this aspect of the history in determining the validity of the symptoms, the severity, and even the psychological aspect of the impairment. Terms do have relationship as to the tissue site of the pain production. A "nerve" pain usually is sharp, precise in its distribution, whereas symptoms from inflammation of soft tissue such as ligaments, muscles, or joint capsule are dull, vague, and nonspecific in their location.

The degree of severity, which leads to impairment, is also valued in depicting the patient's reaction and interpretation of the significance of the pain. Terms such as "excruciating," "devastating," "killing," "unbearable," and "intolerable" indicate a severe emotional component to pain recognition and to the patient's level of tolerance.

The **meaning** of the pain always presents a problem to the examiner. Pain is a symbolic term employed by the patient to denote:

1. Evidence of physical damage.
2. A means of communication.
3. A means of manipulating others, of expressing hostility or anger, or of relieving guilt.

For this section of the text we will discuss pain as it relates to evidence of physical damage or insult and discuss the other meanings of pain later. The description of the pain as relating to a tissue site of a specific area of the lumbosacral spine will take precedence.

The frequency and duration of the pain have both diagnostic as well as prognostic significance. The tissue site of pain influences both of these factors as well as denotes an aspect of patient tolerance.

The **when** and the **how** are significant as is the **where** of the pain. The **when** implies motion, position, action, time of day, state of mind, fatigue, stress, and so on. The **how**, especially in the kinetic spine problem, indicates **the** movement, action, position, and accomplishment of activity that caused or causes the pain.

The history actually denotes whether the pain is **static** or **kinetic**. A static pain needs to be categorized as to whether an increased lordosis is the causative factor or whether excessive forward flexion in daily activities, either personal or professional, contributes to the pain.

In eliciting an accurate history, the state of mind of the patient at the time of injury is important. Distraction, inattention, anger, impatience, depression, to mention a few "distractors," may have led to the "incident." This history documents whether the injury is a normal action imposed on an unprepared yet normal low back.

Of value in taking a thorough history is to allow the patient to be fully expressive and not merely answer in the affirmative or negative. The "check off" questionnaire sheet is a limited method of history taking as is a history taken "by an assistant." The knowledge obtained by these methods is valuable for the chart but limited in aiding the examiner to understand the "problem" and to know the sufferer.

THE PHYSICAL EXAMINATION

A meaningful examination must reveal a significant structural deviation and relate it to the current symptoms. The examination must confirm what the history has alluded to as being a factor causing, maintaining, or aggravating the pain.

A basic axiom of evaluating the functional basis of low back pain follows: **If the characteristic pain can be produced by a position or by a movement, and the precise relationship of that position and movement to the functional anatomy of the part is understood, the cause of the pain becomes clear.**

If, by placing the patient in a specific position or posture, **the** low back pain can be produced or aggravated and the precise anatomic motion produced by that position is understood, the site of pain production and its relationship to that posture become clear.

If, from the history and from resuming the position or performing **the** specific movement described by the patient, **the** pain is reproduced and the precise anatomic motion performed by that motion is understood, **the anatomic site and the precise movement** become clear.

The examination is a tissue analysis as well as a position and movement analysis clarifying where and what tissue is responsible for the pain. The movement analysis deducted from the history and reproduced in the examination reveals the **way** that the patient caused the symptoms.

GENERAL OBSERVATION OF THE PATIENT

The history and physical examination begin immediately on personal contact between physician and patient. The manner in which the patient enters the office, sits or stands, and approaches the examiner is revealing. The attitude of the patient depicted by the posture, the tone of voice, and the visual confrontation begins the examination.

The posture can be immediately observed. The first observation is the erectness of the head posture. A forward head posture "slump" can be observed. The forward head posture with an increase in cervical lordosis indicates the probability of an increased lumbar lordosis. A forward head posture also implies that there is sustained muscle tone to support the entire spine. The posture is a form of "body language" that possibly indicates the patient's emotional status.

The patient must be sufficiently undressed to expose the necessary anatomic positions of the body. Propriety must be observed to avoid embarrassment to the patient. Possibly the best gown for an examination is one that is open behind and covers the front of the patient. A male, to a male examiner, need merely undress to the degree of remaining in shorts.

The fitness of the individual is also indicated by general appearance. The facial characteristics speak a volume as to the patient being in severe pain, being depressed, or merely being concerned.

A handshake is too often omitted in the examination. The handshake offers valuable evidence of the physical and emotional status of the patient. A firm grip conveys cooperation. A limp, cold, clammy, moist hand indicates anxiety, depression, or an excessive vasomotor component to the symptoms. A warm handshake by the examiner can allay the concern of the patient and reaffirm an "interest" that so often is considered not to exist in the examining physician. The history, following a warm, interested examiner introduction, often is facilitated.

The history should include the patient's reaction to the onset of the pain. What, in the patient's opinion, "caused" or was responsible for the pain is important in the history. The number of physicians involved in the patient's search for help needs to be elicited. The attitude toward these physicians and their recommendations should be ascertained. The numbers of and the precise type of treatments attempted should be established. The response to these treatments as to benefit or failure gives a sound basis of the medical problem.

The daily activities of the person, whether personal or professional, give a basis for a possible contributing factor in pain causation.

Every physician will formulate a procedure, a sequence of items, in doing the examination. It is important that every aspect of the examination have a precise meaning and be properly interpreted. A report following a history and an examination must follow an agenda and a complete, comprehensive, detailed analysis from which a diagnosis evolves and on which a meaningful treatment program is based.

EVALUATION OF POSTURE (STATIC SPINE)

The erect posture should be examined before the patient is aware of being evaluated. The examination of the posture begins as the person stands during the introduction. On being subjected to "being examined," the patients assume a posture considered, by them, to be the normal posture. This often conveys, to the examiner, what the patient wishes to portray.

Examined from the side, the relationship of all the spinal curves to the center of gravity is immediately apparent. The head should be directly in the center of gravity. The shoulders should be loosely held at the side with no excessive dorsal kyphosis. The lumbar lordosis should be minimal. The abdomen should not protrude excessively (Fig. 7–1).

Further examination of the static spine as a factor in determining postural pain requires that the postural pain be reproduced. By aggravating the patient's lordosis, if the low back pain is reproduced or intensified, the probabilities are that excessive lordosis is a contributing, if not the causative, factor in the static low back pain.

Increasing lordosis may be accomplished by asking the patient to lean

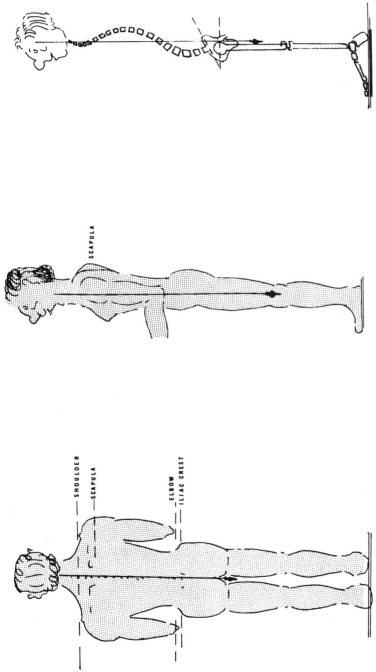

Figure 7–1. Standing posture: center of gravity. An anterior-posterior view of the center of gravity (*left*) should show the plumb line descending from the occiput through the sacrum. A lateral view (*middle* and *right*) should show the plumb line passing through the cervical vertebrae, through the shoulder of the dangling arm, posterior to the hip joint, anterior to the center of the knee joint, and slightly anterior to the ankle lateral malleoli. (From Cailliet, R: Scoliosis. FA Davis, Philadelphia, 1975, p 8, with permission.)

backward to the limit of tolerance or by passively aggravating the lordosis and holding the person in that acquired position.

PELVIC LEVEL: LEG LENGTH

Viewing the patient from behind, the pelvic level can be easily determined. Assuming that there is a leg length discrepancy as a factor in pelvic obliquity is confirmed by appropriate examination of the legs. The suspicion is raised by finding pelvic obliquity.

A pelvic obliquity changes the horizontality of the sacral base and can be the foundation for a lateral lumbar take-off (Fig. 7–2). A segmental scoliosis results causing a "tropism."

The patient must stand without shoes, with legs together, feet facing forward and knees "locked" in extension. The examiner, who stands behind the patient, places the finger tips of both hands on the pelvic brims and sights the equal level of the two hands (Fig. 7–3). This is a gross evaluation of the pelvic level but is reasonably accurate.

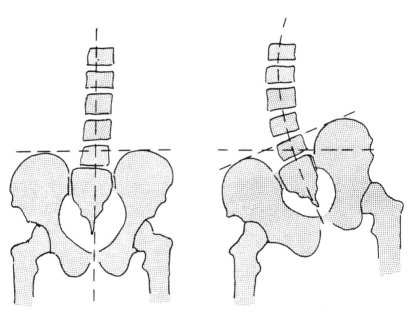

Figure 7–2. Scoliosis due to pelvic obliquity. With a pelvic obliquity due to a unilateral short leg, regardless of cause, the spine can assume a scoliosis (*right*). This is created by the attempt of the spine to assume balance to the center of gravity. (From Cailliet, R: Scoliosis. FA Davis, Philadelphia, 1975, p 38, with permission.)

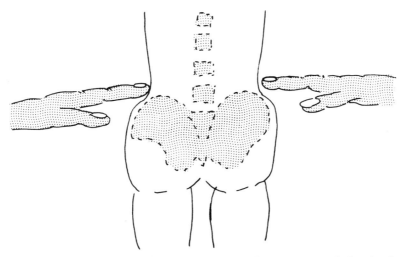

Figure 7–3. Clinical evaluation of pelvic level. With the examiner's hands placed on the brim of the patient's pelvic crests, the patient, while standing erect, is viewed from behind. The level of the iliac crests can thus be determined. An obliquity can be ascertained and its degree determined by placing a board of known thickness under the "short" leg and re-examining the crest level. (From Cailliet, R: Scoliosis. FA Davis, Philadelphia, 1975, p 38, with permission.)

Boards of differing thicknesses of ⅛, ¼, ¾, and 1 inch can be placed under the "shorter" leg and then the pelvic level be reexamined. This gives a measured leg length difference for possible shoe correction prescription. The length of the leg can also be measured by placing a tape measure at the anterior-superior spine prominence and measuring the distance of both legs to the medial malleolus of the ankles. With the patient supine and the legs flexed 90 degrees at the knees and hips, the height of the knee caps can be viewed from above to measure the length of the femora or viewed from below the feet to measure the length of the tibiae.

When a significant leg length discrepancy exists, a further observation will reveal if the discrepancy is due to severe genu valgum or genu valgus. A contracted gastrocsoleus muscle causing a severe foot equinus will lengthen the leg of that side just as a severe genu recurvatum (knee hyperextension) will shorten the leg on that side.

The value of leg length discrepancy is the ascent of the lumbar spine from the sacrum. A segmental functional scoliosis of L5 on S1 results from a significant obliquity of the pelvis. This places lumbosacral stress in the erect static spine, causes asymmetry of the facet joint relationship, and causes a deviation when the spine begins to flex or completes extension.

The flexibility of the hips must also be determined as this may place a stress on the static spine or an impediment upon the kinetic spine. The hamstring range of motion (ROM) is determined by measuring the difference of SLR, one leg against the other leg. This can be done with the patient supine and each leg raised slowly, then measuring the angle at the hips.

The hip flexors also must have equal elongation (the psoas muscles and the hip joint capsule). This is difficult, as the lumbar spine can extend, become more lordotic, and confuse which is being tested — the hip flexors or the lumbar lordosis. With the patient supine and one leg held (by the patient) against the chest, the other leg is lowered from the side of the table.

The hip flexor ROM can be measured with the patient standing, bent over the examining table with one leg extended and on the floor next to the table. The leg to be examined is then flexed at the knee and the thigh moved backward. This tests the hip flexion range and is compared with the other side by the same test.

The hip joint flexibility must be tested to ascertain degenerative joint changes that can influence the static or kinetic spinal movement. With the patient supine each hip is tested by what is termed the Patrick test. One foot is placed on the other knee and the leg lowered to the side. Each leg is so tested and compared as to how far toward the table each leg goes. With joint pathology the leg can only abduct a limited degree. This constitutes a "positive Patrick test."

The neurologic examination will be discussed under the chapter on disk disease. This test includes testing each myotome and each dermatome to localize specific nerve root level.

LUMBAR-PELVIC RHYTHM

With the patient erect and asked to "bend forward **as if** to touch the toes — without bending the knees," the flexion phase of the lumbar pelvic sequence is tested. The quotes of the request are intentional and intended to modify the test and make it realistic and meaningful.

"**As if** to touch your toes" indicates that touching the toes from the erect posture in bending over is not possible for many people nor is it physiologically "normal." Many people have normal spinal flexion and normal hamstring flexibility yet cannot touch their toes.

"With the legs straight . . . without bending the knees" imposes stretch on the hamstrings, and although this is part of the test, it needs clarification.

What this test intends to show is:

1. Determination of the degree the lumbar spine flexes. It reveals the completeness of lumbar flexion **at all spinal function unit levels**. The spine should reverse the lordosis to assume a kyphosis and do so symmetrically

at each spinal level so that when fully flexed, the kyphosis is a normal flexed arch.

2. The flexibility of the pelvis about the hip joints, which should be adequate if both hamstrings are flexible and be symmetrical if each hamstring group of muscles is equally flexible.

Any limitation reveals either soft tissue inflexibility or protective reflex spasm from pain, guarding, or nerve root irritation.

As the person bends over forward, the smoothness of the reversal of the lumbosacral lordosis to kyphosis is observed. The degree of lumbar flexion as compared with the degree of pelvic rotation can be observed. If pain is elicited during this motion, the exact site of pain can be noted by the patient. It can be noted in the low back or down the leg.

The direction of flexion is also noted. If there is a tendency to flex and rotate to one side, this is significant. Flexion with lateral rotation implies either a structural scoliosis, a lumbosacral facet, tropism, or a protective functional scoliosis. The latter will be noted in the discussion of disk disease.

REVERSE LUMBAR-PELVIC RHYTHM

Once totally flexed forward the person is asked to return to the erect position. This is accomplished by gradual decrease of the lumbosacral kyphosis to the erect lumbar lordosis. While this is occurring, there is also gradual derotation of the pelvis. This sequence, to be considered desirable if not normal, should evolve in the sequence of initial pelvic derotation with resumption of the lumbar lordosis occurring after significant pelvic derotation.

A faulty sequence or a limited portion of either aspect of the sequence that is noted may indicate a pattern that has led to pain and impairment. If the person regains the lumbar lordosis while the pelvis is still rotated forward, pain may occur in the low back (Fig. 7–4). This premature lordosis can cause low back pain in that forward flexed position just as it can in the erect posture with the addition of the added weight of the body ahead of the center of gravity.

The patient must also be examined not only in resuming the erect position from the bent-over position but from the bent-over and twisted (rotated) position. This is the sequence of bend over and to one side and return from the position to the full erect posture. The sequence of rotation and flexion followed by extension and derotation has been fully discussed but, during the examination, must be examined and evaluated.

Any pain experienced by the patient during this re-extension–derota-

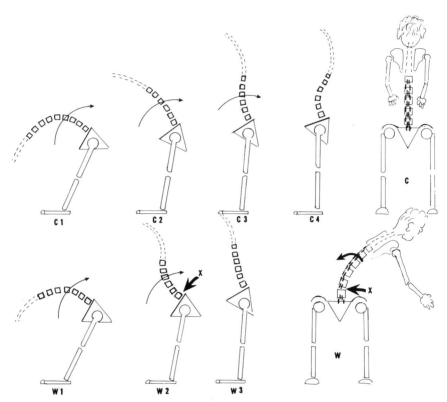

Figure 7–4. Faulty re-extension from the bent-over position. C1 through C4 depict gradual re-extension by simultaneously rotating the pelvis as the lumbar spine moves from reversed lordosis into erect lumbar lordosis. With the spine straight, as in C, the facets move properly. W1 through W3 depict improper re-extension where at W3 the lumbar spine has become already "arched" before the pelvis has adequately rotated in a proper *lumbar-pelvic rhythm*. If the person is also rotated during this re-extension motion, his facets can "jam" during return to erect position, and the disks are subjected to additional stress from the torque motion.

tion must be noted as to **exactly when** in the sequence the pain is noted and **where** in the low back or the leg the pain is felt.

LATERAL ROTATORY FLEXIBILITY

With the patient standing erect, and viewed from behind, the lateral flexibility of the spine can be tested and recorded. With both legs apart a few inches, for balance, the person is passively bent to one side then the other (Fig. 7–5). The patient is also asked to actively bend to one side then the other. The spine is observed and limitation noted. It must be remem-

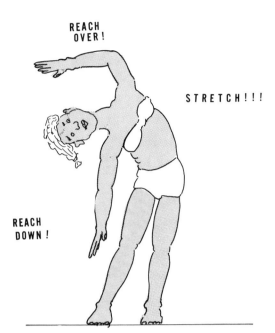

REACH
OVER!

STRETCH!!!

REACH
DOWN!

Figure 7–5. Side bending in evaluation of lateral rotatory flexibility. (Modified from Cailliet, R: Understand Your Backache. FA Davis, Philadelphia, 1984, p 132.)

bered that exclusive lateral spine flexion without rotation is physiologically impossible. Some rotation occurs with lateral flexion; thus, limitation of one-sided lateral flexion indicates restriction from either soft tissue restriction or protective spasm.

SUMMARY OF EXAMINATION

The patient who presents with a complaint of low back pain is evaluated by a history and a physical examination—all based on determining the deviation of normal functional anatomy.

The history is the major portion of the examination. A thorough, meaningful history reveals **where, when,** and **how** the pain occurred. The **static** or **kinetic** aspect of the malfunction is ascertained.

The **where** of the pain furnishes the anatomic location; the **when** indicates the time of the inciting movement with all aspects of location, frame of mind and demands imposed on the person; the **how** is the deduction reached by the examiner who puts the **where** and the **when** into the framework of **functional anatomy** and nociceptive tissue sites.

The **examination** clarifies the structural competency of the structural inadequacies that may contribute to the injury.

The axiom now applies: **if characteristic pain can be reproduced by a position or by a movement and the exact nature of that position or movement is clearly understood, the precise anatomic tissue site responsible is recognized.** The diagnosis, based on this knowledge, becomes meaningful and the treatment appropriate.

CHAPTER 8

Comprehensive Therapeutic Approach to Low Back Pain

After a careful, complete evaluation by history and meaningful examination of the patient with low back pain the causation can be determined. Based on the functional anatomic alteration that has resulted in pain and impairment a correct diagnosis evolves and **meaningful appropriate treatment** results.

The objectives of treatment are

1. Alleviation of pain.
2. Restoration of mobility.
3. Minimizing residual impairment and disability.
4. Prevention of recurrences.
5. Intervention of progression into chronic pain and disability.

TREATMENT OF THE ACUTE EPISODE OF LOW BACK PAIN

It has been aptly stated by many authorities in the diagnosis and management of patients with low back pain that **regardless of what treatment modality is applied, 80 per cent of patients will recover from an acute episode of low back pain within three days to three weeks.**

This being an accepted statement, the basis for instituting appropriate treatment early in the management of patients with low back pain is to hasten recovery, prevent the objectives enumerated above, and ensure that meaningless and possibly harmful treatments are avoided.

It is obvious that any therapeutic modality applied to a suffering patient that affords pain relief and reassurance will be considered specific, precise, and appropriate. **That** treatment will thus be considered **the** basis for the therapeutic success.

116

The modalities used in treating acute low back pain range from bed rest, massage, hot packs, ice brushing, ultrasound, traction, acupuncture, manipulation, oral drugs, psychotherapy, muscle relaxants, injections, surgery, and many others too numerous to itemize.

If any of these modalities are considered to be "**successful**" and are the reason for success, it is apparent that the real basis for relief of pain and impairment is ambiguous. True, many of these modalities can give immediate relief. Some may give complete relief and recovery. Many will at best give temporary relief. Some will afford none of these benefits, yet they continue to be recommended and applied.

The cost in lost time—personal and professional, medical evaluation, and treatment—in emotional distress, and in insurance outlays and disability payments is so exorbitant that **the** appropriate treatment after a meaningful examination requires significant answers.

Frequently, an acute discomfort of the low back suffered by a patient does not permit an immediate thorough examination. The history elicited may cast a light on the cause, the effect, and the meaning of the symptoms. A brief examination of the patient may justify palliative treatment. Often this brief history, brief examination, and palliative treatment do not relieve or clarify the many unanswered questions.

The initial examination too frequently tends to be superficial and not meaningful. "Confirmatory" laboratory tests, such as routine x-rays, often add nothing to the diagnosis. Too often a label, the "diagnosis" given the patient, is a meaningless jumble of terms signifying nothing of value to the examiner or the suffering patient.

Yet we must afford some relief of the painful symptoms in spite of these alleged inadequacies of diagnosis. The patient **must be made comfortable** while the disease process evolves to ultimately assume a firm etiologic and anatomic-pathologic basis. The patient must have minimal discomfort while further examinations are undertaken to reach a more definite diagnosis.

Gross neurologic deficits are immediately easily discernible with a careful comprehensive examination. The presence of abnormal neurologic findings alerts the examiner that mere palliation of pain symptoms is at best temporary.

X-rays taken early in the injury are rarely diagnostic unless a severe injury has precipitated or initiated the symptoms of low back pain or a suspicion of an underlying malignancy is raised from the history.

MODIFICATION OF ACUTE PAIN

As alleviation of pain is the first objective listed in the management of acute low back pain it merits full evaluation.

Reassuring the patient is the most emergent consideration. An apprehensive, concerned patient is prone to magnify the significance of the presenting symptoms. Concern about **what** the illness is and what the ramifications of the outcome may be present a concern to most people no matter how sophisticated they may be. Apprehension augments the severity of any painful condition. Anxiety alters the interpretation of a painful situation regardless of the severity of the organic component.

The relationship of patient to physician is the first aspect of the patient's reaction to the injury. A warm, yet objective approach assures the "injured" individual that there is interest and compassion. The history that is proffered by the patient is more complete and revealing. Here a willing **ear** is appreciated. The doctor who listens is appreciated. The doctor who is "too busy or rushed" to listen is resented and rejected. More patients are "lost" in the first minutes of an examination than many physicians realize.

A diagnostic **word**, unintentionally, may plant a fear in the anxious mind of the suffering patient. An example is the term **degenerative arthritis;** after the patient has viewed the x-rays, this term can conjure the spector of **degeneration** with all its implications of it being unalterable. The term **arthritis** may portray the person with hot painful deformed joints that the patient has observed in other "victims of illness." These are merely gross examples of the misuse of **words** that are not followed by a clarification that can be understood by the average patient. Words, considered as diagnostic labels, are so glibly used in everyday medical practice and accepted by the medical profession, yet instill fear in many patients.

The thoroughness, even though it may be more apparent than real, in the history taking and the examination, can be diagnostic for the physician and reassuring to the patient if it is done in a professional and orderly manner.

REST

Rest has become a controversial subject as to how to implement and how long is desirable and most effective. For decades the advice "go home and rest . . . return in two weeks for recheck" has been almost a printed set of instructions given to patients with complaints of low back pain after "an injury."

Recent studies have documented that "early activity" returns most patients back to work several days to several weeks earlier than complete bedrest. Return to work implies that the painful condition and the restricted flexibility resulting from the acute injury have subsided sufficiently to allow work activities.

Rest must be general and locally specific. Complete bedrest eliminates the effects of gravity. The antigravity muscles allegedly relax in respect to their function of sustaining the erect spine. As a result of injury, the anti-gravity muscles remain contracted in a reflex activity responding to noci-ceptive stimuli, not merely to support the spine. Pain, not gravity, remains the basis of muscle contraction that has been termed "spasm."

DeVries (1966), using electromyographic methods, demonstrated that pain initiated quantitative muscular activity. The intensity of the muscular activity paralleled the intensity of the pain. His studies further showed that **static stretching** of the contracted muscle furnished relief of pain by sig-nificantly decreasing muscular activity.

On the assumption that the injured muscle causes the patient to expe-rience pain from the accumulation of toxic substances and from tears within the muscle-fascial tissues, "resting the part" supposedly decreases this ac-cumulation. The part, being rested, supposedly recovers faster, with less pain and with residual "soreness."

The theory that muscular pain results from ischemia and the accumula-tion of metabolites is undoubtedly partially valid. If this concept is valid, rest (i.e., inactivity) does not have rationality in favorably influencing the pain-spasm-pain cycle. Inactivity can actually enhance ischemia and pro-long pain from the accumulated toxic metabolites.

Rest can have a rational basis for relieving pain occurring from tissue injury with secondary reflex muscle spasm. The injured tissues that can ini-tiate nociceptive stimuli are ligaments, joint capsules, and muscles. The nerve endings of these soft tissues are both mechanoreceptors and nocicep-tive. If these nerve endings are stimulated by irritating nociceptive factors, avoiding motion of the inflamed tissues for a period of time can significantly decrease their irritability.

Avoiding stretching or elongating the capsules of the inflamed facet joints decreases nociceptive stimuli that can originate from the sensory nerve roots of the capsules. The righting reflexes that influence the erector spinae muscles via mechanoreceptors do not get stimulated. The reclining position avoids initiating all these nerve reactions: the nociceptive and the mechanoreceptor of the inflamed tissues. A brief period of rest is thus ini-tially beneficial.

The accepted position for reclining is the so-called "modifed Fowler" position. This a position of the reclining body with the hips and knees flexed and the low back in a slightly flexed position. The flexed position of the hips relaxes the iliopsoas muscle. The iliopsoas muscle originating from the anterior aspect of the lumbar spine increases the lumbar lordosis when it contracts in the act of flexing the hip joint. The flexed knees position per-mits the hamstring muscles to relax. Slight flexion of the lumbosacral spine reverses the lordosis and separates the facet joints. This position of the facet joints avoids approximation of their inflamed synovial tissues.

This semiflexed posture is easily achieved when reclining in a mechan-ical hospital bed. However, as most patients need to be treated at home, the recommended semi-Fowler flexed bed position can be achieved using sofa pillows added to the bed (Fig. 8–1).

Comfortable bedrest demands the use of a mattress sufficiently firm to prevent it sagging in the center. As a mattress primarily cushions the contours of the body, such as the hips, breasts, and shoulders, "firmness" of the mattress must allow this contouring yet give support.

A 4- to 8-inch thick mattress can contour the body and prevent pressure on the bony prominences. A ply board, of approximately ¾- to 1-inch thickness, placed under the mattress prevents the center from sagging.

DESIRABLE BED POSITION

The "proper" position to be assumed by the patient, in bed, is **the position that affords the greatest comfort and permits rest.** It is well documented that in their sleep people change their body position every 90 to 120 seconds. This undoubtedly is a proprioceptively stimulated reflex activity resulting from pressure stimulation of the sensory nerve fibers of the skin over the bony prominences. The bed position intended may persist only briefly as sleep occurs. A change then results.

The flexed fetal position has been accepted universally as an ideal position of comfort. This has physiologic justification in that the hips and knees are flexed, the low back is slightly flexed, and the weight of the legs does not adversely place the low back in an uncomfortable position.

Lying supine often causes the low back to become excessively lordotic due to the weight of the extended legs. In the prone position, the excessive lordosis caused by this posture is also avoided. As many people cannot accept excessive lordosis, it becomes apparent that the flexed posture is the most acceptable. People with symptomatic hiatal hernia have found that lying on one's side improves gastric function.

To assume a flexed, albeit a supine, position, the person can place pillows under the knees. This often is unenforceable as the pillows tend to slip to a wrong position or to compress to the point of not supporting the weight of the legs. The use of sofa pillows as depicted in Figure 8–1 eliminates this defect as they remain firm, of acceptable elevation, and do not slip. The correct number of pillows to assure the correct elevation of the legs can be determined.

Should the side-lying position be chosen, a pillow **between** the legs at the knee level maintains the flexed body position and prevents the upper leg from slipping down to the mattress.

BOWEL-BLADDER CARE

Bathroom privileges must often be modified or curtailed because the position on the toilet is uncomfortable and the distance to the bathroom is

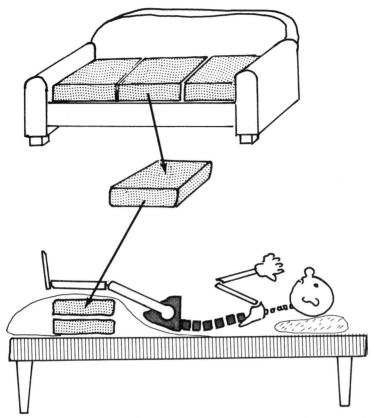

Figure 8–1. Home flexed bed posture utilizing square sofa pillows inserted under bedsheets to facilitate flexed hip and knee posture in lumbar discogenic disease.

long. Many bathrooms are upstairs, and climbing stairs is difficult in the period of acute low back pain. Pain and medication taken for pain may also be constipating. The excessive effort of straining also may aggravate the low back discomfort.

For the male, a urinal used in bed may be acceptable. For women a bedpan may present problems and require assistance. The use of a bedpan may require positions and movements not possible to the acutely impaired person.

A bedside commode is an excellent solution. They are easily available, inexpensive, easily located near the bed, and easily used by the patient.

LEAVING THE BED

Movement from the reclining bed position to the sitting or erect standing position, undertaken without thought when there is no pain, becomes a major ordeal when there is low back pain coupled with low back muscle spasm. There is no one way to move from reclining to the erect, but there are basic principles that facilitate this movement.

1. The patient must **not** come to a straight sitting up position in bed.

2. The patient must roll over to one side using the arms and keeping the knees, hips, and low back flexed.

3. Once rolled over to one's side in the flexed position, the patient must assume the sitting position, moving sideways, using the arms while keeping the low back immobile.

4. Once the patient has his or her feet on the ground, the patient must slowly lean forward until positioned directly above his or her feet.

5. Arising from there is done slowly, regaining the lordosis gradually. The use of the arms during this ascent is desirable.

MEDICATION

Pain is an anxiety-producing event that increases protective tension of the low back muscles. Pain causes anxiety that increases the intensity of the reaction to the pain. A pain medication is of unquestioned value. The brief use of medication does not indicate the advent of addiction. The value of pain relief ensures greater patient acceptance and cooperation.

The increased muscular tension not only compresses all the inflamed tissues and restricts movement but also may become **the** site of pain. The **tension myositis syndrome** of Sarno (1977) implicates muscle tension as a site of pain. This tension can be emotionaly incited, but it can also be protective spasm **aggravated** by anxiety. Either or both respond to relief of pain.

Medication for the relief of pain is best used on a specific basis of every 4 or 6 hours rather than prn, meaning as requested by the patient. The prn basis has been postulated by experts on pain management to increase dependency on drugs rather than merely to decrease nociceptive impulses.

Pain medicine used prn focuses on the "feeling" of pain and its intensity, whereas medicine used on a prescribed specific time schedule allays the build-up of pain sensation.

Oral anti-inflammatory medications have found their proper role in management of nociceptive stimuli. Irritation of soft tissues results in the release of chemical and mechanical substances. These substances, in turn, act on the end organs of sensory nerves that then transmit impulses along the nerve roots to the gray matter of the spinal cord. The route then is via the spinothalamic tracts to the hypothalamus where further transmission to the cortex is interpreted as **pain**.

If peripheral nociceptive chemical and mechanical substances can be prevented from initiating painful stimuli, the sensation of pain and its prolongation with increased intensity can be diminished.

These nociceptive substances are numerous. They include substance P, serotonin, histamine, kinins, and prostaglandin. It has been documented that steroids inhibit the breakdown of phospholipids via actinic acid into prostaglandin B. This steroid inhibition explains why aspirin has proven effective in the treatment of inflammatory diseases. The current nonsteroidal anti-inflammatory drugs (NSAIDs) have provided antiprostaglandin B formation.

When not contraindicated, oral NSAIDs are worth trying early, in adequate doses, for a specific period of time. When there is significant inflammation causing severe pain, the use of oral steroids may be indicated rather than using NSAIDs.

Muscle "relaxants" have been postulated as benefiting the pain caused by muscle spasm. Unfortunately, today, there are no specific muscle relaxants available that inhibit sustained muscle contraction without some sedative effect. It is even considered that much of the "muscular relaxation" induced by drugs occurs because of general relaxation and sedation. When sedation is not contraindicated, there is no reason to withhold muscle relaxants. In treating a patient who must remain ambulatory and in full control of mental acuity, these drugs frequently are ill advised.

Many muscle relaxants, albeit also sedative in their action, have a tendency to be depressants also. Depression, so often associated with prolongation of pain, becomes enhanced by the prolonged use of depressing sedating muscle relaxants. Clinical judgment is required in the use of these drugs.

Patients who have been depressed before the advent of the low back pain episode and who have the potential for becoming "chronic pain" candidates have benefited by the oral use of antidepressants. Antidepressants have also been acknowledged to be creators of endorphin, in itself a potent pain remedy.

MODALITIES

There are many locally applied physical modalities that have been used with varied success. These can be evaluated as to their efficacy and as to their assumed mode of action.

Ice applied locally over the site of low back pain has value if applied properly. Ice applied to the skin acts as an analgesic and also decreases the resultant reflex muscle spasm by desensitizing the nerve endings and nerve conduction. As some of the nociceptive end organ substances are vasodilators (histamine-like in their action), ice decreases this dilation. Further edema from the insult, which becomes a mechanical irritant to the nerve endings, is minimized.

Ice applied indiscriminately, by merely placing an ice pack over the area may cause more pain and spasm by its vasoconstriction properties. Ice

brushing or spraying (vasocoolant [Travel 1952] or ethyl chloride) is beneficial but requires the assistance of another person who may not always be
available or trained.

Ice may be applied to the patient's low back by brushing with an ice
stick that can be made by placing water in a paper cup in the freezer compartment of the ice box (Fig. 8–2). A stick or spoon inserted into the water
will become a handle once the water freezes. This ice stick then is brushed
in long strokes across the area of the low back that is painful. When exercises are used to stretch the low back, to overcome the spasm, ice application of this nature precedes the exercise.

Hot packs have a time-honored place in treatment of inflammation and
spasm. There are many patients who welcome heat rather than ice, and this

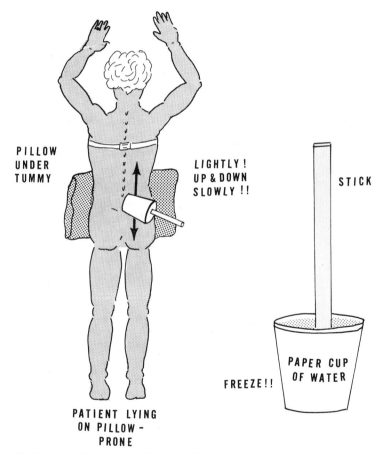

Figure 8–2. Ice application to the acute low backache. This is done several times
daily. (From Cailliet, R: Understand Your Backache. FA Davis, Philadelphia, 1984,
p 110, with permission.)

should be recognized and accepted. Moist heat is preferred as the modality, and this is available in the home. The **hydrocollator pack** is readily available in the local stores and is easy to apply.

Massage is soothing and does decrease spasm and remove nociceptive substances by bringing blood flow to the part. It requires another person, preferably a skilled individual. Massage by a physical therapist is becoming more difficult to attain as many therapists relegate this modality to an assistant as it is time-consuming and not remunerative.

Massages given in a therapy office require travel to the center from home and return, meaning car travel, getting in and out of a car, waiting in a waiting room, dressing, and undressing, etc. The benefit from these modalities, in a professional therapy center, is frequently diminished by these added activities.

LOCAL INTRAMUSCULAR INJECTIONS

The tissues that are innervated by the posterior branch of the lumbar dorsal ramus (Fig. 8–3) have been adequately discussed. These tissues are contained in a region called the **multifidus triangle** (Fig. 8–4). Within this triangle are included the facet joints, the erector spinae muscles, the interspinous ligaments, and the fascia. All these tissues are potential nociceptive sites of inflammation (Fig. 8–5).

The iliolumbar ligament, which connects the transverse process of the fifth lumbar vertebra to the iliac crest, has also been implicated as a site of

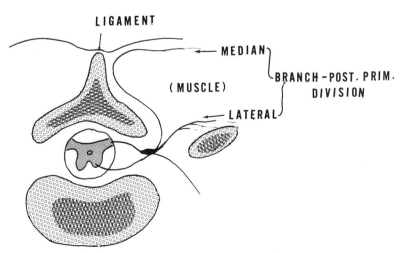

Figure 8–3. Posterior primary division. This demonstrates no innervation to the posterior spinous ligament which is known to be sensitive.

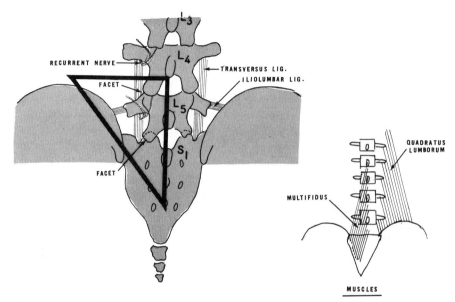

Figure 8–4. Multifidus triangle. This is an arbitrary triangular area extending from L₄ to the iliac crest and down to the sacrum, containing numerous pain-producing tissues, including facets, facet innervation, transversus ligament, quadratus lumborum muscle, multifidus muscle, iliolumbar ligament, and fascia.

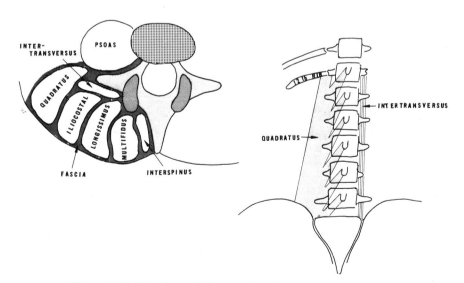

Figure 8–5. Muscles and fascia within the multifidus triangle.

nociceptive irritation. This ligament is also included within the triangle (Fig. 8–6).

An injection of an anesthetic agent with a soluble steroid into this region frequently interrupts the painful low back pain cycle. The exact site of injection effect within this triangle is not clear. To postulate that the innervation of the facet is interrupted is moot. Which muscle is beneficially injected is also unclear. Clinically an injection within this area has been beneficial, but the exact tissue site resulting in the benefit remains unproven. Within the references are listed numerous articles, Kellgren (1939), Pederson (1956), Melzack (1977), Rees (1979), and so on, that reveal the numerous concepts that have been postulated as "the" reason and tissue site of low back nociceptive pain.

An injection given must be within the centrum of this triangle and be sufficiently deep to approach the transverse processes of the vertebrae and the facet joints. The iliac crest can be palpated. The posterior superior spinous process of lumbar five can also be palpated. A point halfway between these two points is therefore superficially injected with an anesthetic agent (forming a skin wheal). A 4-inch spinal needle is then slowly inserted to ultimately hit a bony process. The patient remains awake and must be in-

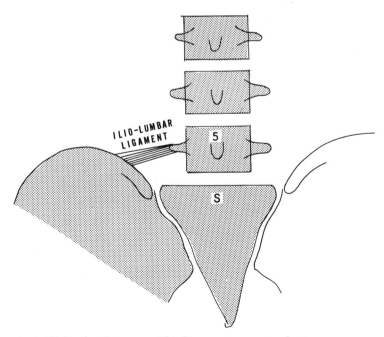

Figure 8–6. Iliolumbar ligament. This ligament connects the transverse process of the fifth lumbar vertebra to the iliac crest. Its function is that of stabilizing the L_5 vertebra.

structed to state any sensation felt so that, if a nerve is approached, immediate partial withdrawal of the needle is indicated. **No injection** must be given along the way. Repeated aspirations must be done along the injection site to assure that no blood vessel has been entered.

Once a bony process has been reached, it must be assumed that this is probably the transverse process. Several cubic centimeters of the anesthetic-steroid solution are then slowly injected after final aspiration has proven that no blood vessel has been penetrated.

The needle can then be withdrawn several centimeters and reinserted at a slight angle—either medially or laterally. The same procedure of inquiring from the patient the sensation and aspirating to verify that no blood vessel has been encroached is repeated and 2 more cubic centimeters of the solution are injected. By the needle being retracted and then reinserted medially, laterally, cephalad, and caudally, through the same skin penetration site, the anesthetic steroid solution has been infiltrated throughout the triangle.

This triangle area is also a common painful site termed **myofascial trigger point**. This concept also remains controversial, but its advocates (Travel 1952; Simon) believe that these areas causing pain exist and can be beneficially treated by vasocoolant spray and stretching of these tissues. They also advocate an injection into the area.

As this is also a "trigger" area (Melzack 1977), and an acupuncture site, the local use of transcutaneous electrical nerve stimulation (T.E.N.S.), acuprobe, or deep pressure over that area has its advocates. Deep low voltage ultrasound, which allegedly partially denervates the sensory nerves, has also been credited with success.

Whether a chemical or mechanical rhizotomy has been accomplished with denervation of the facet with these approaches is conjectural. Facet injection, under fluoroscopy, has been advocated, and there are claims of success, but this procedure should be held for later in the course of treatment when all other approaches have failed.

MANIPULATION

There are numerous practitioners who claim that manipulation of that region "unlocks," mobilizes a "jammed" facet, reflexly releases muscle spasm, elongates the capsule, or realigns a subluxed joint. Manipulation varies from gentle stretching in the correct direction that is restricted, forceful rotation of the flexed spine using long lever or short lever, or "manipulation in the direction of no pain or restriction" (Maigne 1978). The concepts are as numerous as their advocates.

Exactly what manipulation does remains conjectural. That it benefits some patients is evident. That it affords a lasting benefit is less accepted.

When combined with other modalities its effects appear better, but the question remains as to what role the manipulation played.

Of the benefits gained by manipulation some of the concepts are:

1. A facet is immobilized by an acute synovial reaction and "adherence" of the adjacent joint surfaces of the facets. The passive movement of the manipulation separates these surfaces.

2. A meniscus exists within facet joints that becomes entrapped.

3. The capsule of the facet joint becomes lodged between two adjacent articular surfaces.

4. The mechanoreceptors of the joint capsule are desensitized by the abrupt movement of the joint, and reflex protective spasm is eliminated and allows the joint to again move.

5. The spindle systems of the adjacent muscles are reflexly stimulated and reciprocally relax the extrafusal muscle fibers.

6. The "malaligned" spinal segments are realigned to conform to the center of gravity.

7. Manipulation is a placebo, benefiting the patient merely from the "laying on of the hands."

The concept of manipulation is the manual application of a force to the spine to passively regain the normal range of motion lost by the injury or the resultant spasm. Normally a joint moves actively or passively as far as its surrounding soft tissues will permit. These soft tissues are the capsule and the surrounding ligaments or tendons.

The normal joint moves to its soft tissue, capsular, limits. If there has been an imposed limitation, regardless of the cause, the joint is moved to the degree possible, then a small force is applied to increase that direction of movement (Fig. 8–7).

The medically accepted basis for any benefit derived from manipula-

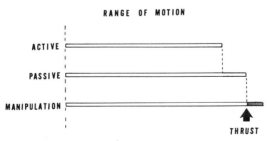

Figure 8–7. Concept of manipulation. A joint has an active range of motion that can passively be physiologically exceeded. When that range is reached, a firm but gentle thrust achieves the desired "joint play" that restores motion that frequently is lost.

tion remains to be confirmed. The numerous techniques of manipulation are well-documented in current textbooks and are beyond the scope of this text.

TRACTION

Traction has enjoyed a range of evaluations ranging from being a "specific" modality for relief of low back pain to merely being a means of "keeping the patient off his or her feet." The precise physiologic benefit gained from traction remains controversial as does the specific manner of applying traction.

Traction applied to the patient in a horizontal manner decreases the effects of gravity. This minimizes the need for the antigravity muscles to maintain erect posture when these antigravity muscles are reflexly splinted to prevent movement of the inflamed vertebral segment. Mere bedrest, in the proper position, probably accomplishes the same antigravity effect.

Distraction of the component parts of the functional units has been claimed to result from traction. In this respect, traction causes some vertebral distraction. A tremendous force of traction, in the hundreds of pounds, would be needed to accomplish significant distraction. A force of this magnitude is not physiologically possible and, today, is accomplished only when the total body weight is applied as the traction force.

More realistically the effects of traction on the lumbosacral spine can be attributed to:

Decreasing the lordosis which
(a) opens the intervertebral foraminae.
(b) separates the facets' joint surfaces.
(c) elongates the erector spinae muscles causing relaxation and release of protective spasm of the erector spinae muscles.
(d) "stiffens" the annular fibers of the disk. This annular effect, along with decreasing the intrinsic force within the nucleus, minimizes the annular "bulging."
(e) decreases the length of the nerve roots and their dura and decreases their tension.

Traction has been applied with the patient in a supine position. A contoured band encircles the pelvis to which are attached straps that continue to attach to a spreader bar and a rope pulley to which variable weights are applied (Fig. 8–8).

The direction the traction is to pull **up** on the pelvis as well as in the direction of elongation (Fig. 8–9). By this pull the lordosis is decreased. This traction is best applied in a hospital environment where the bed can be flexed at the knees and hips and the upper portion also elevated (Fig. 8–10). In the home environment similar traction may be applied using

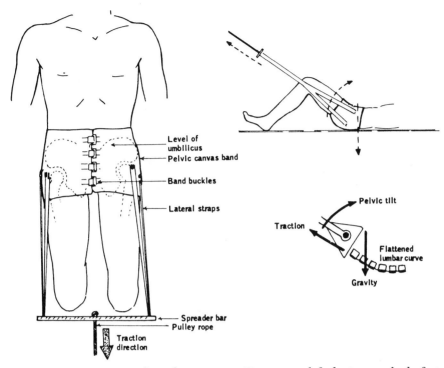

Figure 8–8. Equipment for pelvic traction. Drawing at left depicts method of attaching pelvic traction equipment. The lateral straps are placed to permit leg movements and exercises in bed. Drawing at right discloses the resultant pelvic rotation gained by this method of applying traction.

equipment such as BackTrac. This is a piece of equipment that pulls the pelvis in the same manner as does the above hospital-type traction equipment. This home equipment has the advantage of being used within the home as often and whenever possible with minimal personal displacement and expense.

Recent medical literature has advocated total body weight being used to apply the traction on the lumbosacral spine. It has been assumed that 30 percent of the total body weight is located below the third lumbar vertebra. Thus, if the patient is suspended at the thoracic spine, this amount of total body weight is exerted on the lumbosacral spine.

To apply traction by this method a belt, contoured to fit the rib cage, supports the body, and the portion of the body below the belt furnishes the traction force (Fig. 8–11). One manner of applying this type of traction is within a hospital circular bed (Fig. 8–12).

Another manner of using body weight as the force of traction is the "Gravity Traction Equipment" in which the lower body weight is used as

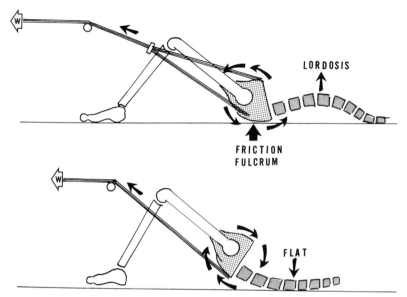

Figure 8–9. Pelvic traction principles. In the upper drawing the friction of the bed with the buttocks acts as a fulcrum about which the pelvis rotates to increase the lordosis. In the lower drawing the strap under the pelvis pulls to elevate the pelvis and decrease the lordosis.

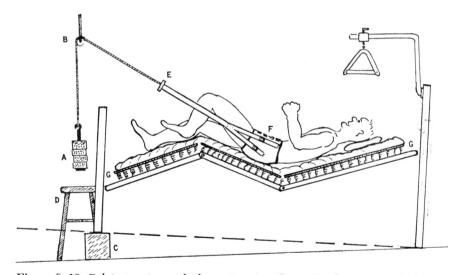

Figure 8–10. Pelvic traction with the patient in a "semi-Fowler position." The patient is wearing a pelvic band with the pull acting so as to flex the lumbar spine.

A. Weights applying the traction, usually 20 lb.

B. Overhead pulley so placed that the pull tilts or lifts the pelvis.

C. Ten-inch block to elevate foot of bed.

D. Stool to support the weights when patient temporarily disengages them.

E. Spreader bar to separate the lateral straps pulling on the pelvic band around patient's pelvis.

F. Pelvic band with buckles to permit easy detachment by patient.

G. Split board between mattress and box springs to prevent sagging.

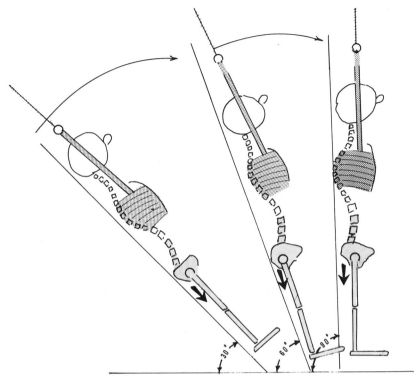

Figure 8–11. Gravity lumbar traction. As the bed (traction) angle is increased from 30 degrees to 90 degrees full upright, the amount of traction increases. The duration of traction can be determined.

depicted in Figure 8–13 or by using the upper body weight and suspending the patient by his or her feet either via boots or dangling at the flexed knees (Fig. 8–14).

The physiologic effects of gravity traction have been studied and found to have a primarily vagal influence from the head-down position (deVries-Cailliet, unpublished paper) which causes relaxation of the musculature. Some elongation from this traction has been verified by x-ray pictures taken with a patient in the equipment.

Medical literature has claimed that there is an elevation of ocular pressure from the upside down posture, which makes this form of treatment contraindicated in patients with glaucoma. This has not been completely verified but should be discussed with one's physician before contemplating gravity traction.

Hypertension has also been claimed to be a contraindication to the use of gravity traction. This also needs confirmation and discussion with one's physician.

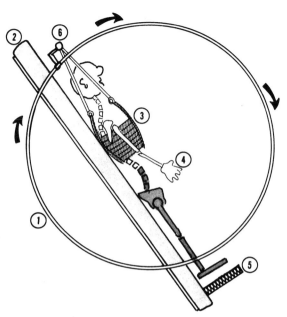

Figure 8–12. Gravity lumbar traction: (*1*) lumbar traction applied in a hospital setting with a circular bed; (*2*) mattress with bedboard within Stryker Circ-O-Lectric bed; (*3*) chest harness with lower straps under the rib cage and upper straps firmly grasping the rib cage; (*4*) bed manually controlled by patient; (*5*) footplate several inches below patient's feet for security; (*6*) snap ring attached to bed frame.

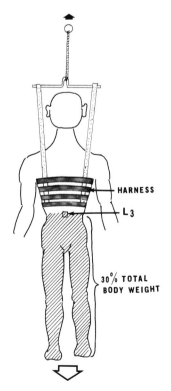

HARNESS

L₃

30% TOTAL
BODY WEIGHT

Figure 8–13. Gravity lumbar traction. Based on 30 percent of total body weight below the third lumbar (L₃) level, traction is applied by supporting the body from a chest harness.

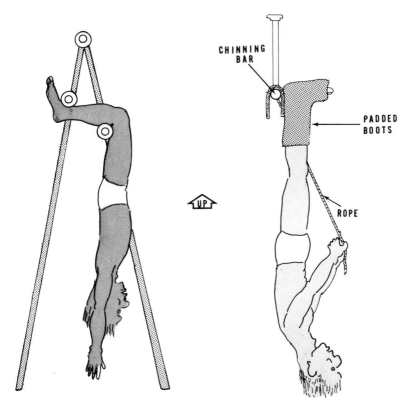

Figure 8–14. "Gravity" traction. There are numerous types of equipment for this traction—hanging from the knees or from the feet via boots. The principle is that the weight of the upper body stretches *all* the tissues of the low back: the muscles, fascia, ligaments, and possibly the disks. (Modified from Cailliet, R: Understand Your Backache. FA Davis, Philadelphia, 1984, p 136, with permission.)

Whether a person hangs passively or actively exercises within the traction varies with the prescribing physician. Both have been expounded by various researchers.

INJECTION: EPIDURAL STEROIDS

The use of local injection of an analgesic substance with or without steroids has been mentioned in the treatment of the acute lumbosacral sprain-strain. In some patients the acute phase persists or during the acute phase there is evidence of nerve root irritation. The physical examination depicts a **positive dural sign** (Fig. 8–15).

As was discussed in the examination of the patient during the acute

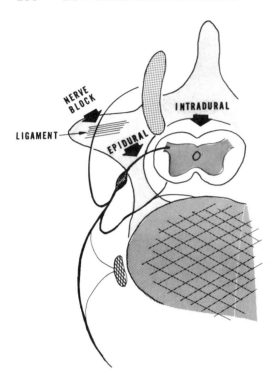

Figure 8–15. Differential diagnosis of site of radicular pain. By getting relief of "sciatic-like" pain from a nerve blocking the posterior primary division at the level of the intertransversus ligament, the site of pain is thus specified as being an irritation of that root. Relief from epidural steroids implicates inflammation of the sinuvertebral nerve. Benefit from intradural steroids indicates nerve root and dural inflammation.

phase of low back pain, performing the straight leg raising (SLR), it was maintained that an abnormal SLR be documented as being **muscular** or **neurologic**.

Pain, from neurologic nerve entrapment, emanates from dural irritation. Thus, after finding a limited SLR it must be determined if the restriction is caused by hamstring muscle limitation or by nerve root inflammation. If muscular, the limitation is felt in both legs as well as in the low back. Once the discomfort behind the legs has been elicited by SLR, the patient's head is flexed (placing the chin on the chest) or the foot is dorsiflexed. If these maneuvers aggravate the referred leg pain, it indicates that the nerve and its dura are the site of the leg pain.

Presence or persistence of this neurogenic pain may be treated by prolonged bedrest, oral NSAIDs, or oral or intramuscular steroids. The blood–spinal fluid barrier restricts a significant strength of steroid being deposited near an inflamed nerve. An epidural approach has been found to be an effective and relatively safe procedure.

Epidural injections for the treatment of **sciatica** have been used for more than 50 years. The injection site varies from the caudal route or at the lumbar level. The former has been less effective as the caudal canal is obliterated in many people whereas the lumbar site is usually patent.

There is a negative pressure gradient within the epidural space so that when a needle, attached to a syringe, reaches this space the plunger is drawn into the syringe barrel. If the needle penetrates the dura, the spinal fluid within the dura is under pressure and the plunger is forced out of the barrel by the spinal fluid. This is the means by which it is determined whether the needle tip is within the epidural or the dural space (Fig. 8–16).

Once into the epidural space a solution of an analgesic and a soluble steroid is inserted into the space. The immediate reaction is anesthetic feel-

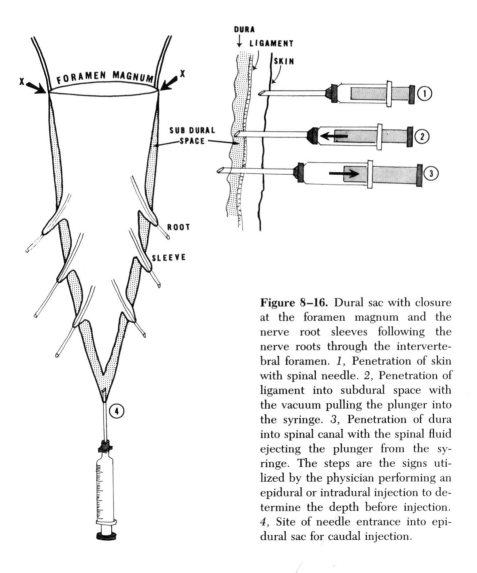

Figure 8–16. Dural sac with closure at the foramen magnum and the nerve root sleeves following the nerve roots through the intervertebral foramen. *1*, Penetration of skin with spinal needle. *2*, Penetration of ligament into subdural space with the vacuum pulling the plunger into the syringe. *3*, Penetration of dura into spinal canal with the spinal fluid ejecting the plunger from the syringe. The steps are the signs utilized by the physician performing an epidural or intradural injection to determine the depth before injection. *4*, Site of needle entrance into epidural sac for caudal injection.

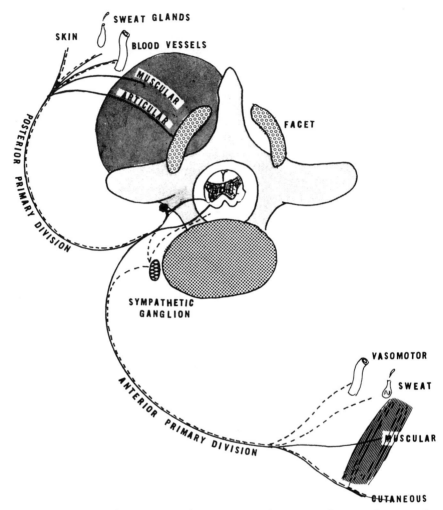

Figure 8–17. Neurologic pain pathways. A simplistic neurologic pathway is depicted, via anterior and posterior primary rami through which pain sensation is mediated.

ing of the dermatome region of the nerves coated and some paresis of the same myotomes. This indicates that the injection has been directed to the proper site. The anesthetic state vanishes within hours and the steroids exert their benefit within several days. The common procedure is to repeat epidural steroid injections at 4 to 8 day intervals for a series of three injections.

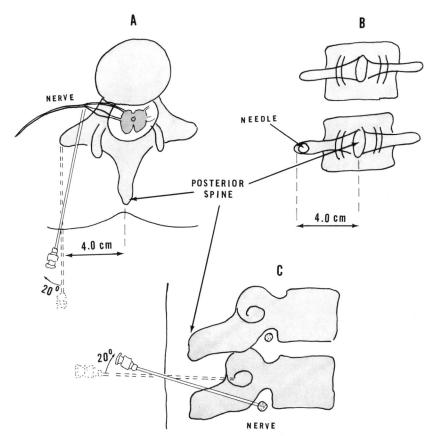

Figure 8–18. Technique for nerve root injection. With the patient in the prone position and with a pillow under the belly, the needle (8–10 cm, 21-gauge) is inserted 4 cm lateral to the *upper* margin of the spinous process until it penetrates to the lower margin of the transverse process (*B*). Upon contact the needle is withdrawn and inserted medially (*A*) and downward (*C*) about 20 degrees. Passing inferiorly to the transverse process (*C*), the needle is inserted until the nerve root is contacted, and the patient feels sudden sharp pain in the distribution of the root dermatome.

INTRADURAL INJECTION

An intradural injection of an anesthetic agent combined with steroids has also been advocated in the treatment of low back pain with radiculopathy. This injection has been used as a diagnostic test to determine whether the patient has "true" organic pain or is "malingering." In this test, a saline solution is injected and the patient's reaction noted. A second injection follows using a 0.2 percent Novocain solution. If there is relief from this solution, and not the saline, sympathetic nerve fibers are considered to be instrumental in the transmission of pain (Fig. 8–17). Relief from injecting a solution of 0.5 percent procaine "verifies" that pain is being transmitted via somatic nerves and is a "true" organic pain. This confrontation test has lost most of its original enthusiasm and is being merely mentioned as a method of treatment and diagnosis that has been employed.

NERVE ROOT BLOCK

The specific nerve root that is involved in a radiculitis may be identified by precise injection of that nerve root. This is a technically difficult injection and must be done under fluoroscopic viewing. The patient must also be awake and be able to identify the precise dermatomal area that becomes "numb" and the muscle (myotome) that becomes weak.

The fifth lumbar nerve is located at the transverse process of the fifth lumbar vertebra but the first sacral nerve (S1) must be reached through the sacral foramen (Fig. 8–18). The use of a specific nerve block is both diagnostic and therapeutic but is used rarely and only after all other modalities of treatment and diagnosis have failed to afford results.

FACET JOINT INJECTIONS

The facet joint has been included in the lumbar dorsal ramus syndrome (LDRS) as a site of local and referred pain in low back pain syndromes. Irritation of the facet joint has also been proven to result in referred pain to the lower extremity.

Denervation of the facet joint(s) has been advocated in the treatment of low back pain, and intra-articular steroid anesthetic injection into the joint apparently accomplishes the same result. This injection must be done under fluoroscopic vision. An "arthrogram" of the facet joint, in which dye is injected into the joint, assures that the joint has been entered. An anesthetic agent, with or without steroid, is then injected via the same needle that has remained within the facet joint.

A beneficial facet joint injection verifies that the facet is the site of pain. Often the injection affords pain relief, albeit temporary. If the facet is recognized as the major source of pain, then denervation of that facet joint is justified.

All the mechanical and tissue aspects of low back pain have now been discussed. All diagnostic procedures have been enumerated. A generalized summary of the **management of acute low back pain** can now be stated.

MANAGEMENT OF ACUTE LOW BACK PAIN

The frequently experienced symptom of **low back pain** has a natural history of being benign and self-limited. It has been accepted by students of this condition that current conventional treatment modalities may alleviate symptoms but fail to significantly influence the outcome of the disease.

In his presidential address to the International Society for the Study of the Lumbar Spine, Mooney (1976) attempted to answer the question "Where is the pain coming from?" The question referred to **low back pain,** which is the plague of the average person, the ubiquitous patient, the frustrated physician, the badgered insurance carrier, and the beleaguered employer or spouse.

In recent medical literature Waddell (1987) discussed the inefficiency of current treatment methods and modalities and Carron (1987) reviewed the current medical literature evaluating the rehabilitation of persons with chronic low back pain. These reports reviewing the current literature and, hence, current medical experience, reveal the frustration of medical experts who are faced with diagnosing and treating this common impairment and disability. These reports cast some sobering light on the current status of knowledge on the subject.

Statistics appear in the literature that, at some stage in life, most human beings (80 percent) will experience low back pain, with 2 to 5 percent of the average population seeking medical attention. It is of interest that disabling low back pain is becoming a "Western disease" in its incidence and prevalence.

Low back pain appears to be most prevalent in the active working years of a person's life, age 30 to 45 years. The cost to society is approximately $25 billion per year for both direct and indirect costs. The incidence of low back pain does not progress with age nor does it particularly correlate with the age-related changes of disk degeneration.

Of significance is the accepted fact that 80 to 90 percent of those suffering acute attacks of low back pain will recover within 6 weeks "regardless of what type of treatment has been undertaken." The majority of patients cope with the symptoms themselves, without medical intervention. Those that do seek medical assistance appear to do so due to their concern about the significance of symptoms, their expectations of the results of medical intervention, and their cultural patterns.

With the discovery of "disk herniation" by Mixter and Barr in 1934, the "cause" of low back pain with sciatic radiation seemed to implicate the intervertebral disk. Key, in 1945, indicated confirmation of the disk being "the lesion" in most low back pains. Surgery of the offending disk became prevalent, yet today's statistics reveal that, whereas 70 to 80 percent of patients carefully screened for radicular symptoms benefit from surgery, only 1 percent of patients suffering from low back disorders have disk herniations.

These statistics emphasize the sobering fact that little is known of the causation of low back pain symptoms and further question the verification of a "specific" type of treatment.

The significance attributed to the symptom of low back pain and its resultant disability is influenced by the statement (complaint) of the patient with, often, little if any, objective documentation as to its cause. It becomes apparent, therefore, that much of the implied discomfort and disability influence the physician by the patient's concern, attitude, belief, coexisting psychological distress, and illness behavior.

The significance of the low back pain symptom is also influenced by how the complaint and the "clinical findings" are interpreted and treated by the physician. Diagnostic procedures and subsequent treatment are influenced more by the patient's discomfort and illness behavior than by the "organicity" of the complaints and physical findings.

Evaluation of the basis for success of "specific" treatment modalities has failed to corroborate the value of any treatment modality over another. Treatment modalities have varied from rest, analgesic medicines, manipulations, heat or ice applications, and traction to corsets, not to mention a myriad of offered nostrums. For the average therapist a full evaluation therefore merits review.

The standard recommendation, in fact, prescription, for the acute low back pain is "bedrest," as if this were a specific, proven modality of anticipated benefit and curative value. The vague advice of a week to 10 days bedrest has actually proven to be not only useless but detrimental.

Inactivity has been shown to cause demineralization of bone and a 3 percent loss of muscle strength per day. The psychological aspects of enforced bedrest also tend to emotional depression and dependency as well as indicating "severity" of the condition to a susceptible person. Tissue healing, if there is any tissue insult, can be delayed by inactivity. Statistics also reveal that "return to work" is impaired by prolonged inactivity. After inactivity, ultimate return to work is permitted with a partially deconditioned person returning to the previous occupation. This enforced inactivity causes disuse, rendering injury-prone workers to be more prone to aggravation or recurrence of symptoms.

There is no scientific basis for assuming that activity during the acute low back symptomatology increases tissue damage. In spite of these questions of the advisability of bedrest, the prescription continues to be issued.

The current prevalent prescription of local ice, heat, ultrasound, and massage, as a precise specific benefit, is not substantiated by fact. Soothing as these modalities may be, possibly acting as placebo, they are at best a modality to assist active movement. Hence these modalities are best used to accompany and ensure exercise.

"Exercise" also does not enjoy standardization. Which type, intensity, frequency, as well as purpose of exercise remain arbitrary. The purpose of exercise can be essentially stated to maintain physiologic flexibility as well as muscle strength and endurance. Joint capsules, ligaments, and tendons also benefit from active elongation. Reparative blood flow is enhanced, and there is evidence that exercise also promotes endorphin formation, which is a psychotherapeutic assist.

The current **back school** concept of low back care is essentially furnishing information to the person who has been injured to assist recovery and prevent recurrence. By having knowledge of "how" the spine mechanically functions the person allegedly assumes control. Exercise in conjunction with education improves the condition of the tissues needed for proper function.

The fear regarding the **low back pain** patient is progression from the acute or the recurrent type into the condition of **chronic pain**. Chronic pain is a completely different problem from acute pain. In the latter, the acute, there is assumed to be transient tissue insult creating nociceptive substances that initiate the symptom of pain. Activity, coupled with all the assistive modalities, can eliminate these nociceptive substances with the relief of pain and elimination of disability.

Once the pain becomes "chronic," the cause becomes dissociated from all the factors of acute pain. There is usually no remaining objective evidence of the factors of nociception. Removal or modification of the acute factors originally considered to have caused the pain is no longer feasible. Chronic pain becomes a self-sustaining "condition" that resists amelioration by any of the standard physical, pharmacologic or even psychological modalities. Depression, dependency, and anxiety prevail as the person gradually assumes an uncorrectable sick role.

It becomes apparent that every effort must be made to curtail and minimize the extent, severity, and duration of the acute episode. In the susceptible person the acute anxiety generated by the acute pain must be addressed early by clearly understood reassurance. Early activity must be ensured. Ill-advised, unnecessary bedrest and complete avoidance of normal activities, such as walking or bending, must not be prescribed. Instruction of the patient in understanding the "how" the low back works, how and what tissues have been insulted resulting in pain, the difference between "hurt" and "harm," and the need for active exercise to ensure this proper function is the desirable management of the acute low back episode.

In summary it can be stated that there is no indication for prolonged bedrest as being specific and beneficial in treating the acute low back pain patient. Early gradual activity including sensible exercise to regain and maintain flexibility and muscle strength is desirable. Dispelling anxiety early is mandatory, and this is best accomplished by understandable discussion and instruction and active exercise early. Early return to work, by this approach, is not only possible but beneficial. Progression of acute pain into chronic pain can also be minimized and possibly prevented for most people.

REFERENCES

Adams, JE and Inman, VT: Stretching of the sciatic nerve: a means of relieving postoperative pain following removal of ruptured lumbar intervertebral disk. Calif Med 91:24, 1959.

Anderson, TP, Sachs, E, Fischer, RG, and Kraut, RM: Postoperative care in lumbar disc syndrome. Arch Phys Med Rehab 42:152, 1961.

Bagley, CE: The articular facet in relation to low back pain and sciatic radiation. J Bone Joint Surg 25:481, 1941.

Barry, PJC and Kendall, H: Coricosteroid infiltration of the extradural space. Ann Phys Med 6:267, 1962.

Bauwens, P and Cayer, AB: The "multifidus triangle" syndrome as a cause of recurrent low back pain. Br Med J 2:1306, 1955.

Bensman, LL and Bensman, AS: Iliolumbar ligament syndrome: a frequent cause of low back pain. Arch Phys Med Rehab 59:11, 1978.

Blau, L and Kent, L: Conservative and surgical aspects of disk lesion management. West J Med 120:353, 1974.

Bogduk, N: Lumbar dorsal ramus syndrome. Med J Aust, Nov. 15:537, 1980.

Bogduk, N and Long, DM: Lumbar dorsal ramus syndrome. J Neurosurg 51:192, 1979.

Bourdillon, JF: Spinal Manipulation. Appleton-Century-Crofts, New York, 1970, pp. 86–89.

Brena, JF and Unikel, IP: Nerve blocks and contingency management in chronic pain states. In Bonica, JJ and Albe-Fessard, D (eds.): Advances in Pain Research and Therapy. Vol 1. Raven Press, New York, 1976.

Burn, JMB and Langdon, L: Lumbar epidural injection for treatment of chronic sciatica. Rheumatol Phys Med 10:365, 1974.

Burton, C and Nida, G: Gravity lumbar reduction therapy program. Sister Kenney Institute Publication No. 731, 1976.

Cailliet, R: Low Back Pain Syndrome, ed. 2. FA Davis, Philadelphia, 1977, p. 76.

Carron, H: Rehabilitation of persons with chronic low back pain. Rehabilitation Research Review, DATA Institute, Catholic University, Washington, DC, 1987.

Dilke, TFW, Burry, HC, and Grahame, R: Extradural corticosteroid injection in management of lumbar nerve root compression. Br Med J June:635, 1973.

Doran, DML and Newell, DJ: Manipulation in treatment of low back pain: A multicentre study. Br Med J 2:161, 1975.

Gentry, WD, Newman, MC, Goldner, JL, and von Breyer, C: Relation between graduated spinal block technique and MMPI for diagnosis and prognosis of chronic low back pain. Spine 2:210, 1977.

Goldie, I, and Peterhoff, V: Epidural anesthesia in low back pain and sciatica. Acta Orthop Scand 39:261, 1968.

Grant, AE: Massage with ice (cryokinetics) in the treatment of painful conditions of the musculoskeletal system. Arch Phys Med Rehab 45:233, 1964.

Green, LN: Dexamethasone in the management of symptoms due to herniated lumbar disk. J Neurol Neurosurg Psychiatry 38:1211, 1975.

Hardman, J, Winnie, AP, Ramaurthy, S, Mani, MR, and Meyers, HL: Intradural and extradural corticosteroids for sciatic pain. Orthop Rev 3:21, 1974.

Heyman, CH: The relief of low back pain and sciatica by release of fascia and muscle. J Bone Joint Surg 23:474, 1941.

Hirsch, C, Inglemark, B, and Miller, M: The anatomic basis for low back pain. Acta Orthop Scand 33:1, 1963.

Hockaday, JM and Whitty, CWM: Patterns of referred pain in the normal subject. Brain. 90:481, 1967.

Kellgran, JH: Deep pain sensibility. Lancet 1:943, 1949.

Kellgren, JH: On the distribution of pain arising from deep somatic structures with charts of segmental pain areas. Clin Sci 4:35, 1939.

Kennedy, B: A muscle bracing technique utilizing intra-abdominal pressure to stabilize the lumbar spine. The Aust J Physiother 11:102, 1965.

King, JS, and Lagger, R: Sciatica viewed as a referred pain syndrome, in Surgical Neurology.

Lidstrom, A and Zachrisson, M: Physical therapy on low back pain and sciatica. Scand J Rehab Med 2:37, 1970.

Lindahl, O: Hyperalgesia of the lumbar nerve roots in sciatica. Acta Orthop Scand 37:367, 1966.

Macnab, I, Cuthbert, H and Godfrey, CM: The incidence of denervation of the sacrospinales muscles following spinal surgery. Spine 2:294, 1977.

Maigne, R: Orthopedic Medicine. Charles C Thomas, Springfield, IL, 1972, p. 379.

Maigne, R: Charniere dorsolumbaire et lombalgier bases. Gaz Med France 85:1181, 1978.

Maigne, R: The concept of painlessness and opposite motion in spinal manipulations. Am J Phys Med 44:55.

Mathews, BHC: Nerve endings in mammalian muscle. J Physiol (Lond.) 78:1, 1933.

Matthew, BR: Manipulative treatment, Br J Phys Med 13:241, 1950.

Melzack, R, Stillwell, DM, and Fox, EJ: Trigger points and acupuncture points for pain: correlation and implication. Pain 3:3, 1977.

Mennell, JM: The therapeutic use of cold. J Am Osteopath Assoc 74:1146, 1975.

Mooney, V: Where Is Pain Coming From? Presidential Address, International Society for Study of the Lumbar Spine, Dallas, 1986, Annual Report 2075.

Mooney, V and Robertson, J: The facet syndrome. J Clin Orthop 115:149, 1976.

Moore, D: Sciatic and femoral nerve block. JAMA 150:550, 1952.

Murray, DG (ed): Instructional Course Lectures: The American Academy of Orthopedic Surgeons. CV Mosby Company, St. Louis, 1981, pp. 457–83.

Nachemson, A: The load on lumbar disks in different positions of the body. Clin Orthop 45:107, 1966.

Nachemson, A: The lumbar spine: an orthopedic challenge. Spine 1:59, 1976.

Nachemson, A: Work for all, for those with low back pain as well. Clin Orthop Oct. 1983, vol. 179, JP Lippincott, Philadelphia, 1983.

Natchev, E and Valentino, V: Low back pain and disk hernia observation during auto-traction treatment. Manual Medicine 1:39, 1984.

Newton, MJ, and Ruhl, D: Muscle spindle response of body cooling, heating and localized muscle coolant. J Am Phys Ther Assoc 4:91, 1965.

Oudenhoven, RC: Paraspinal electromyography following facet rhizotomy. Spine 2:299, 1977.

Oudenhoven, RC: The role of laminectomy, facet rhizotomy and epidural steroids. Spine 4:145, 1979.

Parsons, WB and Boake, HK: Manipulation of backache and sciatica. App Therap 8:954, 1966.

Pearce, J and Moll, MH: Conservative treatment and natural history of acute lumbar disc lesions. J Neurol Neurosurg Psychiatry 30:13, 1967.

Pedersen, HE, Blank, CFJ, and Gardener, E: Anatomy of lumbosacral posterior rami and meningeal branches of spinal nerves. J Bone Joint Surg 35-A:377, 1956.

Pere, ER: Mode of action of nociceptors in Hirsch, C, and Zatterma, Y (eds.): Cervical Pain. Pergamon Press, Oxford, 1972.

Ray, MB: Manipulative treatment. Br J Phys Med 13:241, 1950.

Reese, WS: Multiple bilateral subcutaneous rhizolysis of segmental nerves in the treatment of intervertebral disc syndrome. Ann Gen Prac 26:126, 1974.

Sarno, JE: Psychosomatic backache. J Fam Prac 5:353, 1977.

See, DH and Kraft, GH; Electromyography in paraspinal muscles following surgery for root compression. Arch Phys Med Rehab 56:80, 1975.

Shealy, CN: Technique for percutaneous spinal rhizotomy. Radionics, Burlington, 1974.

Shealy, CN, Prieto, A, Burton, C, and Long, DM: Radio frequency percutaneous rhizotomy of the articular nerve of Luschka—an alternative approach to chronic low back pain and sciatica. Paper presented to the American Association of Neurological Surgeons, Los Angeles, April 9, 1974.

Sinclair, DC, Feindel, WH, Weddell, J, and Falconer, MA: The intervertebral ligaments as a source of segmental pain. J Bone Joint Surg 30-B:515, 1948.

Steer, JC and Horney, FD: Evidence for passage of cerebrospinal fluid along spinal nerves. Can Med Assoc J 98:71, 1968.

Steindler, A: The interruption of sciatic radiation and the syndrome of low back pain. J Bone Joint Surg 22:28, 1948.

Steindler, A, and Luck, J: Differential diagnosis of pain low in the back. JAMA 110:108, 1938.

Stoddard, A: Manual of osteopathic technique, ed 3. Hutchinson, London, 1980.

Travel, J: Ethyl chloride spray for painful muscle spasm. Arch Phys Med Rehab 33:291, 1952.

Waddell, G: A new clinical model for the treatment of low back pain. Spine 12:632, 1987.

CHAPTER 9

Prevention of Recurrence of Low Back Pain

Low back pain can be envisioned in three phases: (1) acute, (2) recurrent, or (3) progression into chronic pain and disability. The acute phase has been discussed and its management outlined. It has also been stated that 80 percent of acute low back pain episodes subside within a 3-day to 3-month period regardless of the prescribed treatment program.

Unfortunately, many patients who have recovered from the acute episode are candidates for recurrence. Some residual impairment also may remain even though symptoms have subsided. Prevention of recurrence must reveal and overcome or remove the residual factors that led to the first episode or may remain after the acute phase has subsided.

There undoubtedly were factors that predisposed the patient to sustain the initial acute episode. If these factors had been recognized and addressed, the acute attack might have been avoided. Some of these factors may not have been under the control of the patient and thus were not completely avoidable. If recognized, however, their presence in the future would be recognizable and avoided.

The controllable factors that can be recognized can be addressed and effort expended to avoid recurrence of low back pain. These factors can be itemized in the following categories:

The person must

1. Regain or acquire adequate flexibility of the pertinent **soft tissue** of the lumbosacral spine and the pelvic region.

2. Acquire or regain adequate strength of the pertinent muscles related to low back function.

3. Learn or relearn proper posture in everyday activities.

4. Learn or relearn and implement into everyday activities the proper manner of bending, stooping, lifting, pushing, pulling, turning, twisting, and sitting.

5. Recognize, then control or avoid, any interfering psychosocial, professional, or personal emotional factor that can impair low back function.

Structural damage may have resulted from the acute injury. Structural abnormalities may have preceded and contributed to the acute initial injury. These must be identified.

Correction, or at least modification, of any or all of these factors must be addressed to prevent recurrence of low back pain. Correction and modification must be achieved if chronic pain is to be avoided. Chronic pain will be addressed in a subsequent chapter, but the avoidance of recurrence will be highlighted here.

STATIC SPINE: PROPER ERECT POSTURE

The correction of faulty posture appears relatively easy if appropriate concepts are accepted. Proper posture requires that all curves—lordosis, kyphosis, cervical thoracic, and lumbar—are held at a minimum. All curves must conform to decreasing their distance from the center of gravity. In essence all curves must be minimized in their arc (Fig. 9–1).

For centuries the concept of decreasing the lumbar lordosis was considered **the** manner of minimizing static low back pain. To accomplish this decrease of lumbar lordosis, exercises and the concept of "pelvic tilt" were advocated. More recently (McKenzie 1980) a degree of lordosis was advocated as desirable and physiologically sound. The pelvic tilting exercise was replaced by the encouragement of lordosis.

The final answer as to which is the most desirable for the majority of people has not yet been accepted. There is good clinical evidence that both concepts have merit, depending on which presents the painful problem to the patient.

If the clinical story and the physical examination reveal that, by accentuating the lordosis, **the low back pain** can be reproduced, then lordosis is not desirable. If the history and examination reveal benefit from acquiring and holding an accentuated lordosis, then this increased lordosis is desirable.

In the case of the undesirable excessive lordosis the "pelvic tilt" exercise is frequently advocated. In the vernacular this is termed "tuck in the pelvis," which implies that the pelvis is voluntarily rotated to decrease the

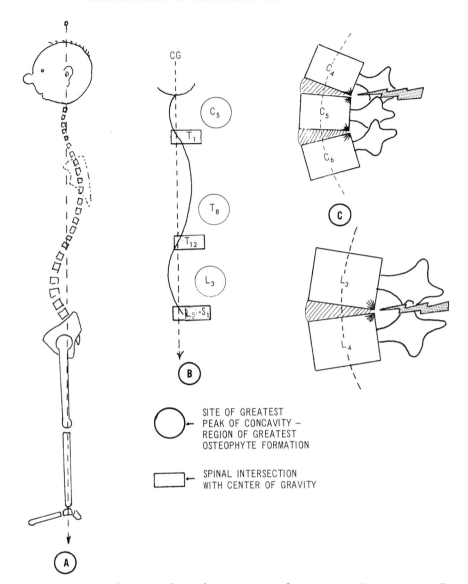

Figure 9–1. Spinal curve relationship to center of gravity. *A*, Erect posture. *B*, Transection of the spinal curves to the center of gravity (CG). *C*, Potential injury to the spinal joints from excessive lordosis.

lumbosacral angle (Fig. 9–2). The muscles that allegedly rotate the pelvis are the abdominals in front and the gluteal muscles behind (Fig. 9–3).

The patient is literally told to "tighten" the abdominals and "pinch" the buttock muscles together. By doing these muscular activities the patient "gets the feeling" of the decreased lordosis.

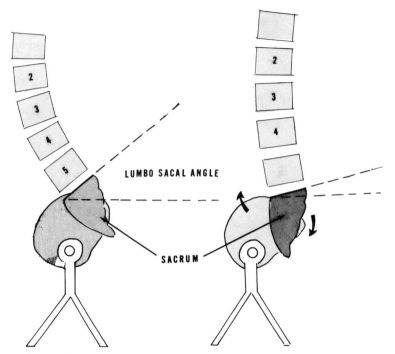

Figure 9–2. Lumbar lordosis, modified by lumbosacral angle. Figure on *left* indicates that as the pelvis descends anteriorly the lordosis increases. In the *right* figure, the pelvic muscles depress the posterior pelvic brim and decrease the lordosis. (Modified from Cailliet, R: Understand Your Backache. FA Davis, Philadelphia, 1984.)

To accomplish an adequately rotated pelvis the erector spinae muscles must have reasonable flexibility and the abdominal muscles adequate strength and endurance. To maintain this posture requires continuous concentration until the decreased lordosis is acquired. This effort is unrealistic and is one of the factors that leads to failure.

A more realistic and efficient manner of decreasing excessive lordosis is to concentrate on the neck position. When the cervical lordosis is decreased and the head is held directly above the center of gravity, the lumbar lordosis simultaneously decreases. The pelvic tilting exercise is valuable in elongating the erector spinae muscles and strengthening the abdominals, but the concentration on the cervical lordosis implements the proper posture with minimal effort.

An exercise that accomplishes this total postural effort is to stand with the shoulder blades to the wall and the feet some 6 inches from the wall base. The back of the head is pressed to the wall and the neck is gradually "forced" toward the wall. With an increased cervical lordosis, three or

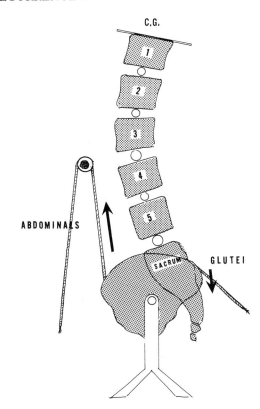

Figure 9–3. Lordosis, dependence upon sacral angle. The pelvis rotation about the hip joints determines the extent of the superincumbent lumbar lordosis. (Modified from Cailliet, R: Understand Your Backache. FA Davis, Philadelphia, 1984, p 27.)

more fingers can be placed between the neck and the wall. When only two or fewer fingers can be placed between the neck and the wall, the lordosis is optimal. The intent of this exercise is "pushing the head toward the ceiling," "tucking in the chin," thus veritably standing "taller." Not only the cervical but the lumbar lordosis is decreased, and posture is improved (Fig. 9–4).

The factors that led to the formation of the undesirable posture are numerous, well established, and not easily broken. Family posture may be considered as the patient's "destiny." Professional occupational attitudes may initiate and prolong this abnormal posture. Emotional posture is "body language" where depressed or anxious persons unwittingly depict their attitudes via their posture.

All these must be recognized and modified or corrected. However, even if these factors are influenced, the physical posture must be corrected and this can be done only by a conscientious exercise effort and implementation during everyday activities.

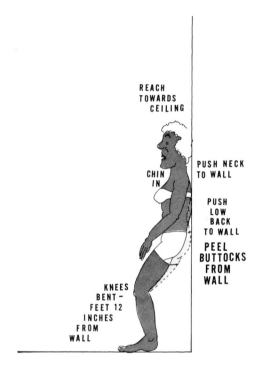

REACH
TOWARDS
CEILING

PUSH NECK
TO WALL

CHIN
IN

PUSH
LOW
BACK
TO WALL

PEEL
BUTTOCKS
FROM
WALL

KNEES
BENT -
FEET 12
INCHES
FROM
WALL

Figure 9–4. Postural exercise. With shoulders to the wall and feet some 6–12 inches from baseboard, the head is pushed toward the ceiling and back to the wall. Chin is "tucked in." The neck should be within two fingerbreadths from the wall. The pelvis may also be "pulled" slightly from the wall and the low back pressed toward the wall. (Modified from Cailliet, R: Understand Your Backache. FA Davis, Philadelphia, 1984, p 120.)

LOW BACK FLEXIBILITY EXERCISES

A tight low back implies lack of flexibility. This manifests itself in that the lumbosacral spine does not fully flex either forward or sideways. This limitation can be a complaint by the patient and can be observed during the examination.

Limitation symptoms may be merely a feeling of "tightness" or may be considered a result of pain. Limitation is a manifestation of restriction of elongation of the soft tissues of the lumbosacral spine. These tissues are the erector spinae muscles, the lumbosacral fascia, the ligaments, and the facet joint capsules. Each manifests itself differently and evokes different symptoms.

A muscle that elongates on passive stretching does so gradually with eccentric relaxation until the fascia has been stretched to its maximum. At this point no further stretching is permitted and an "endpoint" sensation is experienced. This endpoint sensation is not a pain or a discomfort unless an effort is made **by** the patient or **to** the patient that exceeds normal range of motion. If the patient is poorly conditioned and has not kept limber, this endpoint is reached sooner than anticipated in attempting flexion movement. This is evident from the history and from the examination.

The lumbosacral spine reverses its lordosis symmetrically and equally at each functional unit. The lordosis is viewed as gradually forming a symmetrical kyphosis. Once reached, the pelvis has also fully rotated to the extent that is permitted by the flexibility of the hamstring muscles. All this has been determined during the examination.

If there is a painful condition of the low back, the muscles react by going into "spasm." This spasm is essentially a limited elongation of the muscle fibers because they remain in a state of isometric contraction and will not eccentrically elongate.

The neurologic mechanism that results in this "spasm" is considered to be mediated via the intrafusal and extrafusal system depicted in Figure 9–5. The nociceptive stimuli released by tissue trauma initiate a mononeural reflex from the dorsal roots to the anterior horn cells that initiate contraction of the extrafusal muscle fibers.

As a "painful patient" attempts forward flexion, only the pelvis rotates and the lumbar spine bends forward without reversal. Some clinicians claim that "spasm" can be palpated but this is a moot question. What is

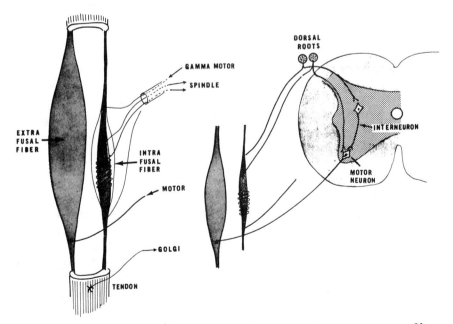

Figure 9–5. Intrafusal and extrafusal system. The extrafusal system consists of large muscle fibers under voluntary control. The intrafusal fibers consist of gamma motor neurons that "set" the muscle length for reflex action. The spindle cells report the muscle length and tension to the central nervous system. The Golgi neurons respond to the length and tension within the muscle tendon.

noted is inflexibility and subjective pain from the attempt. The muscles are palpably "taut," which is what is termed "spasm."

Spasm may be reflex from nociceptive irritation or may be unwillingness on the part of the patient to move the painful region, thus "splinting" the muscles. Both manifest themselves in the same manner.

At first the protective spasm is beneficial in that it prevents further liberation of nociceptive tissue elements at the site of irritation. If allowed to persist, there is contracture of the soft tissues—the fascia, the ligaments, and the joint capsules. The edema, at this tissue site, contains protein and can "organize" into inflexible tissue. Gradually this sustained muscular contraction becomes "the" tissue site of pain and limitation.

Sustained tissue tension is aggravated by fear and emotional tension that further the "spasm." A vicious cycle evolves.

TREATMENT PROTOCOL

Active and passive stretch is the mainstay of relaxing muscles and regaining elongation. Prior to exercise, the tissues of the low back may be prepared for the elongation forces needed to accomplish its goal.

Ice is probably the best modality for this purpose. Ice is a local anesthetic and decreases pain and apprehension. Ice decreases further formation of kinins, histamine-like substances, and other nociceptive tissue metabolites. Ice decreases the nerve conduction of sensory fibers.

Ice can be applied by ice packs, by ice brushing, or with vasocoolant spray of the area (see Fig. 8–2). This ice is applied for 10- to 15-minute periods several times a day for 2 days, after which heat packs are beneficial. These heat packs can be thermofor, Hydrocollator packs, electric pads, or even a hot shower. Moist heat penetrates better and is more desirable than dry heat.

The best low back exercise is to achieve the "fetal" position. The legs are used for the fulcrum leverage. This position is the knee-chest attitude with the instruction that the patient "feels" the low back being stretched gently but definitely (Fig. 9–6). The buttocks must be raised from the floor. Merely bringing the knees to the chest may not stretch the low back.

The knees (each separately) are brought to the chest slowly and for several repetitions (five at first; gradually twenty). After the knees are brought to the chest, they should be held there for a few moments. This stretch exercise "unloads" the spindle system of the intrafusal system.

To avoid abrupt extension of the low back after this flexion exercise, each leg must be lowered slowly to place the foot on the ground, maintaining the bent knee and hip position. Lowering one leg at a time is preferable to lowering both legs simultaneously (Fig. 9–7).

Gradual flexion of the low back should be accompanied by flexing the

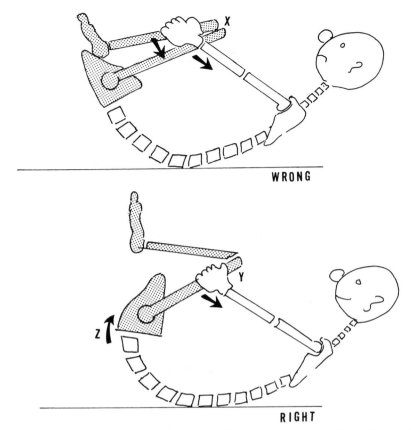

Figure 9–6. Low back flexibility exercises. The legs are used as a lever to flex the lumbar spine, as depicted in the lower drawing. The upper drawing shows the knees being hyperflexed, which stresses the knees without flexing the lower back.

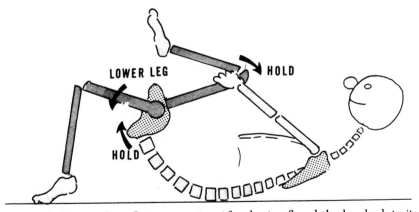

Figure 9–7. Descent from flexion exercise. After having flexed the low back to its maximum, *one* leg should be returned to the floor while maintaining a flexed pelvis. This prevents the return of lordosis during the descent of both legs, which may be painful.

neck, bringing the chin on the chest. This stretches the neck extensors and strengthens the neck flexors. Care must be exercised in the early phase not to cause neck discomfort in the attempt to stretch the low back. Holding the breath while exercising also may initiate a Valsalva effect, which is uncomfortable.

The low back muscles that get stretched from this exercise are the erector spinae as well as the spinalis, longissimus, and iliocostalis muscles extending to the thoracic spine. These muscles are also lateral flexors (Fig. 9–8) and thus can, and should, be stretched by lateral flexibility exercises (Fig. 9–9).

The shoulder muscles—the latissimus dorsi and the trapezius—also attach to the pelvis and spine and are considered important spine muscles. They too must be stretched so that in lateral trunk stretching the upper arm reaches overhead toward the other side and the lower arm reaches across the pelvis.

A low back stretch exercise that eliminates the hamstring muscles can be performed in the sitting or modified "Yoga" position (Fig. 9–10). In the sitting position the person, seated with feet on the ground, gently bends forward in an attempt to place the head between the knees or fingers to the floor.

The exercise frequently advocated to stretch the low back is that of standing, with legs extended, then **bouncing** down to **touch the floor with the fingertips**. This is a good example of the adage **no pain-no gain**. Noth-

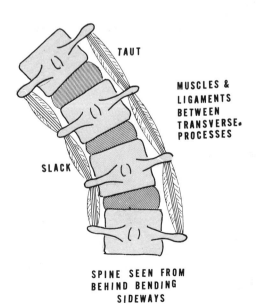

TAUT

MUSCLES &
LIGAMENTS
BETWEEN
TRANSVERSE.
PROCESSES

SLACK

SPINE SEEN FROM
BEHIND BENDING
SIDEWAYS

Figure 9–8. Lateral ligaments of the spine. These lateral ligaments allow side bending but must be kept flexible by exercise. (From Cailliet, R: Understand Your Backache. FA Davis, Philadelphia, 1984, p 131, with permission.)

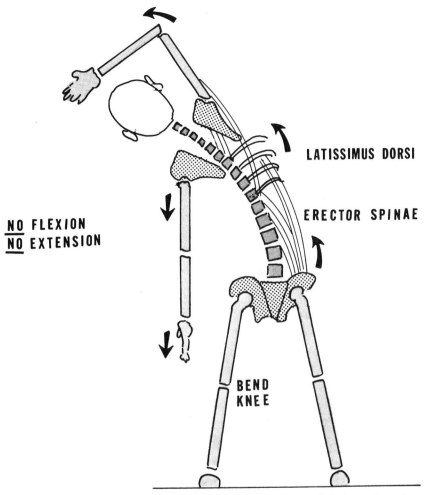

NO FLEXION
NO EXTENSION

LATISSIMUS DORSI

ERECTOR SPINAE

BEND KNEE

Figure 9–9. Lateral flexion exercises. With both legs apart slightly and one knee bent, the trunk is gently and progressively flexed laterally *without forward or backward flexion.* The unilateral erector spinae muscles and their fascia are stretched. As the scapular muscles also attach to stabilize the spine, they too must be stretched by placing the arms overhead.

Figure 9–10. "Yoga" exercise. With the patient in a squat position, with the knees and hips flexed, the low back is gradually flexed until the head approaches the floor or the toes. This exercise fully stretches the entire spine.

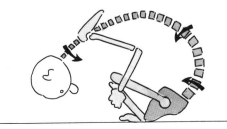

ing could be more contraindicated. This is an exercise that should be prohibited and avoided.

The position of standing with feet erect ensures that the low back will be **overstretched** because the hamstrings, in this position, have limited flexibility. When they have elongated to their limit, the pelvis no longer rotates and all further flexion occurs in the lumbosacral spine. Often, this flexion exceeds normal.

To touch the floor with the fingertips implies that this is a normal criterion of flexibility. This is an error. Not everyone can **normally** touch their toes, and many who can have low back problems, just as many who cannot have normal spine flexibility.

"Bouncing" to regain flexibility defeats the purpose of a stretch exercise. The abruptly stretched muscles, from bouncing, merely irritate the proprioceptors of the ligaments, the tendons, the joint capsules, and the muscles and initiate a reflex contraction with increased irritability of these soft tissues. There is more spasm than increased flexibility.

A simple exercise that can be done in the home that will stretch the low back and simultaneously strengthen the abdominal muscles is the **prone arch and sag** exercise (Fig. 9–11). Being up on one's hands and

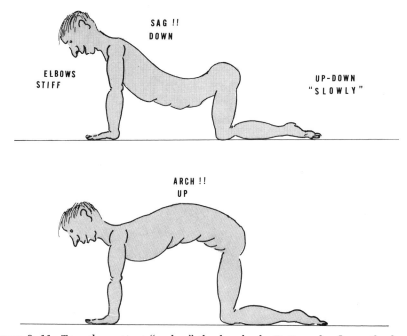

Figure 9–11. *Top*, the patient "arches" the low back. *Bottom*, he flexes the back, strengthening abdominal and buttock muscles. (From Cailliet, R: Understand Your Backache. FA Davis, Philadelphia, 1984, p 129, with permission.)

knees causes the low back to sag, which extends the low back. The low back then is elevated to its fullest, which stretches the back extensor tissues. This exercise also instills the concept of "pelvic tilting."

TRACTION

During the acute phase the question of the value of traction is often raised as to eliminating any residual impairment that could result in recurrence of low back pain. Traction has been discussed in the previous chapter.

During the acute phase and for periodic use in convalescence or minor recurrence, a simple home traction position is possible until the low back muscles become adequately stretched (Fig. 9–12). Lying on one's back and using a chair to support the legs at a height elevates the low back from the floor. This reclining position decreases the lumbar lordosis and elongates the erector spinae muscles.

Gravity traction, which has also been discussed in a previous chapter, elongates the low back and increases flexibility. While in traction the pelvis can be tilted (flexed), which adds strengthening along with increasing flexibility.

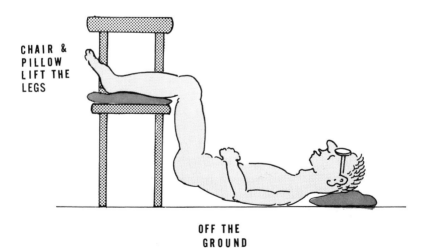

CHAIR &
PILLOW
LIFT THE
LEGS

OFF THE
GROUND

Figure 9–12. Pelvic traction. By placing legs on chair and sufficient pillows, the body is lifted from the floor. This flexes and stretches the low back. Remain in this position as long as possible. (From Cailliet, R: Understand Your Backache. FA Davis, Philadelphia, 1984, p 134, with permission.)

LOW BACK STRENGTHENING EXERCISES

Regardless that a controversy exists as to the desirable lordotic posture versus lumbar kyphosis in the erect posture, pelvic "tilting" exercises for preventing recurrences have a proven benefit. These exercises, along with others to be enumerated, increase flexibility and increase the strength of the pertinent low back musculature.

In bending forward and resuming the erect posture, the need for flexibility of the low back has been discussed. The need for strength of the appropriate muscles now must be addressed.

The "flat back" position is indicated in posture and in proper bending and lifting and thus should be mastered by the patient. Pelvic tiling influences several tissues involved in the function of the lumbosacral spine. To "tilt" the pelvis requires (1) flexibility of the lumbosacral spine; (2) strengthening of the abdominal muscles; (3) strengthening of the buttock muscles; and (4) the concept of "flattening" the lumbar lordosis. All of these activities are instrumental in regaining a properly functioning low back.

PELVIC TILTING EXERCISES

Pelvic tilting initially can best and most easily be taught with the patient in the supine position with the knees and hips flexed and the feet on the ground. The patient must be comfortable; this requires an adequate amount of cushioning behind the head for comfort, allowing no straining of the neck flexors during the exercise.

The exercise is performed in the following sequence:

1. The low back is pressed on the floor.

2. Once pressed to the floor, it must not be allowed to raise from the floor.

3. The buttock is raised **slowly and gently** from the floor. The distance the pelvis is lifted differs with each individual, but must never be done to the extent that the low back leaves the floor.

The first step may be facilitated by placing one's hand between the floor and the low back and ensuring that the hand remains compressed during the entire exercise. If the low back raises from the floor, it is the equivalent to a "wrestler's bridge," which arches the low back.

The second step, that of raising the buttocks, may be enhanced by concentrating on the sensation of the buttock muscles contracting and the abdominal muscles tightening.

A question arises whether this tilting must be done rhythmically or merely done, sustained, then released. There is no value to alternating rhythmically this movement and, in fact, this repeated movement fre-

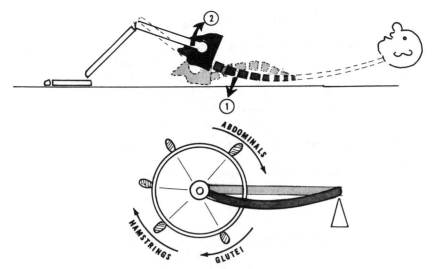

Figure 9–13. Concept of pelvic tilting. *Top,* (1) Pressing the lumbar spine against the floor, table, or bed; (2) gentle gradual lifting of the pelvis from the floor, table, or bed. *Bottom,* The musculature involved in pelvic tilting.

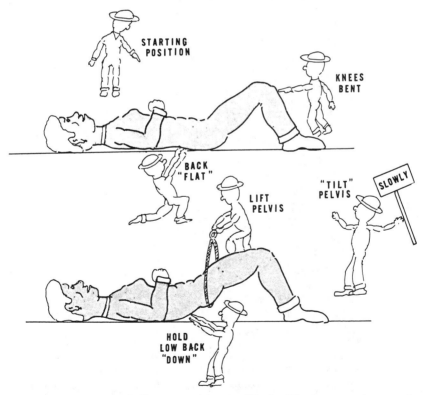

Figure 9–14. Pelvic "tilting" exercise. This is a "flat back" exercise to decrease lumbar lordosis and strengthen the abdominal and buttock muscles. It also teaches this "concept" to the patient.

quently leads to raising the low back from the floor. Holding and sustaining adds strength and endurance to the participating muscles.

Figure 9–13 depicts the pelvis as a nautical wheel that, when it rotates, causes the connected flexible board (the low back) to bend. Figure 9–14 shows the technique of pelvic tilting.

One of the benefits of pelvic tilting is the stretching of the iliopsoas muscles. The iliopsoas muscle attaches from the lumbar spine and inserts into the anterior femur. Its function is to flex the hips and to increase the lordosis. When the exercise is begun with the hips flexed, the psoas relaxes. By pressing the low back to the floor, the psoas muscle undergoes some stretch.

ERECT PELVIC TILTING EXERCISE

The pelvic tilting exercise has been advocated as being best done in the supine position. But, as the "flat low back" becomes a desired position

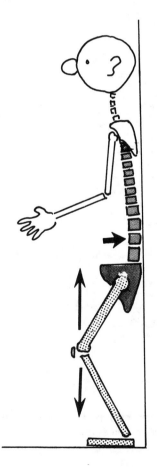

Figure 9–15. Erect pelvic tilting training. With the patient standing against a wall with feet slightly forward, the pelvis is "flattened" against the wall as it is against the floor in the supine exercise. This trains the patient to feel the position of the "flat" lumbar spine.

in the erect posture, the exercise should also be done in that erect stance position. By doing it in the erect position it also means that the exercise can be done frequently, in everyday activities, without needing to assume the supine position.

This exercise has been mentioned in the section on posture where the neck component of the erect posture was stressed. In the pelvic tilting exercise the routine is the same, merely concentrating on the pelvis.

Standing up against a wall with the feet 6 to 12 inches from the wall, the low back is pressed against the wall until only a few fingers can be placed between the back and the wall. To do this the pelvis must be pulled away from the wall while keeping the low back pressed to the wall (Fig. 9–15).

Further modification of this exercise should progress. The low back can be pressed against the wall as the feet are slowly brought closer to the wall. Ultimately the low back can be "flattened" with the feet completely against the base board of the wall.

A slow deep knee bend with the low back in this position is also a good adjunct to the exercise. This strengthens the quadriceps muscles. As instruction in proper bending and lifting advocates lifting with the bent knees, the quadriceps muscles need to be strengthened.

As advised in the section on posture, a weight perched on the head that is "pushed toward the ceiling" improves the posture, decreases the lordosis of the neck and the low back, and helps impart the concept ("feeling") of proper posture (Figs. 9–16 and 9–17).

STRENGTHENING OF APPROPRIATE MUSCLES

As stated regarding the factors needed to prevent recurrence of low back pain, there is need to strengthen the **appropriate** muscles to ensure proper lumbosacral function. These "appropriate" muscles are the abdominals, the erector spinae, and the quadriceps muscles.

It has been aptly, and correctly, stated that "a low back is as strong as are the abdominal muscles." This truism has been universally expounded but its veracity never explained.

The need for strong abdominal muscles has been explained in the following manner:

1. The abdominal muscles contain the contents of the abdominal cavity, which forms an "air bag" that unloads pressure on the spine.

2. Strong abdominal muscles balance the forces of the erector spinae muscles on the spine.

3. The abdominal muscles strengthen the fascia of the erector spinae muscles.

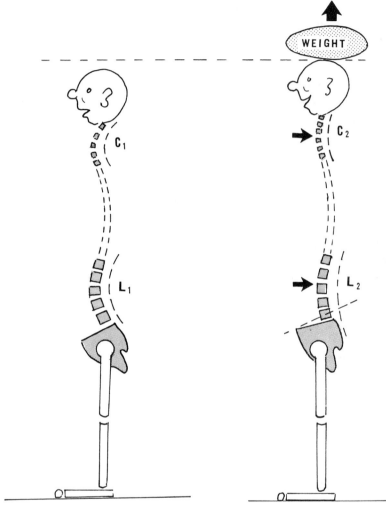

Figure 9–16. Erect posture concept training: *"distraction."* Placing a balanced weight upon the head and "pushing upward" (being taller) decreases the cervical and lordotic curves. The posture improves without the patient's awareness of any specific action of the pelvis or the shoulders. The "concept" of erect posture is gained unconsciously and can become habit.

The "air bag" concept has recently been questioned and even refuted because significant intra-abdominal pressure to neutralize the forces on the low back would overwhelm the venous and arterial pressures of the intra-abdominal blood vessels.

The proponents of the concept that the value of the abdominal muscles

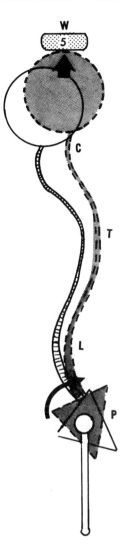

Figure 9–17. Mechanism of distraction exercise. By distracting the spine, elevating the weight upon the head, the cervical and lumbar curves decrease and the pelvis rotates.

exert their effect on the erector spinae fascia claim the following: The abdominal muscles that affect the low back extensors are the abdominal obliques, which originate from the fascia of the rectus abdominus and insert on the fascia of the erector spinae group. By strengthening the fascia of the erector spinae muscles, they reinforce the tissue that is used by the low back in resuming the erect posture.

To review this concept let us review how the lumbosacral spine resumes the erect lordotic position from the forward flexed kyphotic position. As the attempt is made to begin returning to the erect position the first movement is derotation of the pelvis. The lumbar spine returns to the erect position without altering its kyphosis until 45 degrees of forward flexed position has been reached. The return to the erect thus has, to this point, been achieved by the pelvic muscles (the gluteus maximus). Little, if any, erector spinae muscle contraction has been invoked. The stress on the lumbosacral spine has been borne largely, if not exclusively, by the erector spinae fascia and the superior spinous ligaments.

By improving the contractile strength of the oblique abdominal muscles, the erector spinae fascia has been reinforced. The erector spinae fascia has also been widened (i.e., pulled laterally). This widened and reinforced fascia becomes more efficient to support the lumbosacral spine and spares the erector spinae muscles.

The erector spinae muscles cannot adequately extend the forward flexed spine by pulling on their points of attachment between adjacent vertebral laminae and posterior spinous processes. These muscles have proven to be incapable of extending the spinous functional elements in this spinous position. The angle of pull is mechanically inadequate and the strength of muscle contraction insufficient through this small angle of pull about the axis of rotation. To expect muscle to resume the flexed (lordotic) position in the forward bent forward position is to ensure muscular failure. The fascia and the posterior ligamentous structures spare the muscles.

The value of strengthened abdominal muscles therefore must emphasize the oblique abdominal muscles. The standard "sit up" or "sit back" exercises are valuable, but they particularly strengthen the rectus abdominus flexor muscles—not the obliques. They should be done, as they do cause some contraction of the obliques, but, the latter, the obliques, must, in addition, be stressed.

ABDOMINAL STRENGTHENING EXERCISES

It has been conventional thinking to advocate the "sit up" or the "straight leg raises" as **the** ideal method of strengthening the abdominal muscles. Both may have a place in the regimen of abdominal exercises, but both must also be tempered as to their rightful role.

The abdominal rectus muscles, by their site of origin and insertion, elevate the anterior portion of the pelvis and depress the lower portion of the rib cage. Acting on the basis of a string in a bow, they also decrease the lumbar lordosis. The obliques, by virtue of their origin and attachment, pull on the fascia of the erector spinae muscles, but they also rotate the trunk upon the pelvis. The obliques also laterally flex the trunk on the pelvis. All of these functions must be considered in advocating muscle strengthening exercises.

Let us dispel the value of SLR exercises as an abdominal strengthening exercise. The legs are very heavy and flexing them at the hips, which is what is done in SLR, is done primarily by the iliopsoas muscle group.

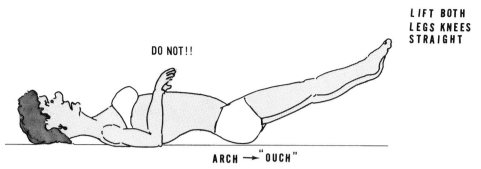

Figure 9–18. Straight leg raising is *not* advised. Straight leg raising tends to arch low back, which is a no-no. (From Cailliet, R: Understand Your Backache. FA Davis, Philadelphia, 1984, p 125, with permission.)

The iliopsoas muscle originates from the anterior portion of the lumbosacral spine as well as the inner aspect of the ilia. Due to the angle of pull, the iliopsoas muscle pulls the anterior aspect of the lumbosacral spine forward and **increases the lordosis** if the abdominal muscles are not sufficiently strong to prevent arching the low back. In a person with very strong abdominal muscles, this SLR is permitted and can be beneficial but, as the vast majority of people do not have strong enough abdominal muscles, this is not a recommended exercise (Fig. 9–18).

SIT-UP EXERCISES

From the supine position the gradual curl-up to reach a full flexed position exercises the abdominal muscles **if done properly**. If attempted with the legs fully extended, the iliopsoas muscle, again, is predominant in flexing the spine. It has been demonstrated that the first 30 degrees of trunk flexion occur from iliopsoas muscle contraction; after 30 degrees, the abdominal muscles become the prime flexors (Fig. 9–19).

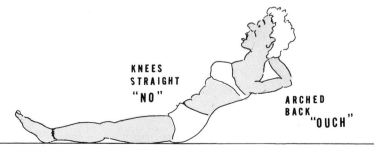

Figure 9–19. Wrong abdominal exercise. Situps with legs straight are a no-no. In this exercise, there is a tendency to arch the low back. (From Cailliet, R: Understand Your Backache. FA Davis, Philadelphia, 1984, p 125, with permission.)

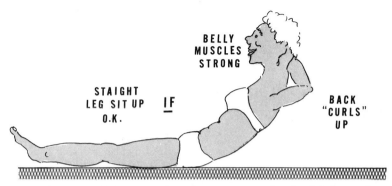

Figure 9–20. Setup with legs straight. This is permitted *only* if abdominal muscles are strong enough to permit patient to *curl* up and back and *not* arch low back. (From Cailliet, R: Understand Your Backache. FA Davis, Philadelphia, 1984, p 126, with permission.)

BACKACHE

Again, it may be stated that if a person has adequately strong enough abdominal muscles that he or she can prevent lumbar lordosis while gradually assuming a flexed position during sit-ups, this exercise may be permitted (Fig. 9–20).

It becomes apparent that the sit-up exercise advocated to strengthen the abdominal muscles must be done with the hips and knees flexed (Fig. 9–21). In doing the exercise properly, the lumbar spine must be "peeled"

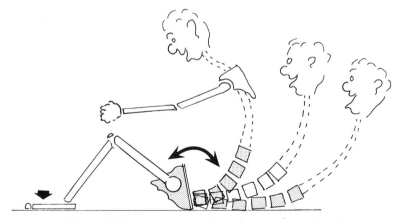

Figure 9–21. Abdominal flexion exercises from shortened position. Beginning in a full-flexed position, the body is gradually lowered, the position sustained and returned to upright position, permitting full flexion gradually from supine position. Arms are held near knees to prevent excessive extension.

from the floor. By "peeling" means that each vertebra, from the sacrum gradually and progressively to the first lumbar vertebra, must be flexed before the next is flexed. In this sequence there is gradual lumbar kyphosis evolving from the physiologic lordosis.

Depending on the original conditioning of the individual the exercise is best done in gradual stages:

1. Stage one is merely raising the head and shoulders from the floor. This is done with the arms on the floor at the person's side, gradually sliding them down toward the feet.

2. Stage two requires raising the shoulders further from the floor.

3. The next stage is raising the shoulder blades from the floor with the arms extended forward toward the feet.

4. While coming to a full flexed position the hands are placed behind the head with elbows forward. This arm position assists sitting up with the forward held arms placing weight ahead of the center of gravity.

5. Finally the sit-up is done with the hands behind the head and the elbows held behind the head. This arm position places added resistance to the abdominal muscles by adding weight behind the center of gravity.

In doing a sit-up with hips and knees bent the feet may be placed under a supporting structure if the legs are of insufficient weight to permit the sit-up without support.

Repeated sit-ups gradually increase strength. Endurance can be added if an isometric component is added to the sit-up exercise. This can be simply done by "holding" at various degrees of flexion (Fig. 9–22). The obviously easiest degree of flexion at which "holding" is easiest is at full sit-up position. With less complete flexion more upper body weight is imposed on the abdominal muscles and more resistance thus imposed on these muscles.

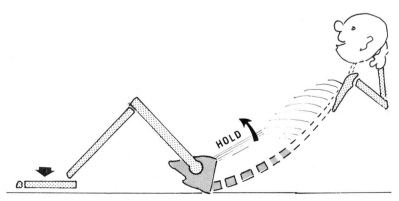

Figure 9–22. A partial flexed position to strengthen pelvic muscles isometrically.

"SIT-BACK" ABDOMINAL EXERCISES

It has been postulated that "sit back" exercises are as, if not more, effective in strengthening the abdominal muscles as are sit-up abdominal exercises. For the person with weak abdominal muscles even the slow gradual sit-up previously postulated may not strengthen the muscles comfortably or rapidly enough. In these patients the "sit back" abdominal exercises are valuable.

From the seated position with both hips and knees flexed and the hands behind the head and (at first) the elbows forward, the person slowly leans back a few degrees. The person holds at the point that is possible with comfortable effort. Initially the person has gotten to the full sit-up po-

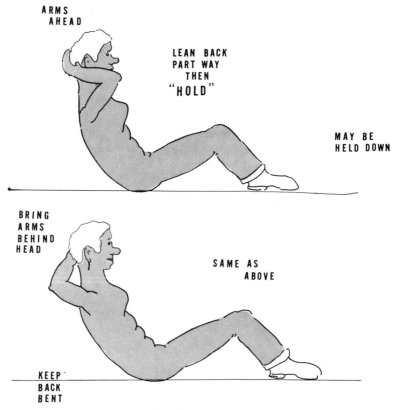

Figure 9–23. "Reverse isometric" abdominal exercises. Person "leans" back about 25 to 30 degrees, then "holds." This contracts abdominal muscles. At first, arms with hands behind head are held in front of body. Gradually, arms are brought "behind" the head. This increases the demand on the abdominal muscles. Hold briefly at first, then longer, to tolerance. (From Cailliet, R: Understand Your Backache. FA Davis, Philadelphia, 1984, p 123, with permission.)

sition with the use of the hands so no abdominal muscle strength is needed to assume the starting position.

Gradually a few degrees more of leaning back are attempted and held at this newly acquired position (Fig. 9–23). Ultimately a full leaning back followed by "sit up" is possible as the strength increases. The arms behind the head position held initially with elbows forward is gradually changed to placing the elbows behind the head. This position adds more resistance to the abdominal muscles.

Sit-back exercises to strengthen the oblique abdominal muscles can easily be added to this exercise by rotating the trunk to the left (or the right) and holding. The exercise is done with rotation to either or both directions (Fig. 9–24).

Another oblique abdominal muscle strengthening exercise is to lie on one's back with knees flexed and one foot placed on the opposite knee. Once in this position, with hands behind the head, the head and shoulder

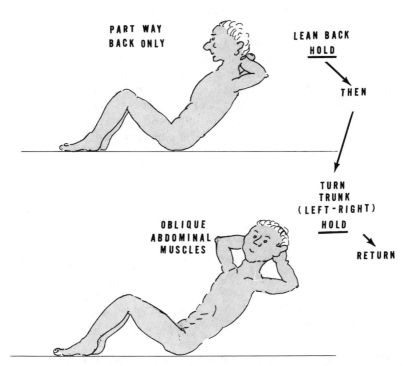

Figure 9–24. Oblique abdominal muscle exercise. This exercise begins as noted in Figure 9–23, but once held at 25 to 30 degrees, the trunk is rotated, held, then returned to straight ahead. The one arm comes forward and the other behind. Trunk must remain "flexed." (From Cailliet, R: Understand Your Backache. FA Davis, Philadelphia, 1984, p 124, with permission.)

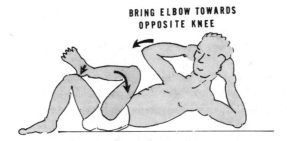

BRING ELBOW TOWARDS
OPPOSITE KNEE

Figure 9–25. Oblique abdominal muscle exercise. Lying supine with one leg bent and the opposite foot placed upon the knee, the low back is slightly flexed and the iliopsoas muscle is relaxed. From this position the person raises the opposite elbow from the floor and attempts to touch the knee. This attempt contracts the oblique abdominal muscles. Once the full flexed position has been reached it is held to that point for a slow count of three.

are lifted with the elbows of the raised arm reaching toward the opposite knee. When the elbow has reached as far to the knee as is possible, this position is held for 3 sec and released. The total exercise is repeated 10 times—to the right then to the left (Fig. 9–25).

The advantage of this exercise is that it stresses the oblique abdominal muscle, and the initial flexed knee and opposite foot on the knee decreases the lumbar lordosis and relaxes the iliopsoas muscles.

This oblique abdominal muscle exercise can be varied by the person lying supine and both legs slightly bent at the knees. Both feet are crossed, then the head and one shoulder are lifted and the arms reach across the chest and over the knees (Fig. 9–26). The person reaches as far as possible, then holds for a slow count of three. The exercise is done to the left then to the right.

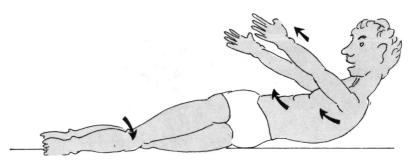

Figure 9–26. Oblique abdominal muscle exercise. Lying supine with both legs slightly bent at the knee, the upper leg is crossed over the lower. From this position the arms are raised forward and across the chest, reaching over the knees. This position is held for a slow count of three and released. The exercise is repeated in the opposite manner.

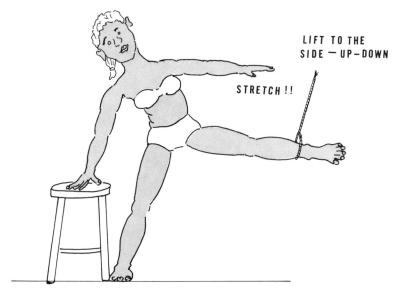

LIFT TO THE
SIDE — UP-DOWN

STRETCH !!

Figure 9–27. Side bending exercise. This exercise strengthens the side-back muscles and the lateral thigh muscle. The leg must *not* be brought *backward* too far, as that would arch the low back.

LATERAL TRUNK MUSCLES

It is unfortunate that the lateral trunk flexor muscle strengthening exercises are often overlooked, as these exercises for strengthening lateral trunk flexors also strengthen the abdominal oblique muscles. A simple exercise that accomplishes this is to stand, maintaining balance by holding on to an object, such as a stool or chair, and raise the opposite leg to the side as far as possible and hold it (Fig. 9–27). A weight can be fastened to the lifted leg for added resistance. This exercise also strengthens the hip abductors—the glutei—which are also pelvic rotators.

WALKING: THE BEST LOW BACK ABDOMINAL EXERCISE

There are numerous schools of thought regarding the optimum exercise to strengthen the low back and the abdominal muscles. All have validity but it can be correctly accepted that **walking** is probably the best exercise for maintaining a healthy low back (Fig. 9–28).

When Saunders and colleagues (1953) postulated their Determinants of Gait, they established that pelvic motion was an important aspect of nor-

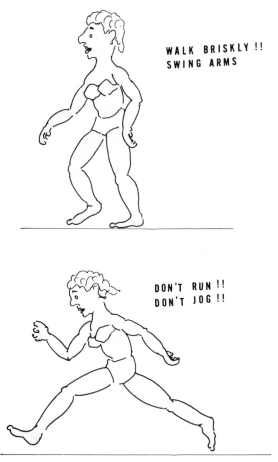

Figure 9–28. Walking: good. Jogging: bad. Running: acceptable.

mal gait to decrease the energy requirements of ambulation. They revealed that, in locomotion, the pelvis rotates in a horizontal plane. They also described pelvic "list" and lateral displacement. All these pelvic motions had to occur about the lumbosacral junction and require muscular action. Gracovetsky and Farfan (1986) carried the concept further to postulate that gait actually occurred and resulted secondary to lumbar pelvic movement.

It has been well documented that the nucleus of the intervertebral disk, under compression, causes the annular fibers, being of viscoelastic material, to become less taut because their angulation changes. With relaxation more rotation is thus possible before annular fiber failure. The vertical compressive forces narrow the disk space, which allows the annular fibers to become slack, but due to nuclear pressure there is an outward bulging, which "takes up the slack" of the annular fibers.

Three to 5 degrees of rotation has been postulated as being the "limit" to fiber elongation before failure. A pressure of 20 nm in the disk has been estimated during walking, which is the equivalent of 3.5 degrees of rotation.

Gait analysis has revealed that during walking there is a lateral bend of 7 degrees for the entire spine. This lateral bend combined with normal lordosis invokes a corresponding rotatory torque of less than 5 degrees.

To analyze the muscular effect on the pelvis and thus the lumbar spine in walking, the following may be extrapolated. As the left leg advances (swing-through phase), the right leg remains in extension. The pelvis elevates on the left during this phase of swing. The lateral trunk flexors contract and bend the spine.

Left lateral flexion of the spine engages the facets on the left side, which flex the spine and reduce the lordosis. Viewed from above, as the left leg swings forward, the pelvis rotates clockwise. The trunk shoulders and upper extremities rotate in the opposite (counterclockwise) direction. The left shoulder rotates backward (Fig. 9–29). The annular fibers become taut and store energy to initiate the reverse rotation on the next phase of ambulation.

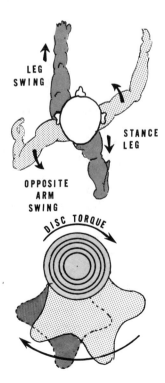

Figure 9–29. Physiologic effect of walking upon the intervertebral disk. The determinants of gait specify that as the forward leg swings, the hind leg remains stance and the arms swing in the opposite direction. This imposes a rotational torque upon the spine of an estimated 8 degrees of rotation. The vertebral disk undergoes torque (rotation) with simultaneous compression (body weight bearing). This imposes torque upon the annular fibers and enhances their "rigidity" (strength). Walking is thus a beneficial exercise for the health of the intervertebral disk.

As the right leg "pushes off" in moving from stance phase to swing through, the spine has been "wound up like a spring" and must rotate in the opposite direction during the next phase of ambulation. The spine becomes more lordotic due to the spine ligament action and the muscular effect of the (right) psoas muscle. This psoas muscular action initiates lateral flexion of the spine to the right to complete the cycle. Throughout both phases of gait it is apparent that the intervertebral disk is exposed to minimal compression but also to slow undulating rotation within the limits of annular elongation.

The erector spinae muscles and the psoas muscles thus control the lateral bend of the spine and therefore the degree of torque, with the latter (psoas) the more adequate from its point of attachment and insertion. The control of the extensor muscle is via its fascia; thus the oblique abdominal muscles are also vitally involved.

There is a neurologic mechanism that alternates the function of the ligamentous structures with the muscular. This neurologic mechanism is identical to that which operates during the process of lifting a heavy object in the sagittal plane. During the lift the fascia-ligaments work and the muscle "takes over."

HAMSTRING STRETCHING EXERCISES

It has been shown that with restricted hamstring flexibility and forward flexion, such as reaching to touch one's toe or bend over, the low back is subjected to excessive stretching. "Tight" hamstring muscles thus place added stress on the lumbosacral spine, including excessive disk posterior annular stress, and posterior ligamentous and erector spinae muscle strain. Once discovered by a careful examination these muscles must be stretched by proper exercise.

There is an inclination to stretch both hamstring groups simultaneously by sitting supine with the legs straight out and "bouncing" in an attempt to touch one's toes (Fig. 9–30, *top*). This is to be condemned, as doing this exercise actually imposes stress on the low back with little effective stretch of the hamstring muscles. "Bouncing" is also to be condemned, as this places abrupt stretch on the spindle system of the muscles with reflex extrafusal muscle contraction that makes the muscle more irritable rather than more relaxed and elongated. The fascial tissues of the muscle bands also respond bettter to a gentle sustained stretch rather than forceful "bouncing."

This exercise has been advocated being done in the standing position with both legs extended and bending forward to "try and touch the toes." For the same reason as in the supine position with both legs extended, this is also to be condemned.

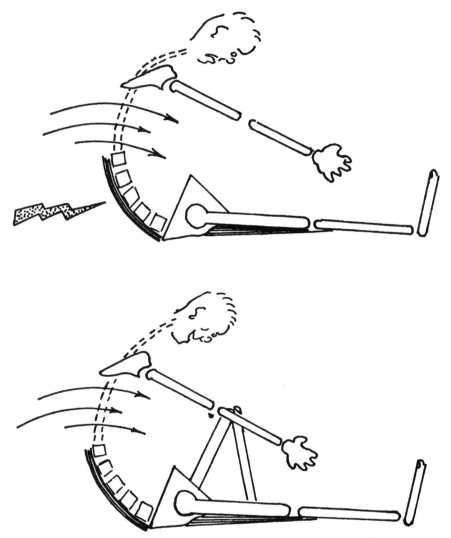

Figure 9–30. Protective hamstring stretching exercise. *Top*, The method of stretching both hamstrings simultaneously, which results in overstretching the low back. *Bottom*, Pelvic immobilization by flexing one hip and then stretching the other hamstring.

The proper manner to stretch is by the "protective" hamstring stretch (Fig. 9–30, *bottom*). The beginning position for doing this exercise is to sit supine with one leg flexed with that foot on the ground and the heel near the buttocks. The other leg to be stretched is held extended. Slow gradual forward body flexion, reaching toward the toes, stretches the hamstrings of

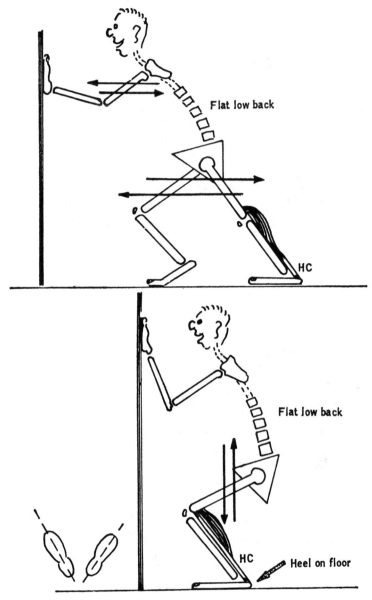

Figure 9–31. Exercises for heel cord stretching. *Top,* The manner of stretching a bilateral heel cord by leaning against a wall and moving back and forth. The rear foot is kept flat against the floor, which insures stretching of the heel cord. The forward leg is flexed to permit to-and-fro rocking. The lumbar spine must be prevented from arching. *Bottom,* Bilateral heel cord stretching is performed by squatting and sitting on both heels. The feet are placed slightly apart and externally rotated. The stretching motion is a rhythmic up-and-down bounce with balance maintained against a wall or chair.

the extended leg. The flexed leg "protects" the low back by avoiding excessive flexion of the lumbosacral spine.

A note of caution must here again be repeated that pain down the leg may be irritability of the sciatic nerve root and not of the hamstring muscle. In this case, the leg pain from sciatic neuropathy, there is a positive "dural sign," which has been discussed in the chapter on examination. When there is nerve stretch pain, the stretch exercise, done either with both legs extended or in the protective manner, **must be avoided**. Stretching an irritable nerve causes damage and there is no benefit from the simultaneous hamstring muscle elongation.

It must be remembered that a unilateral hamstring tightness (limitation) causes asymmetrical restriction on the pelvis and causes pelvic rotation and lateral flexion to result. This is transmitted onto the lumbosacral spine and has been considered a mechanical cause ("tropism") or aggravation of low back pain. The limited hamstring elongation must be stressed in doing the protective exercises.

HEEL CORD STRETCHING EXERCISES

The presence and importance of tight heel cord in relationship to low back pain is that the "tight" heel cord places excess stress on the hamstrings and ultimately on the lumbosacral spine in bending forward. Bilateral heel cord tightness causes general lumbosacral stress. Unilateral heel cord limitation causes asymmetry and ultimate pelvic rotation and lateral flexion.

There are two exercises advocated to gently stretch the heel cords (Fig. 9–31). Care must be considered in doing these exercises that there is slow gradual stretching and no "bouncing." Care must also be taken that the low back not be arched.* This is most prevalent in the standing and leaning into the wall exercise (see Fig. 9–31, *top*).

HIP FLEXOR STRETCHING EXERCISES

The hip flexor muscles, the iliopsoas group predominantly, when limited in extensibility, exert an adverse action on the pelvis and lumbosacral spine. This is evident from the fact that the iliopsoas attach from the anterior aspect of the lumbar spine as well as the inner aspect of the ilia. From their attachment to the anterior position of the femorae they can increase lordosis and prevent lumbosacral kyphosis in daily activities.

The presence of hip flexion limitation must be ascertained during the examination but must also be associated with the functional diagnosis as being related to the particular symptoms of the low back pain.

---

*Even in performing the MacKenzie extension series of exercises, this type of extension is not advisable.

An exercise for stretching the iliopsoas is depicted in Figure 9–32. The position assumed by the patient protects the low back by the opposite leg being held to the chest. This decreases the lordosis. The leg to be stretched may so be by placing a heavy object on the anterior portion of the thigh, tying the thigh down by straps, or having the leg held by an assistant.

The exercise causes the hip flexors to be stretched as the opposite leg is slowly, gradually, and gently brought to the chest and held there. This opposite leg manuever obviously stretches the "held down" hip flexor.

A modification of this exercise may be implemented by assuming the same position but with the opposite leg held to the chest which, with a tight hip flexor, causes the contracted leg to remain flexed. This leg is slowly and gently flexed, lifting the weight placed on the thigh. After a few degrees of flexion the leg is allowed to descend, which stretches that hip flexor. By contracting the extensors of that leg (the glutei) the hip flexors are passively stretched and simultaneously reciprocally relaxed.

It must be remembered that many activities of daily living require the average person to be seated, which maintains hip and knee flexion. There is adaptive shortening of the soft tissues which, in this case, are the hip and knee flexors. The advocated "minute break exercises" have the patient stand briefly and frequently during the day. In standing with the low back "tucked in," which decreases the lordosis, and simultaneously leaning backward gently, the adaptive shortening of the hip flexors is minimized.

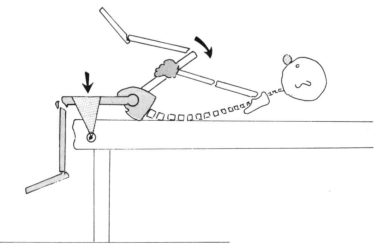

Figure 9–32. Hip flexor stretching exercise. With the hip held down, flexing the opposite hip to the chest tilts the pelvis and stretches the opposite hip flexor.

BRACING AND CORSETING

Occasionally low back "support" in the form of corseting or bracing seems to be indicated. A rationale and indication must, as in all other forms of treatment, exist to justify corseting.

The basis for corseting has evolved to accomplish the following effects:

1. It may decrease the need for the presence of "spasm," which occurs to splint the inflamed injured low back. As this "spasm" is usually self-limited and of brief duration, the purchase and use of a corset for this purpose is rarely indicated. Many people who have frequent recurrent low back pain episodes and have experienced relief from briefly wearing a corset may have its use justified. There is a psychological basis, a sense of security, for wearing a corset that, if it does not lead to dependence, may also justify its use.

2. The corset that "uplifts" and supports the abdomen is claimed to "unload" the gravity effects on the disks. This implies the acceptance of the "air bag" concept of unloading the spine.

3. The corset improves the posture by decreasing the lordosis.

4. The corset restricts the movement of the lumbosacral spine, allowing the pelvis and hip joints to perform the major portion of bending and lifting activities.

These factors are itemized in Figure 9–33. A corset must be custom-fitted to the specific individual. A "standard" corset picked from the shelf may not be the precise size or shape for that particular individual. It is also very apparent to people who wear corsets that they fit in one position and not the other. In essence, because the spine has a different conformity in standing than in sitting, from lordosis to kyphosis, no corset can conform to both (Fig. 9–34).

Certain principles for corseting apply:

1. The uplift of the abdomen with a degree of compression of the abdominal cavity is necessary. Where the anterior portion of the corset applies, the abdomen is therefore vital.

2. The contour of the hind portion is also important if a specific contour of the lumbosacral spine is required. Stays are frequently inserted for that purpose. Recently the use of stays has been unacceptable to many patients as the low back varies during daily activities. Except in spondylolisthesis, where greater restriction is required, the author rarely prescribes stays.

3. A corset or a brace must never be worn as a final modality but merely as a means to an end. Total dependency on a corset allows the soft tissues, the ligaments, the capsules, and the muscles to relinquish their function, and when the corset is removed the spine can literally fail. If the

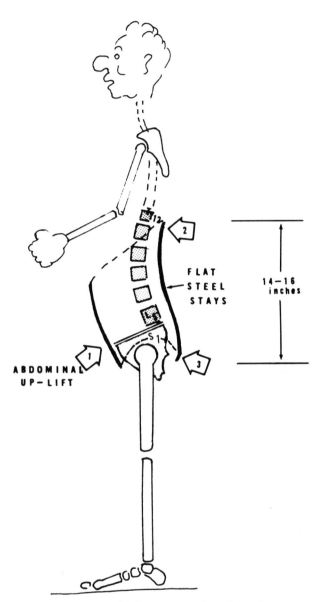

Figure 9–33. Corseting. Proper back support is based on three points of contact: (1) firm, uplifting abdominal support; (2) contact at the thoracolumbar junction; and (3) contact over the sacrum. Points 2 and 3 insure that the lumbar curve is "flat," indicating that lordosis is decreased.

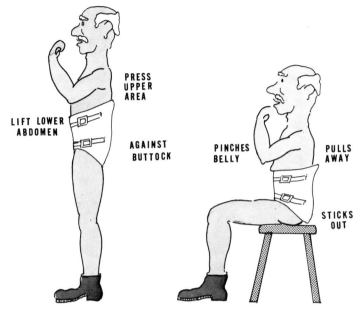

Figure 9–34. Lumbosacral corset. *Left,* Desirable features of corset, but there are also undesirable features (*right*) of most corsets. (From Cailliet, R: Understand Your Backache. FA Davis, Philadelphia, 1984, p 137, with permission.)

purpose of the corset is fully explained to the patient and **an exercise program is simultaneously implemented**, then such a prescription is justified.

The use of a corset to assist the patient's proper use of the low back in bending or lifting obviously also implies that it must be a means to an end during the instruction phase of proper body mechanics.

SUMMARY

The intent of this chapter has been the **prevention of recurrence of low back pain** with the emphasis on conditioning or reconditioning the tissues of the low back that must be adequate for normal spine function.

Posture needs no justification. All that remains to be clarified is what is the proper physiologic posture? The degree of lordosis, in the erect position and especially in bending and lifting, remains to be clarified. Insofar as the accepted posture remains unclear, a precise program to achieve "this" posture also remains unclear but certain principles are evident and acceptable.

Flexibility is unquestioned. As the spine must be flexible to accomplish daily activities, this characteristic of its tissues is unquestionably desirable. It is also apparent that the nociceptive stimuli originate within the soft tissues that require flexibility.

What remains unclarified is not only what physical tissue changes occur that impair flexibility but what psychological, hormonal, endocrine, and mechanical factors lead to inflexibility and thus must be addressed in its remedy.

Muscular function must also be addressed. Muscles act to elongate in a synchronous manner and must contract with strength and endurance to activate daily functions. This, therefore, implies **neuromuscular** function with the muscle merely the end organ performing the task that has been desired, initiated, and performed by the central nervous system. Exercise intended for improvement of this **neuromuscular** function must address all these factors.

What role exercise plays in back health has been the basis of controversy throughout the medical world and still remains unresolved. Not only the type and the manner of exercise but the benefit is being debated. Unbiased and objective studies to determine what type of exercise is best are not fully documented.

How a person uses the low back or misuses the lumbosacral spine is less controversial than are the methods of "conditioning" the tissues. It cannot be questioned that a **machine must have proper working parts but how that machine is used ensures the job being efficiently done and the machine not breaking down or prematurely wearing out.** Malfunction is a sequence of faulty use leading to failure of the functional parts of the machine.

Chapter 12 relates to proper function.

REFERENCES

Cailliet, R: Minute Breaks: The Rejuvenation Strategy. Doubleday, New York, 1987.
Inman, VT, Ralston, HJ, and Todd, F: Human Walking. Williams & Wilkins, Baltimore, 1981
Gracovetsky, S and Farfan, H: The optimum spine. Spine 11:543, 1986.
Saunders, JB, Inman, VT, and Eberhart, HD: The major determinants in normal and pathological gait. J Bone Joint Surg 35-A:543, 1953.

CHAPTER 10

Back to School

All the exercises to regain flexibility, improve strength, and improve posture are of **no practical value** if the person does not put them to daily use in sitting, standing, bending, and lifting. All the value of exercise and training would also be wasted if the person inadvertently misuses or abuses his or her low back.

An acute injury may inevitably occur in spite of all preceding conditioning exercises and functional training from a situation beyond a person's control (Figs. 10–1 to 10–3). Once injured a low back may be made more

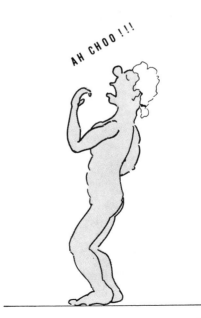

AH CHOO!!!

Figure 10–1. A sneeze may "catch the back unprepared for the stress" and cause low back strain. (From Cailliet, R: Understand Your Backache. FA Davis, Philadelphia, 1984, p 73, with permission.)

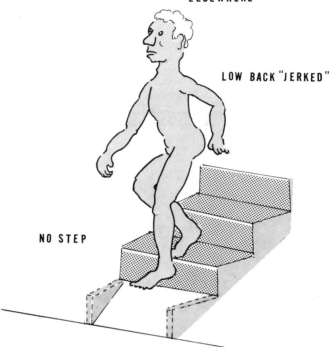

MIND
ELSEWHERE

LOW BACK "JERKED"

NO STEP

Figure 10–2. The absent step. Stepping down upon a step that is not there can jar the back. This is another example of the mind being upon a "task" and the wrong, unexpected task being performed, resulting in a low back strain/sprain. This back injury can occur from stepping into an unseen hole, stepping off a curb of unexpected height, and other similar situations. (From Cailliet, R: Understand Your Backache. FA Davis, Philadelphia, 1984, p 74, with permission.)

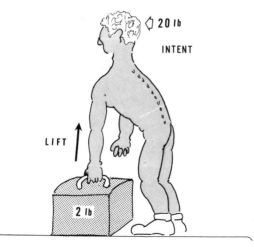

20 lb

INTENT

LIFT

2 lb

Figure 10–3. Miscalculation of lifting effort. If the person intends to lift an object considered to weigh 20 lb that weighs only 2 lb, the person *overlifts* and thus can injure the back. The opposite, an *intended* lift of 2 lb that is actually 20 lb, can equally cause a low back *underlift* injury. (From Cailliet, R: Understand Your Backache. FA Davis, Philadelphia, 1984, p 68, with permission.)

186

susceptible but, again, even being reconditioned but untrained in proper function, reinjury is more apt to recur.

In summary, at the end of Chapter 9, all the unknown and confirmed factors of reconditioning were enumerated. It was aptly stated that proper **function** is the major aspect of **prevention of recurrence of low back pain**. The **how** to stand, sit, bend, stoop, and lift and the **how not to** are the emphases of prevention of recurrence.

The current approach to restoring proper low back function has been termed the **low back school**. The "student" (the patient or potential patient) is taught **how** the low back is structured and **how** the low back works.

Where in the low back structures of pain and impairment may occur is clarified. **How** a person must **properly** stand, sit, bend, stoop, lift, push, pull, etc. is also described. **How** person may overuse, misuse, or abuse the low back is also discussed. The effect on the low back function of the **state of mind** is included. The role of the physical status of the environment as it contributes to permitting proper low back function also is covered during the school course.

The student is thus exposed to knowledge that, if properly applied, should improve function, decrease pain, and prevent recurrence of impairment. All correctable or alterable factors are remedied. It is now up to the students to implement all the factors regarding which they have been instructed.

Failure may, and unfortunately does, occur with resultant recurrence of pain and impairment or a persistence of pain and impairment in spite of proper education. These will be discussed, but it behooves us now to enter the **school** and learn its agenda and instructions.

A significant portion of the curriculum as to how the low back functions, which tissues are susceptible, and how to recondition these tissues has been discussed in previous chapters. Let us turn to training in proper **function**. **Body mechanics** is an appropriate term for the proper use of the movement of the lumbosacral spine.

Learning has also been discussed. The learned facts form the basis of education, but practice is its implementation. Constant practice leads to proper **habit**. Prevention of the proper implementation from fatigue, anxiety, impatience, or distraction must always be a major concern.

THE "SCHOOL" CURRICULUM

Posture has been adequately discussed. The methods of influencing posture also have been enumerated. It must be stated that static postural pain can be reproduced easily and the exact mechanism ascertained. Correction must therefore be to alter, change, or correct the postural component that reproduces **the** static erect low back pain that has been created during the examination.

In this context the adage: **to reproduce the pain by position or movement and knowing what is being done that causes the pain reveal the mechanism of the pain**, becomes informative.

The posture of the complaining person can be observed either from the side or from the rear. The examiner can manually increase or decrease the lordosis of the patient. By reproducing the complaint from that posture the examiner gets clarification of which of these positions are causative of low back pain.

Of greater value from the examination and history is the factor of **when** this static (postural) low back pain occurs. **When** indicates the daily activity or the implicated movement that is responsible. If the activity is clarified and correctable, a valuable aspect is learned.

If increased lordosis is considered causative (Fig. 10–4) and prolonged standing is a factor, this can be corrected by instruction as to standing with one foot on an elevation (Figs. 10–5 and 10–6).

The static postural low back pain, as stated, can be reproduced by the

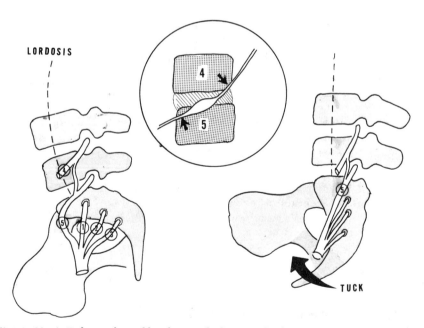

Figure 10–4. Relationship of lumbosacral plexus to lordosis. In the drawing at left, the lumbar lordosis has an angled L_5 root, owing to its attachment to the sacrum. With decrease of the lordosis, the L_5 root straightens and thus is under less tension.

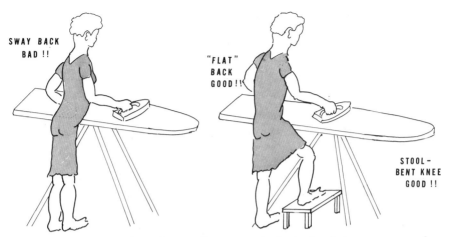

Figure 10–5. Prolonged standing with excessive lordosis plus fatigue may cause low backache. This can be eliminated by placing one foot up on a small stool. (From Cailliet, R: Understand Your Backache. FA Davis, Philadelphia, 1984, p 56, with permission.)

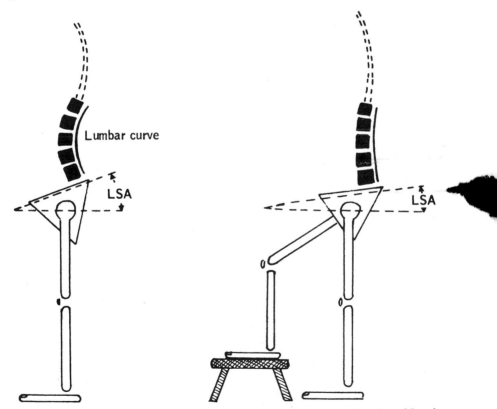

Figure 10–6. Relaxed, prolonged standing posture. A small foot stool enables the hip of one leg to be flexed, thus relaxing the iliopsoas and "flattening" the lumbar curve. This method is advisable for dentists, housewives, and barbers, among others.

examiner and its occurrence from a daily activity ascertained. Once so diagnosed, a correction is possible.

A person not only must stand properly but must sit properly. There are numerous sitting postures (Fig. 10–7), but there are certain principles of sitting that must be observed.

1. The height of the chair should permit the feet to be firmly on the ground (Fig. 10–8).

2. The legs should be at an angle so that the knees are slightly higher than the hips.

3. There should be supported low back **slight** lordosis. A **small** pillow at the lower lumbar area may be needed.

4. The object of manual activity must not mandate "leaning forward" for long periods. It must be remembered that sustained lumbar forward flexion causes a posterior "oozing" (migration) of the disk fluid in the lower lumbar functional units, which weakens the disk.

5. Frequently during the day a "1-minute break" should be instituted when the person "pulls" away from work and stands, changes posture, or does an exercise in the seated position.

6. Whenever possible the arms should support the body, as it has been shown that arm support decreases pressure on the lower disks by 50 percent.

The vast majority of injuries to the low back are, however, from faulty movement. This can be termed **kinetic** low back injury.

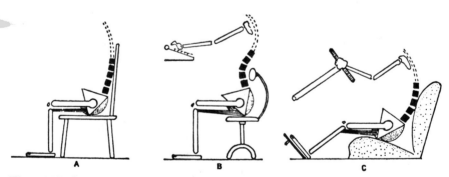

Figure 10–7. Sitting postures. *A*, Correct sitting posture in a firm, straight-back chair in which the seat has the proper width and height to allow hips and knees to be flexed with no strain and with both feet touching the floor. The back of the chair supports the low back 4 to 6 inches from the seat and permits a "flat" lumbar curve. *B*, The chair back increases the arch and causes a hamstring strain and a fatiguing low back posture. *C*, The hamstrings are taut and place traction on the pelvis, causing rotation and ultimately strain on the low back.

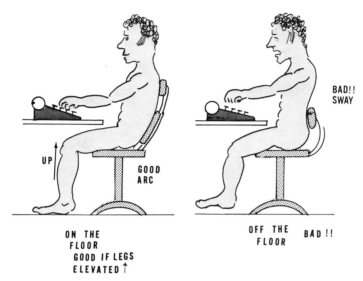

Figure 10–8. Faulty sitting posture may cause low backache. The proper low back support, feet on the floor with legs slightly elevated, table and typewriter at the right level—all must be proper to avoid low back strain. (From Cailliet, R: Understand Your Backache. FA Davis, Philadelphia, 1984, p 58, with permission.)

KINETIC LOW BACK FUNCTION

The accepted "proper" manner of bending over and returning to the erect posture has been amply discussed. It can be summarized in the following (Fig. 10–9):

1. Bending forward must be done in a sequence of **gradually** reducing the lumbar lordosis into a lumbar kyphosis.

2. Pelvic rotation must occur synchronously with the lumbosacral rotation.

3. Once fully flexed, return to the erect position (be it merely resuming the erect or the process of lifting an object) must do the exact opposite with the following sequence:

   (a) The pelvis must derotate until the upper body is flexed ahead of the center of gravity by 45 degrees.

   (b) During this pelvis rotation the lumbar spine must not begin significant return to lordosis. As stated, there are several schools of thought as to whether the stress on the lumbosacral spine in resuming the erect position is borne by the ligamentous fascial sheath or by the contracting erector spinae muscle. If the former is accepted, the lumbosacral spine should remain fully

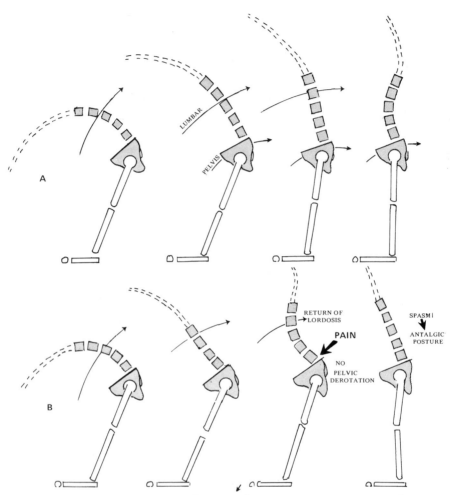

Figure 10–9. Proper vs. improper flexion and reextension. *A,* Proper simultaneous resumption of the lumbar lordosis with pelvic rotation. *B,* The regaining of pelvic lordosis with no pelvic derotation, thus causing painful lordotic posture with the upper part of the body held ahead of the center of gravity.

flexed. If the latter is correct, a small degree of lordosis should be initiated. In either case **only a slight degree** of lordosis should be assumed and thus the major degree of return to the erect must be from pelvic rotation.

4. The return to the erect position must not allow significant and uncontrolled rotation. This implies that little if any rotation of the spine must be allowed in bending forward, thus requiring little or no derotation to resume the erect position.

5. Any object lifted, regardless of weight or size, should be picked up "close" to the body (Fig. 10–10). This is exemplified in Figure 10–11, and the gravity factors that justify this lifting and holding ahead of the body are clearly depicted in Figures 10–12 and 10–13.

The proper way to lift is depicted in Figure 10–14, and the improper way to lift in Figure 10–15. The cause of any low back kinetic injury is accepted to be the regaining of the lordosis prematurely during the sequence of resuming the erect posture from that of being bent over (see Fig. 10–15, number 3).

Failure to properly derotate when resuming the erect position from the bent-over position is even more frequently the cause of low back injury (see Fig. 10–15, number 4). To prevent such an undesirable bending, turning, and returning to the erect posture in everyday activities, each activity

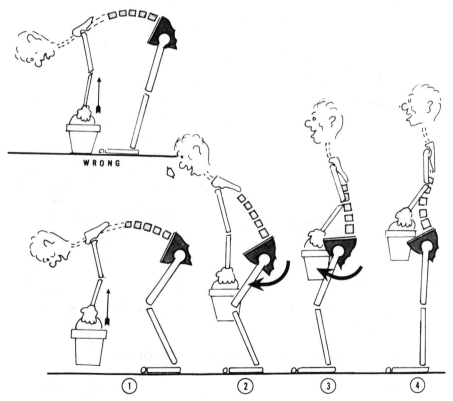

Figure 10–10. Proper method of lifting. The wrong way to lift is shown with the weight ahead of the body and the legs straight, causing strain. In proper lifting (lower drawing) the weight is brought close to the body while the pelvis tilts. The lumbar spine then gradually resumes the erect lordosis upon the tilted pelvis.

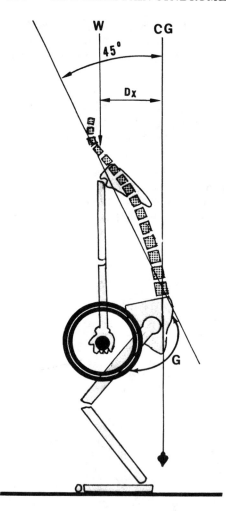

Figure 10–11. Heavy weight-lifting. With the weight close to the body (D_x) the fulcrum is more efficient. The muscles of the back (erector spinae) contract to elevate the spine during the last 45 degrees of extension. Until 45 degrees the fascia and ligaments of the lumbar spine carry the burden with the pelvic muscles rotating the pelvis.

of daily living may need to be explained. Several examples of the "correct" way to use the low back need to be explained, as shown in Figures 10–16 and 10–17.

Many factors must be kept in mind when explaining the physiology of the low back in relation to posture, movement, and exercise; recent studies of intradiskal pressure of the lumbar spine have added to current knowledge. How these facts add to understanding normal and abnormal physiology leading to "failure" of the spine remains unresolved.

There is no doubt that intradiskal pressures are vital in spinal function. There is no doubt that variations in intradiskal pressure occur from numer-

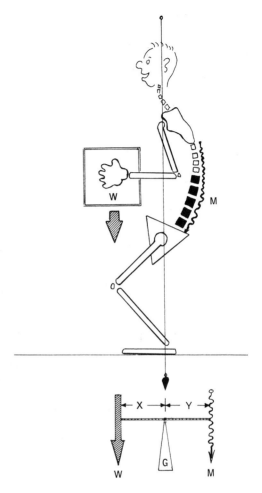

Figure 10–12. The relationship of the distance of a carried weight from the center of gravity and the resultant tension on the spinal musculature is expressed by the equation $W \times X = M \times Y$, where W = the weight of the object carried; X = the distance the weight is held from the center of gravity; Y = the distance of the spinal musculature from the center of gravity; and M = the tension developed by the musculature. In a simple lever system the weight supported by the fulcrum (G) is the sum of the weights acting at each end of the lever bar: 100×10 inches = 100×10 inches, thus G = 200 lb; 100×20 inches = 200×10 inches, thus G = 300 lb.

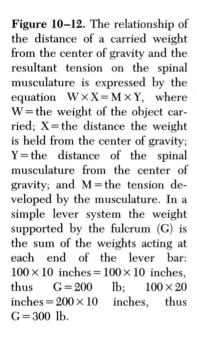

ous positions and activities and that the intradiskal pressure acts on the tension of the annular fibers. It must be accepted that failure occurs from failure of the annular fibers that encircle the nucleus and modify the intrinsic pressures. The current research is directed to evaluating these variations influenced by various movements, various positions of the spine, and various metabolic factors that also influence intradiskal pressure.

Complete reliance on intradiskal pressures does not take into consideration the muscular, ligamentous, and capsular stresses that are also invoked in daily spinal activities. The intradiskal pressure, by separating the adjacent vertebral body endplates of each functional unit, also impose tension on the posterior spinal elements wherein reside these ligaments, erector spinae muscles, and facet capsules. Approximate load measured in the L3 disk of a 70-kilo individual has been estimated as shown in Table 10–1.

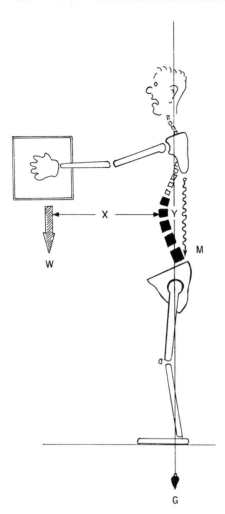

Figure 10–13. The increase of strain imposed upon the erect spine when an object of the same weight is held at arm's length. Using the formula $W \times X = M \times Y$, if $W = 100$ lb, $X = 24$ inches, and $Y = 6$ inches, then $100 \times 24 = M \times 6$; thus $M = 400$ lb, and $M + W = 500$ lb. By increasing any component of a simple lever arm, the total weight superimposed on the supporting structure can be altered. Either changing the weight of the object held or increasing the distance from the body will increase the gravity (G) strain and will concurrently increase the muscular stress (M) as the distance (Y) changes little if at all. The M stress is a muscular compressive force on the vertebral disks.

The method of teaching proper lifting technique has been amply discussed, but a brief addendum is warranted. Lifting with a fully flexed lumbosacral spine, allegedly to impose all the stress on the fascial sheath of the erector spinae muscle group, has not been completely refuted. The erector spinae muscles have been considered to be inadequate to sustain the load being lifted with the small fulcrum about the axis of rotation of the involved functional units.

This is exemplified in Figure 10–18, which shows why premature regaining of full lordosis in the process of returning to the erect posture leads to failure of the soft tissues and the disks of the lumbosacral spine.

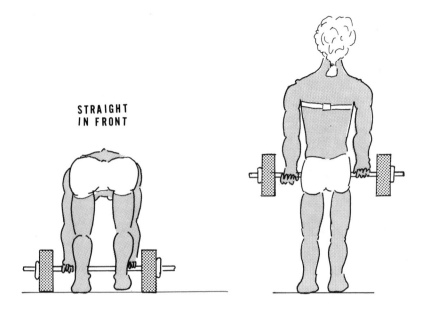

STRAIGHT
IN FRONT

GOOD!

SLOWLY

TUCK

BEND
KNEES

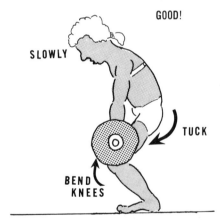

Figure 10–14. Proper bending and lifting. (From Cailliet, R: Understand Your Backache. FA Davis, Philadelphia, 1984, p 65, with permission.)

The value of strong abdominals to unload the spine, originally declared to be the effect of "air bag" principles, is no longer totally acceptable, as this intra-abdominal pressure would constrict vital intra-abdominal blood vessels beyond their tolerances. The increase in abdominal tension has been postulated to increase the fluid content of the erector spinae fascial

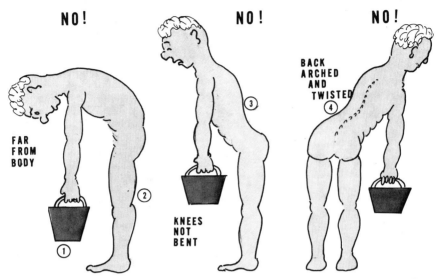

Figure 10–15. Improper aspects of lifting that can injure the low back: (*1*) Object lifted far from body; (*2*) lifting without bending knees; (*3*) regaining lordosis prematurely; (*4*) bending and twisting and returning to erect position improperly. (From Cailliet, R: Understand Your Backache. FA Davis, Philadelphia, 1984, p 146, with permission.)

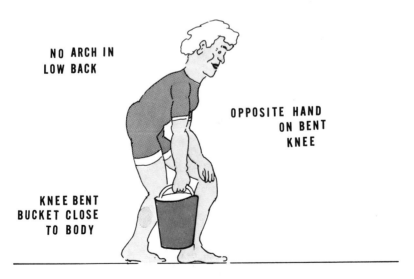

PROPER ONE-ARM LIFT

Figure 10–16. Proper one-arm lift. (From Cailliet, R: Understand Your Backache. FA Davis, Philadelphia, 1984, p 144, with permission.)

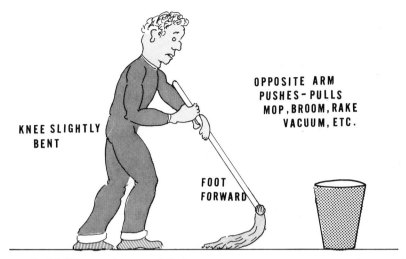

Figure 10–17. "Diagonal principle" of proper mopping, vacuuming, raking, and so forth. (From Cailliet, R: Understand Your Backache. FA Davis, Philadelphia, 1984, p 145, with permission.)

Table 10–1. LOAD MEASUREMENTS IN THE L3 DISK OF A 70-KG INDIVIDUAL

Supine in traction	10 kg
Supine	30 kg
Erect with corset	30 kg
Erect standing	70 kg
Walking	85 kg
Twisting (erect)	90 kg
Bending sideways	95 kg
Upright sitting with no support	100 kg
Isometric abdominal exercises	110 kg
Coughing	110 kg
Jumping	110 kg
Straining	120 kg
Laughing	120 kg
Bending forward 20 degrees	120 kg
Bilateral straight leg raising in supine position	120 kg
Hyperextension exercise (prone)	150 kg
Sit-up exercises (knee extended)	175 kg
Sit-up exercises (supine with knees bent)	180 kg
Bending forward 20 degrees with 10 kg	185 kg
Lifting 20 kg with back straight and knees bent	210 kg
Lifting 20 kg with back bent but knees straight	340 kg

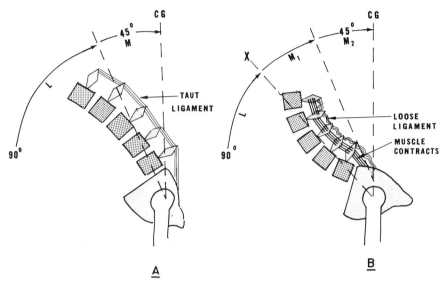

Figure 10–18. Faulty reextension of lumbar spine. *A,* Correct reextension. Until the last 45 degrees, the lumbar spine is supported (L) by supraspinous ligaments requiring no muscular effort. Muscles normally become active in the last 45 degrees (M) when the carrying angle is close to the center of gravity (CG). *B,* Premature lumbar lordosis with pelvis not adequately derotated causes the erector muscles (M_1) to contract before having reached the last 45 degrees. The ligaments loosen, and the muscles take the brunt and contract inefficiently and forcefully, resulting in pain.

sheath (Figs. 10–19 and 10–20). Abdominal muscles, especially the obliques, also probably exert lateral pull on the erector spinae fascia, thus increasing its mechanical efficiency in the lifting process.

Involvement of the erector spinae muscles in lifting, however, is becoming more accepted from kinetic electromyographic studies. "Some" degree of muscular contraction is known to occur in the process of lifting objects of some weight from below the waist level. It is probable that this muscular contraction is a coordinated reflex activity to defray excessive strain on the fascia and ligaments.

The exact mechanism of this neuromuscular reflex activity remains obscure, but its failure may be the causative factor in many low back injuries. To pursue this concept an example can be offered:

A person lifting a heavy object from the floor, possibly even to one side of center, may be lifting "properly" in that there is minimal lordosis and the object is reasonably close to the body, yet there results a "back strain" with resultant pain and impairment. The fascia, in this case, was not

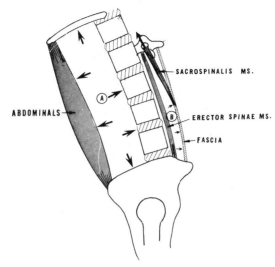

ABDOMINALS

SACROSPINALIS MS.

ERECTOR SPINAE MS.

FASCIA

Figure 10–19. Increase in abdominal tension causes pressure posteriorly against the dorsolumbar fascia, causing it to become tense and thus relieving the tension upon the erector spinae muscles. The sacrospinalis muscle, by its attachment to the fascia, also increases its tension.

fully employed as there was "minimal lordosis" (thus requiring some isometric erector spinae muscle contraction).

How much isometric erector spinae muscle contraction was engendered is a delicate neuromuscular action computed instantaneously from the mechanoreceptors of the ligaments, the joint capsules, and the erector muscle mediated through the spindle system. Too much or too little muscular contraction can, obviously, disrupt the delicate mechanical function of the spine. Malalignment of the functional units, albeit temporary from the position of lifting, is now subjected to inappropriate muscular contraction. Failure, of varying degree, of the annular fibers of the disk, the ligaments of the functional unit, and erector spinae muscles results. Low back pain and impairment result.

What has impaired the **proper** neuromuscular reaction to the intended lifting or bending over?

1. Faulty training.
2. Faulty "habit" from inadequate practice.
3. Fatigue.
4. Distraction, anxiety, tension, depression, anger, and numerous other psychophysiologic factors that distract.

All these latter factors must be discussed with the patient to minimize their presence or their effect on daily activities. This is why relaxation tech-

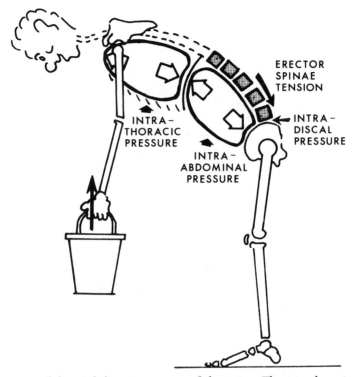

Figure 10–20. Abdominal-thoracic support of the spine. The intrathoracic and intraabdominal pressures created during the act of lifting decrease the pressure exerted by stress forces upon the intervertebral disks. This substantiates the efficacy of a corset, a brace with an abdominal support, and the need for strong abdominal muscles to insure a strong back.

niques such as biofeedback, stress management, psychotherapy, meditation, relaxation, and the like, are incorporated in the School agenda.

A hypothetical concept of causation diskogenic syndrome has been postulated by the author that remains to be confirmed and thoroughly researched. This concept can be briefly summarized:

For years psychological factors have been incriminated in the causation of pain, often with ultimate diskogenic disease. The diskogenic factor has varied from bulging, herniation, to inevitable degeneration. Being aware, clinically, of the frequent relationship of anxiety, emotional tension, and even depression to the occurrence of lumbar and sciatic nerve root pain in this entity led me to a search of the literature that revealed many factors that need correlation and confirmation.

The role of the intervertebral disk has been accepted as hydrodynamic. The fluid in the disk (88 percent) is accepted as being balanced by imbibition and osmotic factors. Both are dependent on ionic (sodium and potassium) transfer of fluid across a permeable membrane. Both of these ions are controlled largely by adrenocortical pituitary control, which in turn is directly related to the emotions.

The concept postulated is that during severe, chronic, or recurrent emotional stresses there is a concurrent adrenocortical reaction that affects the osmotic imbibitory balance of the disk, thus altering the mechanical stability of the disk. The disk, thus affected, is subjected to added mechanical stresses such as faulty lifting, bending, and twisting. Failure results from the combination.

This concept also alleges that degradation of protein polysaccharides comprising the annular fibers leading to disk degeneration (Naylor 1976) may be adversely influenced by emotional as well as metabolic factors.

The normal neuromuscular activities (such as bending, lifting, and stooping) are also influenced by the emotional "tone" of the individual. This added hormonal influence from the emotions contributes to spinal failure from disk metabolism and enforces the need for the psychological education and correction aspect in the **school** curriculum.

More will be discussed in the chapter on **chronic pain**.

REFERENCES

Bartelink, DL: The role of abdominal pressure in relieving the pressure on the lumbar intervertebral disks. J Bone Joint Surg 39-B:718, 1957.

Brown, T, Nemiah, JC, Barr, JS, and Barry, H: Psychological factors in low back pain. New Eng J Med 251:123, 1954.

Cappen, A: Disorders of mineral metabolism in depressive patients. Psychiatri Neurologi Neurochirugi 72:f89, 1969.

Cappen, A and Shaw, DM: Mineral metabolism in melancholia. Br J Med 2:1439, 1963.

Charnley, J: Fluid imbibition as a cause of herniation of the nucleus pulposus. J Bone Joint Surg 33B:472, 1951.

Chetty, et al: Stress factor in the disk syndrome. J Bone Joint Surg, 37-B:107, 1955.

Davis, PR: Posture of the trunk during lifting of weights. Br Med J 1:87, 1959.

Fraioli, F, et al: Physical exercise stimulates marked concomitant release of B endorphins and adrenocorticotropic hormones (ACTH) in peripheral blood in man. Experientia 36:987, 1980.

Goodard, MD and Reid, JD: Movements induced by straight leg raising in the lumbosacral roots, nerves and plexus, and on the intrapelvic section of the sciatic nerve. J Neurol Neurosurg Psychiatry 28:12, 1965.

Gracovetsky, A, Farfan, HF, and Lamy, CB: A mathematical model of the lumbar spine using an optimized system to control muscles and ligaments. Orthop Clin North Am 8:135, 1977.

Jonck, LM: The influence of weight bearing on the lumbar spine: A radiological study. S Afr J Radiol 2:25, 1964.

Keegan, J: Alterations of the lumbar curve related to posture and seating. J Bone Joint Surg 35-A:589, 1953.

Knutsson, B, Lindh, K, and Telbag, H: Sitting: An electromyographic and mechanical study. Acta Orthop Scand 37:415, 1966.

Kraemer, J, Kilditz, D, and Gowin, R: Water and electrolyte content of human intervertebral discs under variable loads. Spine 10:69, 1985.

Levine, ME: Depression, back pain and disc protrusion. Dis Nervous System 3:41, 1971.

Meeham, JR: Stress, vascular changes and the potential for behavioral modification. J SC Med Assoc 10:535, 1963.

Morris, JM, and Lucas, DB: Biomechanics of spinal bracing. Arizona Med. March:170, 1969.

Morris, JM, Lucas, DB, and Bresian, B: Role of the trunk in stability of the spine. J Bone Joint Surg 43-A:327, 1961.

Nachemson, A: Pathophysiology and treatment of back pain. In Buerger, AA, and Tabis, JS (eds): Approaches to the Validation of Manipulation Therapy. Charles C Thomas, Springfield, IL, 1977.

Nachemson, A, and Elfstrom, G: Intravital dynamic pressure measurements in lumbar discs. Scand J Rehab Med (Suppl. 1), 1970.

Nachemson, A, and Morris, JM: In vivo measurements of intradiscal pressure. J Bone Joint Surg 46-A:1077, 1964.

Naylor, A: Intravertebral disc prolapse and degeneration. Spine 1:108, 1976.

Naylor, A, and Smare, DL: Fluid content of the nucleus pulposus as a factor in the disk syndrome: Preliminary report. Br Med J 2:975, 1953.

Scheldkraut, JJ, Davis, JM, and Klerman, GL: Biochemistry of depression. In Efson, DM (ed): Psychopharmacology: A review of progress, 1957–1967. U.S. Government Printing Office, Washington, DC, 1968.

Scott, JC: Stress factor in the disc syndrome. J Bone Joint Surg 37B:107, 1955.

Watson, FMC, Henry, JP, and Haltmeyer, GC: Effects of early experience of emotional and social reactivity in CBA mice. Physiol Behav 13:9, 1974.

CHAPTER 11

Disk Disease

The term **disk disease** has become synonymous with the major cause of low back pain and sciatic radiculopathy. **Disk disease** has veritably become a specific organic disease entity. The involvement of the intervertebral disk in spinal function and thus its involvement in spinal malfunction has become legend.

Terms such as disk bulging, herniation, rupture, slipping, and degeneration have been bandied about in medical terminology and literature until these terms have become considered as fully understood and unequivocally accepted.

There is need to assess the true role of the disk in spinal function and, more important, its actual role in spinal malfunction, pain production, and functional impairment. Only by so clarifying its role and also clarifying the other contiguous and related tissues involved within the functional unit can the true role of the **disk** be accepted. By such clarification more meaningful treatment can evolve.

Very few, if any, measures actually alter the natural history of herniated disks. There are undoubtedly many factors of treatment that moderate the symptoms of disk herniation. By understanding the mechanical aspects of disk herniation and the manner in which the herniation causes symptomatology, the basis for treatment will evolve.

The space available within the functional unit for the nerve roots that mediate pain, hypalgesia, hyperanesthesia, and motor deficit must remain patent. This patency is related to the intervertebral disk and is thus related to the extent of herniation. The basis of treatment is thus to understand the site, the extent, the direction, and the duration of encroachment on the nerve roots within the foraminae by the disk herniation. The movement and position of the functional unit in everyday activity thus play a major role in the temporizing treatment of disk herniation.

Much is known and being learned about the structure, anatomic and chemical, of the intervertebral disk. Its physiology and its pathophysiology are also being better evaluated. Its mechanical function is engendering mechanical analysis with greater clarification of its weight-bearing and kinetic role.

As **pain** is undergoing more attention and evaluation the part that the disk plays in the production of nociception from the low back is also under scrutiny. The evolution of disk tissue changes is receiving much needed attention and "aging" versus damage residual is being clarified. The constituent tissues forming the intervertebral disk are better understood and thus so are changes attributable to aging, wear and tear, and injury.

The intervertebral disk thus must be reviewed as to a normal functional system, an impaired system, and a source of pain and disability.

THE NORMAL FUNCTIONAL DISK

The intervertebral disk has been fully discussed in previous chapters. It need not be again completely considered other than to highlight salient and pertinent factors in its function and its potential failure.

The disk is a hydrodynamic system composed of a centrally situated nucleus wherein resides the pressure gradients that maintain separation of the opposing endplates of the vertebrae that form the functional units. The nucleus is a mucopolysaccharide matrix with intrinsic pressure that is contained by encircling annular fibers.

The annual fibers are layered in sheets that criss-cross between the opposing endplates in an oblique direction. These annular fiber sheets are enclosed within a mucopolysaccharide matrix and have limited elongation. The annular fibers, collagen in nature, by virtue of their angulation and their intrinsic limited elasticity offer resistance to separation of the endplates and restraint to the contents of the nucleus within its central region.

The disk, mechanically, acts as a shock absorber and allows some compression, flexion, and limited rotatory torque. It is an avascular tissue that maintains its nutrition by imbibition and, to a lesser degree, by osmosis. Being so dependent on mechanical forces for its nutrition, these forces must be permitted and maintained yet guarded against excesses that result in injury and malfunction.

There currently is controversy as to the presence of nerve supply to the disk that would allow it to be a site of nociceptive impulses when stressed, damaged, or disrupted. How the disk tissues repair after damage or respond to aging changes remains unknown.

The function of the intervertebral disk between the adjacent vertebral bodies also assures that the posterior neural canal bony contents remain separated and functional. The facets are inexorably dependent on anterior disk function and simultaneously are instrumental in furnishing disk protection in daily function. The disk, by separating the vertebral endplates, influences the patency of the intervertebral foramen and the patency of the spinal canal with its contained nerve roots and cauda equinal contents.

Obviously, any impairment of the intervertebral disk results in impairment of the total functional unit. To deny a role of the disk in low back symptomatology is untenable as is also attributing **all** low back pathology and symptoms to malfunction of the intervertebral disk. It also is apparent that **all** low back **pain**, acute, recurrent, or chronic, is **not** the direct and total result of tissue damage causing nociceptive stimuli but, if the adage that "most low back pain symptoms are attributable to mechanical derangement etiology" is true the disk's role must be ascertained. The differential diagnosis of causation of low back pain resulting from joint, muscular, or disk prolapse has been aptly summarized by Mennell (Table 11–1).

**Table 11–1. CLINICAL FEATURES FOR
DIFFERENTIAL DIAGNOSIS OF BACK PAIN**

| | Trauma | | Disk Prolapse |
	Joint	*Muscle*	
Onset	Sudden During movement With snap or lock	Sudden With lifting With tearing feeling	Sudden With stressful move With lock
Effect of rest	Relieving	Stiffening	Relieving, especially with partial flexion
Effect of activity	Aggravating	Aggravating	Aggravating
Location	Over junction or sacroiliac joint	Over muscle	Over junction
Architectural changes	Segmental alteration of normal curve Curve convex on side of pain Iliac crest raised on side of pain	No change in spinal curve — —	Segmental alteration of normal curve Curve concave on side of pain Iliac crest lower on side of pain
Mobility	Localized loss Recovery straight	Less well localized Recovery tortuous or straight	Localized loss Recovery straight

(*continued*)

Table 11–1—*continued*

| | Trauma | | Disk Prolapse |
	Joint	Muscle	
Percussion	Short sharp pain	—	Short sharp pain, often with radiation
Obvious physical signs	One joint One level Unilateral Pain may be referred No neurologic signs	No joint No area Unilateral Pain in muscle No neurologic signs	One junction Same level joint Bilateral Radiating pain Mixed neurologic signs
General observations	Patient lies still No signs of systemic disease No fever	Patient varies position No signs of systemic disease No fever	Patient lies still No signs of systemic disease No fever
X-ray findings	Negative	Negative	Negative except with special techniques
Laboratory findings	Negative	Negative	Negative except CSF protein often increased

Modified from Mennell, JM: Differential diagnosis of visceral from somatic back pain. J Occup Med 8:477, 1966.

LUMBAR DISK HERNIATION

The term "herniation of a disk" enjoys a common usage often unwarranted and misunderstood. Herniation is by definition (Webster, 20th Century Dictionary, Collins World 1978) "a rupture; a protrusion of all or part of an organ through a tear or other abnormal opening in the wall of the containing cavity."

By "herniation of a disk" it must be understood that the material herniating is **nuclear** material that has herniated through the confines of its annular container. This can occur but does so in varying degrees as illustrated in Figures 11–1 to 11–3.

Torn annular fibers allowing the nuclear material to emerge from

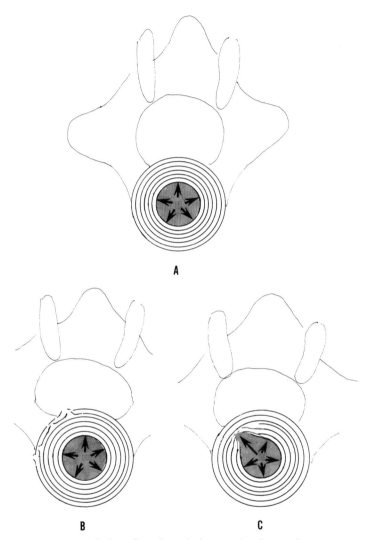

Figure 11–1. *A*, Intact disk and nucleus (schematic). The nucleus is intact and its intrinsic forces (*arrows*) are expended equally in all directions. *B*, Intact nucleus with disruption of outer annular fibers (schematic). The outer annular fibers have been disrupted but there are sufficient annular fibers to contain the intact nucleus. The *arrows* indicate intrinsic forces within the nucleus but no annulus bulging. *C*, Intact annulus (no bulge) but extrusion of the nucleus (schematic). The nucleus has extruded from the inner annular fibers but there are sufficient intact outer annular fibers to prevent significant extrusion of the annulus into the canals.

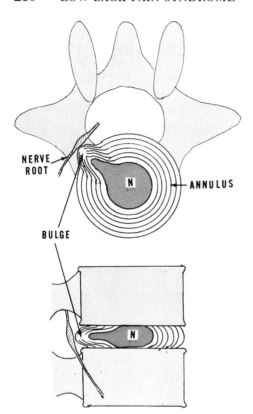

NERVE
ROOT

ANNULUS

BULGE

Figure 11–2. Central extrusion of nucleus causing external extrusion of annulus. *Top,* Internal extrusion ("rupture") of the nucleus in a posterior lateral direction. The weakened and torn annular fibers permit external extrusion of the overlying annular fibers causing pressure upon the nerve root (*bottom*).

within its container into one of the adjacent canals can be construed as a true herniation: a ruptured disk.

Partial tearing of annular fiber sheets with some degree of emergence of the nuclear material from its center region, but remaining within the confines of the total disk, is not true disk herniation (see Fig. 11–1B). The case of the extruded nucleus, where the pressure of the nucleus exerts outward pressure on the weakened annular fiber container causing the annulus to "bulge," can be construed as a disk **annulus** herniation because the intervertebral disk has passed by the borders of the vertebral body into or encroaching on the adjacent foramen (see Fig. 11–2).

This arbitrary differentiation may appear to be trivial pursuit, but because it has clinical significance it will be pursued.

There is recent evidence that the outer annular disk fibers are innervated, containing end organs of unmyelinated nerve fibers. Whether these end organs are within the outer annular fiber layers or are intrusions from the end organs of the adjacent longitudinal ligaments is redundant, as they can transmit nociceptive impulses when injured or irritated. By their pres-

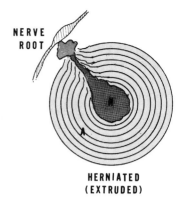

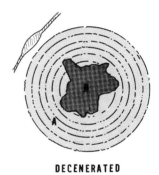

Figure 11–3. Herniation of nuclear material into the foramen against the nerve root. *Top,* This can be construed as true "herniation." The nuclear material has veritably extruded out of the annulus container and into the foraminal cavity. *Bottom,* Degeneration of nucleus into annular fibers.

ence, injury to the outer annular layer can transmit an ultimate sensation of pain (see Fig. 11–1*B*).

Injury to the outer annular layers can "weaken" the annular container and allow the nucleus, being under intrinsic pressure, to extrude from its central position but not herniate the outer annular fibers. This can be termed a **herniation** of the nucleus within the annular layers but not herniation of the disk annulus within its confines (see Fig. 11–1*C*). Admittedly this is a moot point, but the symptoms vary depending on the site, the degree, and the specific tissue of the disk "herniation."

It has been stated that the annular fibers oblique across the disk space in sheets, with each contiguous sheet crossing in the opposite direction as the next outer layer. By this criss-cross intertwining, the annulus has intrinsic strength that permits compression (approachment of adjacent vertebrae in a sagittal direction) and flexion-extension with safety. The only vulnerable factor within the disk that can lead to "failure" is the extent of extensibility of the component collagen fibers comprising the annulus.

The tubular configuration of the disk from the outer layers to the inner layers has been depicted in Chapter 1. It has been clarified that compression of the disk in a sagittal plane adds structural "rigidity" to the annular fibers. Only rotation exceeding 5 degrees of torque is considered to be potential force unaccepted by the annular fibers.

Injury to the disk within the functional unit causing pain and impairment can thus be simplistically stated as: a rotatory torque of the functional unit exceeding 5 degrees of rotation, which elongates the annular fibers within the layered sheets to the point of failure. The annular collagen fibers thus become disrupted and can no longer retain the contents of the nucleus. The nucleus, having its own intrinsic pressure, thus escapes its confines and "extrudes" in an outward direction.

SYMPTOMS IN CLINICAL SITUATION OF DISK "HERNIATION" OUTER ANNULAR TEAR

A low back injury may occur in a person who inadvertently bends forward and simultaneously turns to one side (rotates). This bending may occur in the process of bending forward or returning to the erect posture **with improper simultaneous twisting**. This movement can disrupt the **outer** annular fibers of the disk (Fig. 11–4). If, as stated, this inappropriate action is done without mental (conscious) awareness and is done in an abrupt or in an inappropriate manner, the muscles and ligaments of the functional unit are "caught unaware." The burden of the force is borne essentially, if not completely, by the annular fibers.

In this type of injury to the lumbosacral spine the injury to the intervertebral disk may be restricted to the outer annular fibers. The nucleus is spared injury and extrusion from its surrounding annulus as the inner annular fibers remain intact (see Fig. 11–1B).

The clinical picture of tearing of the outer annular fibers is that of low back pain, if we can assume, as we must, that the outer annular fibers are innervated. The resultant pain is mediated via the recurrent nerve of Luschka (nervus sinu vertebralis) (Fig. 11–5) and is transmitted to the low back via the posterior primary division of the nerve root. The intrinsic pressure within the nucleus may expand the nucleus because there is a resultant weakness of the surrounding annulus. The annulus does not protrude, however, because there are sufficient intact annular fibers remaining to retain the intrinsic pressure of the nucleus. Pain, from a nociceptive source, must be considered to occur from these outer annular nerve endings and not from encroachment on the sensitive posterior longitudinal ligament.

The clinical manifestation of this tear of outer annular fibers is limited trunk flexion, as this motion (trunk flexion) causes the annulus to migrate posteriorly (Fig. 11–6). This posterior nuclear migration may increase the

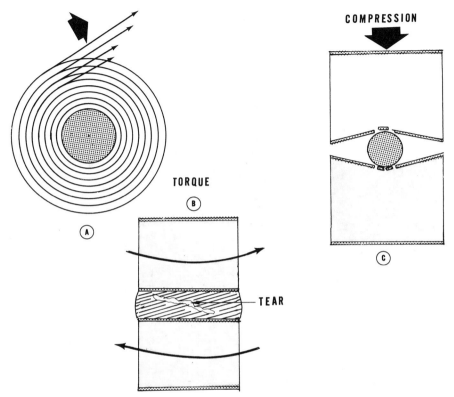

Figure 11–4. Compression versus torque effect upon annulus. A, Annular fibers. Because the outer fibers are longer and more distant from the axis of rotation, they sustain greater torque force in rotation (*arrow*) and thus can tear more easily (*B*). C, Compression force can damage the vertebral body before damaging the disk. The endochondral plates can be penetrated by the nucleus.

pressure on the sensitive posterior longitudinal ligament, but the probabilities are that it merely causes pressure on the outer impaired annular fibers.

Straight leg raising (SLR) is "positive" but of muscular and not neurologic cause. This "muscular" SLR positive test results from elongating (stretching) the hamstring muscles, which causes the pelvis to rotate. This pelvic rotation causes a concomitant flexion of the lumbar spine, which increases the posterior migration of the nucleus. As the adjacent nerve roots as well as the posterior longitudinal ligament are not entrapped from this nuclear extrusion, there is no sciatic radicular pain and no positive dural sign can be elicited from SLR with simultaneous nuchal flexion.

As the pathology is internal extrusion of the nucleus with no outer annular effect route, x-rays are negative. Computed tomography (CT) scan or magnetic resonance imaging (MRI) should also be normal except for the

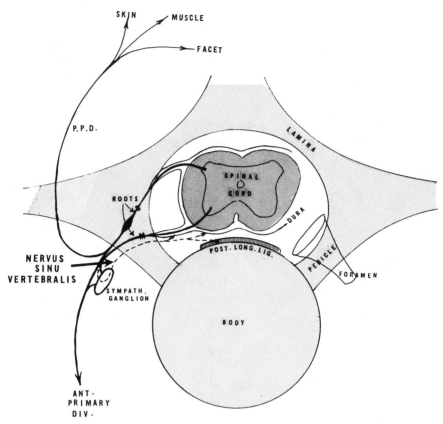

Figure 11–5. Sinu vertebralis nerve. The recurrent nerve of Luschka is considered to convey sensory fibers to the posterior longitudinal ligament, the dura, and reaching to the outer border of the annulus.

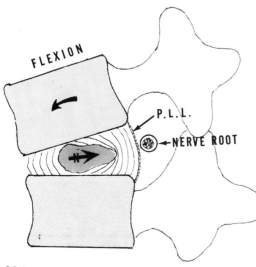

Figure 11–6. Disk nucleus posterior protrusion (schematic). This presents the concept of posterior nuclear migration from the flexed spine position. The nucleus (N) is mechanically extruded posteriorly against the posterior longitudinal ligament (P.L.L.) and the annulus against the nerve root. The nerve root is stretched from the flexed position and cannot escape the protruding disk material.

possibility of a "mild central bulge" because of concurrent protective erector spinae muscle spasm.

Treatment is that of initiating gentle extension exercises and avoidance of flexion and rotation. The other modalities, such as local ice application, massage, and oral anti-inflammatory medication, may be employed to shorten the symptomatology of the acute episode, but time is of the essence as this condition is self-limited with expected recovery. The main concern is to understand that an **annular injury has occurred and predisposes to ultimate further annular insults from a lesser type of injury**. Proper conditioning exercises and especially proper body mechanics are mandatory.

INNER ANNULAR TEAR

A similar injury to that which caused an **outer annular tear**, namely, an inadvertent, improper, or excessive flexion and **rotation**, either in the act of flexion or in the act of returning to the erect position, usually can be considered as causative. As stated, re-extension to the erect position from the flexed and rotated position can cause this type of injury as can the act of flexion.

The symptoms of an inner annular tear are the same as those of the outer annular fibers. The inner annular fibers are not innervated, but with this type of injury they may not cause pain, but they do not remain completely intact. From this injury they create an intrinsic "weakness" and allow a slight protrusion of the nucleus through the torn annular fibers. This causes external pressure that is expended against the outer "sensitive" annular tissues (see Fig. 11–1C).

The diagnosis of a suspected **inner annular tear** cannot be verified by x-rays as these are "negative" except for possible nonspecific disk mild "bulge" on MRI myelogram or CT scan. A diskogram conceivably would reveal the injury.

Treatment of an inner annular tear is as for the outer annular tear. The reason for emphasizing that these tears can occur is that when they are repeated, as in recurrent low back injuries, more accumulative injuries occur to the annular fibers that weaken the disk and lead to degeneration or frank nuclear herniation when an insult may be greater or repeated.

NUCLEAR INNER EXTRUSION WITH
OUTER ANNULAR PROTRUSION

As depicted in Figure 11–2, sufficient annular fibers become disrupted to allow the nucleus to escape from its container (central nuclear extrusion).

If the nucleus extrudes in a posterior lateral direction, the annulus may also so protrude. It has been stated that the vast majority of disk annular disruptions occur in the posterior and posterior lateral areas of the intervertebral disks, so the following clinical conditions may occur.

CENTRAL ANNULAR PROTRUSION

A central disk protrusion encroaches on the posterior longitudinal ligament. There are no radicular signs or symptoms unless the protrusion is so massive as to encroach on a lateral contiguous nerve root dura.

The posterior longitudinal ligament is innervated by the recurrent meningeal (nervus sinu vertebralis) nerve (see Fig. 11–5); because it is sensitive, there is resultant low back pain from its being irritated. Trunk flexion, in either bending forward or sitting, is limited as this position causes further posterior extrusion of the nucleus with a concurrent posterior annular "bulge." The spine is held in the antalgic posture (Fig. 11–7). The SLR test

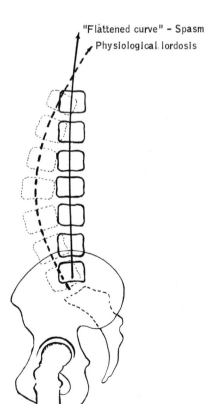

"Flattened curve" – Spasm

Physiological lordosis

Figure 11–7. Lumbar spasm with resultant "flattening." The spasm resulting from nerve root irritation causes a protective spasm. This spasm, rather than increasing the lordosis, results in straightening the lumbar curve. Further forward flexion of the lumbar curve is prevented by this spasm.

is "muscular," not neural. There are no "dural" signs. SLR testing is limited bilaterally with the resultant pain—that of discomfort in the low back region. The neurologic tests are also "negative" as to root sensory or motor impairment, as there is no nerve root entrapment or tension.

Laboratory confirmation by CT scan, myelography, or MRI may reveal the "bulging" disk at a specific level. Electromyelograph (EMG) tests are normal. A diskogram would reveal nuclear extrusion and annular invasion.

Treatment of an inner annular tear with external annular "protrusion" is the same as that indicated for the inner or outer annular tears but without annular protrusion with an expected longer period of recovery. The paraspinous muscle spasm, which occurs in the erector spinae muscles, is "protective." This spasm will probably persist for several days. This spasm and its resultant pain enhancement usually respond well to applications of local modalities such as ice, acupressure, massage, and later local heat. Anti-inflammatory medications are valuable. The "exercises" that are of value in this pathologic condition are those of lumbosacral **extension** and avoidance of flexion-type exercises.

ANNULAR TEAR WITH EXTRUSION OF NUCLEAR FRAGMENT

If the injury is such that there results disruption of the remaining annular fibers between a canal (central or foraminal) and the extruded nucleus, a true "herniation" of the nucleus has occurred. This can be the condition that is termed a "ruptured disk." More accurately this pathologic condition should be termed "a ruptured (herniated) nuclear fragment with or without nerve root entrapment" (see Fig. 11–3).

Symptoms of Extruded Nuclear Material

Low back pain is experienced, as the nerve roots that are entrapped by the extruded nuclear material may include the posterior primary division. The entrapment of the posterior primary division refers the pain in the posterior erector spinae-ligamentous-fascial region.

CENTRAL EXTRUSION

Extrusion of the nucleus through a central annular tear presses against the posterior longitudinal ligament. This ligament is amply innervated by the recurrent nerve of von Luschka. As confirmed by clinical experience, pain from this encroachment is felt in the low back (lumbosacral area). Some pain may also be felt in a nonspecific region of the posterior triangle and buttocks' muscles.

The low back becomes "splinted" and assumes the antalgic posture. Forward flexion is prevented and sitting thus is also limited and painful. After the patient flexes as far as possible before low back pain is elicited, nuchal flexion (bringing the chin down to touch the chest) aggravates the low back pain.

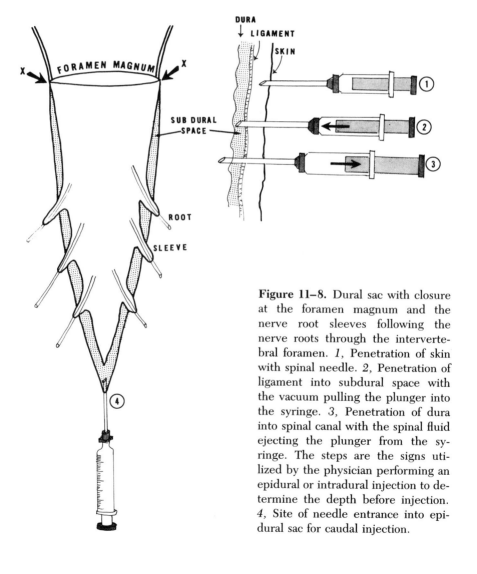

Figure 11–8. Dural sac with closure at the foramen magnum and the nerve root sleeves following the nerve roots through the intervertebral foramen. 1, Penetration of skin with spinal needle. 2, Penetration of ligament into subdural space with the vacuum pulling the plunger into the syringe. 3, Penetration of dura into spinal canal with the spinal fluid ejecting the plunger from the syringe. The steps are the signs utilized by the physician performing an epidural or intradural injection to determine the depth before injection. 4, Site of needle entrance into epidural sac for caudal injection.

The SLR test is termed "positive" in that raising **both** legs in SLR causes pain **in the low back**, but the test is "muscular" and not nerve: the dural sign of SLR test is negative. Any pain felt down the back of the legs is that of muscular stretch sensation. The remainder of the neurologic test is negative.

Routine x-rays are normal but may show a "straightening" of the lumbar lordosis (see Fig. 11–7). A CT scan, myelogram, or MRI may show a central "bulge of the disk," but the nerve roots are not displaced or invaginated. A myelogram, CT with dye, or MRI may actually reveal the presence of a fragment and its location. An EMG is normal.

Treatment

Treatment of a herniated nuclear fragment in a central direction is as in the other disk herniations outlined earlier, **but** extension exercises or extension positioning are to be avoided. Extension can entrap or further protrude the nuclear fragmentation. Flexion exercises are also to be avoided as excessive flexion can herniate more nucleus. In summary: **No exercises** are valuable, in fact, they may be detrimental. Rest in a comfortable reclining position is desirable. No weight bearing except for bathroom privileges for a week or so, until the symptoms subside.

To minimize the inflammatory reaction, oral steroid or oral nonsteroidal anti-inflammatory medication is of value. Persistence or intensification of low back pain may indicate epidural steroid injection (Fig. 11–8).

A corset to immobilize the spine when the patient becomes ambulatory may minimize flexion or extension of the spine during early healing and permit earlier ambulation (see Fig. 9–34). The basis for immobilization of the spine is to prevent further potential herniation and migration of the extruded fragment laterally to possibly encroach on a nerve root.

Manipulation is contraindicated as potentially causing further fragmentation of the extruded nucleus and damage to the longitudinal ligament.

EXTRUSION OF A NUCLEAR FRAGMENT AGAINST A NERVE ROOT

Posterior or posterolateral extrusion of a nuclear herniation through a rent in the longitudinal ligament may encroach on a passing nerve root. This is a major complication or resultant injury engendered by a herniated nuclear fragment. Nerve damage is the feared end result of a disk herniation and is **the major reason for recognition and proper treatment of "disk" herniation**.

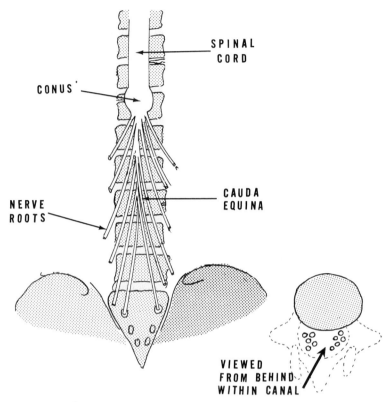

Figure 11–9. Cauda equina viewed from behind. The spinal cord descending within the spinal canal branches out into many nerve roots as it reaches the first lumbar vertebra. These nerves resemble a horse's tail, and hence are called cauda equina. (Modified from Cailliet, R: Understand Your Backache. FA Davis, Philadelphia, 1984, p 46.)

The nerve roots extend laterally and distally from the cauda equina to ultimately exit the spinal canal via the foraminae (Fig. 11–9). On exit, the sensory and motor nerve fibers merge to form a segmental nerve root. This root then divides into a posterior primary division and an anterior primary division (Fig. 11–10). The anterior primary division descends to form either the sciatic nerve (L4-S1) or the femoral nerve (L3-4), depending on its segmental level (Fig. 11–11).

As the nerve enters the foramen, it is contained within a dural sac that in turn contains spinal fluid, venules, capillaries, lymphatics, and nervous nervosus fibers. The dura is attached by fibrous fibrils at its cervical orifice and at its point of emergence (Fig. 11–12).

By these attachments no significant movement of the nerve root and

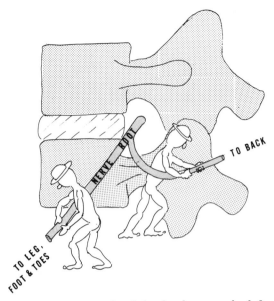

Figure 11–10. Nerve root. At each of the lumbar vertebral functional units, a branch of the cauda equina (termed a root) goes out to the specific area of the leg or foot through its specific intervertebral foramen. Each root then divides into a branch going down the leg and a branch to the low back. (From Cailliet, R: Understand Your Backache. FA Davis, Philadelphia, 1984, p 47, with permission.)

its dura is permitted; therefore, any pressure on the nerve root or traction on the root (Fig. 11–13) may cause vascular impairment to that nerve root.

The symptoms of a specific nerve root impingement may be sensory or motor (Table 11–2). The sensory patterns termed dermatomes are illustrated in Figure 11–14 and the myotomes (motor innervation) and reflexes are summarized in Figure 11–15.

THE CLINICAL MANIFESTATIONS OF SEGMENTAL NERVE ROOT ENTRAPMENT

Every segmental level at which a herniated nuclear fragment occurs has generalized symptoms and findings and, for each level, specific symptoms and findings for that particular nerve root. The clinical complaints and physical findings of general and specific nerve root entrapment can be summarized as follows:

1. Pain is felt in the low back by virtue of the fact that **any** disk herniation into a foramen or the spinal canal involves the posterior primary division of the nerve root involved. Pain in the low back is nonspecific; it is felt

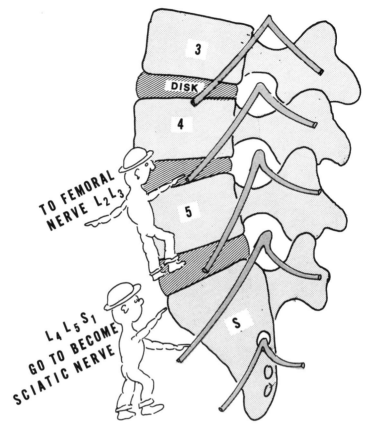

Figure 11–11. Sciatic nerve roots. The fourth and fifth lumbar nerves and the sacral nerve form the sciatic nerve. This nerve goes down the back of the leg to the foot and toes. The second and third lumbar nerves do *not* go into the sciatic nerve. They merge to form the femoral nerve, which goes down the *front* of the thigh to the thigh muscles. (From Cailliet, R: Understand Your Backache. FA Davis, Philadelphia, 1984, p 57, with permission.)

generally in the lumbar region in the so-called triangle of the low back (Figs. 11–16 and 11–17).

2. Pain, hypalgesia, and/or paresthesia is noted down the distribution of that particular nerve root (dermatome) (see Fig. 11–14). The dermatome area may be the site of "numbness" claimed by the patient and may be reproducible by pin scratch or light touch by the examiner. This test, unfortunately, is often not very accurate in localizing a specific nerve root or intervertebral disk space.

3. Weakness of a specific myotome. A "myotome" is the medical term given the muscle group innervated by a specific nerve root. As most mus-

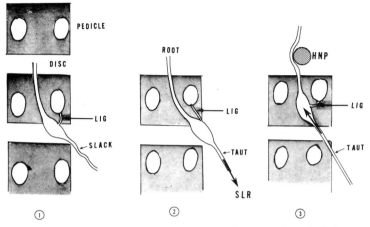

Figure 11–12. Nerve root traction. *1*, The normal root with a slack ligament and full flexibility. *2*, With straight-leg raising, the nerve root dura becomes taut. *3*, With a herniated disk pressing upon the nerve root, the root is pulled cephalad and increases the tautness distally.

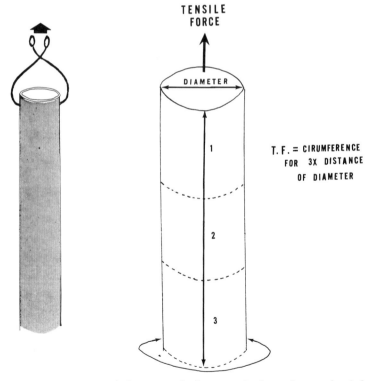

Figure 11–13. Saint-Venant's law. Tensile force applied in a longitudinal direction is distributed uniformly around the circumference for a distance equal to three times the diameter of the tube. Tension thus applied to the nerve root dura is transmitted as a compression force for a distance of three times the diameter of the root, both cranially and caudally. This explains radicular pain caused by an HNP, SLR, and nuchal flexion.

Table 11–2. SCHEMATIC DERMATOME AND MYOTOME LEVEL OF NERVE ROOT IMPINGEMENT

Nerve Root	Inter-vertebral Space	Subjective Pain Radiation	Sensory Area	Bladder Bowel Dysfunction*	SLR†	Ankle Jerk‡	Knee Jerk‡	Motor Dysfunction (Myotome)§
L3	L2-L3	Back to buttocks to posterior thigh to anterior knee region	Hypalgesia in knee region	+/−	Usually −	+	+	Quadriceps weakness
L4	L3-L4	Back to buttocks to posterior thigh to inner calf region	Hypalgesia inner aspect of lower leg	+/−	Usually − Maybe +	+	−	Quadriceps and possible anticus weakness
L5	L4-L5	Back to buttocks to dorsum of foot and big toe	Hypalgesia in dorsum foot and big toe	+/−	++	+	+	Weakness of anterior tibialis, big toe extensor, gluteus medius
S1	L5-S1	Back to buttocks to sole of foot and heel	Hypalgesia in heel or lateral foot	+/−	+++	−	+	Weakness of gastrocnemius, hamstring, gluteus maximus

*Bladder and bowel dysfunction can occur at any level.
†Related to extent of nerve root movement at each level.
‡Ankle jerk is absent only at L5-S1; knee jerk at L3-L4.
§Only the more obvious and functional muscles are listed.

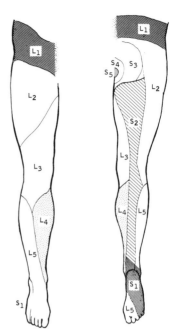

Figure 11–14. Sensory dermatome area map. The areas mapped out are the areas of hypalgesia to pin-scratch testing. Because of patient variation, the areas at best are general and overlapping.

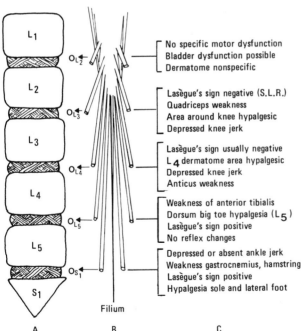

No specific motor dysfunction
Bladder dysfunction possible
Dermatome nonspecific

Lasègue's sign negative (S.L.R.)
Quadriceps weakness
Area around knee hypalgesic
Depressed knee jerk

Lasègue's sign usually negative
L4 dermatome area hypalgesic
Depressed knee jerk
Anticus weakness

Weakness of anterior tibialis
Dorsum big toe hypalgesia (L5)
Lasègue's sign positive
No reflex changes

Depressed or absent ankle jerk
Weakness gastrocnemius, hamstring
Lasègue's sign positive
Hypalgesia sole and lateral foot

Filium

A   B   C

Figure 11–15. Clinical localization of dermatome-myotome level of disk herniation. *A,* Lateral view of the spine showing the nerve root relationship to the intervertebral disk (e.g., S_1 nerve root at level of disk between vertebra L_5 and first sacral vertebra S_1). *B,* Indication of the level at which the cord becomes the cauda equina (L_1). Below this level any nerve injury is equivalent to a peripheral nerve injury. *C,* The clinical manifestations of the various nerve roots as found on neurologic examination.

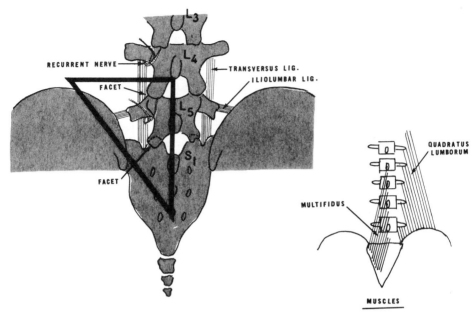

Figure 11–16. Multifidus triangle. This is an arbitrary triangular area extending from L₄ to the iliac crest and down to the sacrum, containing numerous pain-producing tissues, including facets, facet innervation, transversus ligament, quadratus lumborum muscle, multifidus muscle, iliolumbar ligament, and fascia.

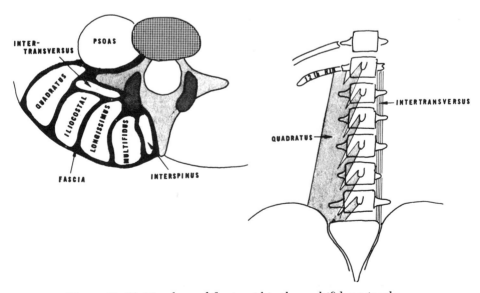

Figure 11–17. Muscles and fascia within the multifidus triangle.

cles are innervated by more than one nerve root, the interpretation of "which nerve root" must be extrapolated (see Table 11–2).

As all muscles are innervated by peripheral nerves that in turn are comprised of numerous nerve roots, the compositions of the peripheral nerves must be fully understood by the examiner (Table 11–3).

In testing for the integrity of nerve roots or peripheral nerves, not only the strength but the endurance of the muscle resisted must be determined manually. Endurance (i.e., repeated contraction against resistance) is a more precise test for intact innervation than is merely testing strength of one or two contractions against resistance. An example is the testing of S1 root (the gastroc-soleus group). A person may arise up on the toes several times or walk a few feet on the toes and depict no weakness, but, on arising many times up on the toes fatigue will manifest nerve impairment.

4. Test for tenderness of the muscle innervated by a specific myotome or dermatome will also reveal localization. It is accepted that some 30 percent of the fibers of a motor root are also sensory, thus a muscle may be tender within a specific area, and eliciting this tenderness may be of further diagnostic value (Fig. 11–18).

5. In a patient suspected of having a disk herniation, whether extrusion or internal nuclear extrusion with annular protrusion and encroachment on a nerve root (Fig. 11–19), the findings reveal the following:

(a) Limited trunk flexion. In attempting to bend forward, such as attempting to touch one's toes, there is no significant reversal of the lumbar lordosis and no acquiring of a lumbar kyphosis. All flexion occurs from rotation of the pelvis about the hip joints.

(b) A "functional" scoliosis may exist. The term "functional" implies that the scoliosis is transient and not from structural vertebral spine changes. The exact mechanism by which scoliosis occurs remains unproven.

There are numerous theories, among which is the tendency for the spine to laterally flex **away** from the nerve entrapment. If the nerve root is under pressure from a medial nuclear bulge, the nerve will move laterally. This lateral movement results from lateral erector spinae muscle contraction (Fig. 11–20). The lateral erector spinae muscles allegedly contract in a reflex manner from irritation of the posterior primary division of the same nerve root being entrapped.

(c) A positive SLR with positive dural sign **must** exist if the diagnosis of nerve root entrapment is entertained. The common terminology of "positive straight leg raising," "SLR," or "positive Lasègue test" is a specific organic neurologic sign and merits full understanding and thus full discussion.

If a nerve root is inflamed or entrapped, regardless of by what tissue, a disk herniation, a facet arthritis process, or a tumor, any tension on the dura of the involved nerve will elicit pain or paresthesia in its dermatomal distribution.

Table 11–3. RELATIONSHIP OF SPECIFIC ROOTS,
MUSCLES, AND PERIPHERAL NERVES

Root	Muscle	Peripheral Nerve
L2	Sartorius (L2-3)	Femoral
	Pectineus (L2-3)	Obturator
	Adductor longus (L2-3)	Obturator
L3	Quadriceps femoris (L2-3-4)	Femoral
L4	Quadriceps femoris (L2-3-4)	Femoral
	Tensor fascia lata (L4-5)	Superior gluteal
	Tibialis anterior (L4-5)	Peroneal
L5	Gluteus medius (L4-5 S1)	Superior gluteal
	Semi-membranosus (L4-5 S1)	Sciatic
	Semi-tendinosus (L4-5 S1)	Sciatic
	Extensor hallucis longis (L4-5 S1)	Deep peroneal
S1	Gluteus maximus (L4-5 S1-2)	Inferior gluteal
	Biceps femoris—short head (L5 S1-2)	Sciatic
	Semi-tendinosus (L4-5 S1)	Sciatic
	Medial gastrocnemius (S1-2)	Tibial
	Soleus (S1-2)	Tibial
S2	Biceps femoris—long head (S1-2)	Sciatic
	Lateral gastrocnemius (S1-2)	Tibial
	Soleus (S1-2)	Tibial

The SLR test is done in several ways:

1. With the leg fully extended at the knee it is flexed upon the pelvis.

2. With the leg at the hip the test then requires extending the lower leg on the upper leg. This can be done with the patient in the supine position or in the seated position.

Because the nerve root, per se, is not sensitive but the dural sac is, pain can be elicited only when the inflamed dura is stretched. Hence, for an SLR test to be considered "positive," and thus implying compression of the nerve root, the dura of that nerve root must be involved. For a positive SLR test to be a positive neurologic test, it must also be a "positive dural sign."

The dural radicular pain test is probably the most significant neurologic test performed; thus it must be performed properly. Most important, however, it must be interpreted properly.

There are numerous names given to the so-called sciatic nerve stretch

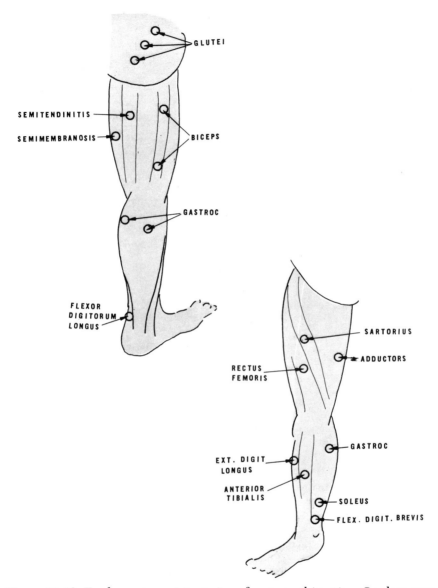

Figure 11–18. Tender motor points at sites of myoneural junction. On deep pressure, these sites of tenderness conform to the muscles innervated by the root at a specific intervertebral space.

test. Lasèque is the most prevalent name given. Lasèque discussed the subject of sciatica in 1864 but did not describe the stretch test that now bears his name. It was Forst (1881) who first described and discussed the SLR test in which he advocated raising the fully extended leg. Pain re-

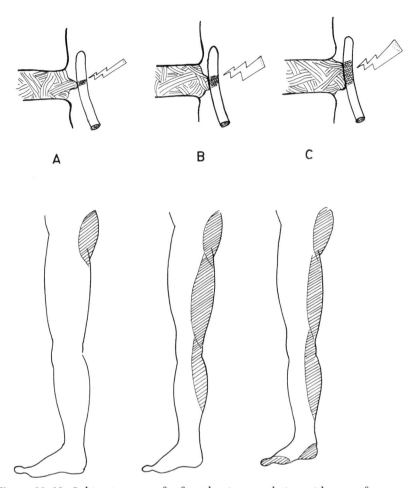

Figure 11–19. Subjective area of referred pain: correlation with area of nerve contact. *A*, A slight degree of nerve contact will cause the patient to claim pain that is referred to the buttocks region. *B*, Pain claimed to radiate down the posterior thigh, with or without buttocks pain, implies a greater degree of nerve contact. *C*, Pain referred to the foot region implies a larger area of nerve contact and also gives an indication of the root spinal level. The amount of pressure is not so important as is the extent of the nerve contact at the foraminal level.

sulted after only a few centimeters of leg raising. It is interesting that in the original illustration of this test **the patient had his neck flexed**. Both Lasèque and Forst claimed that the pain response was the result of stretching the inflamed posterior thigh muscles (hamstrings) and not the sciatic nerve root.

Numerous authors later described this test but much credit must go

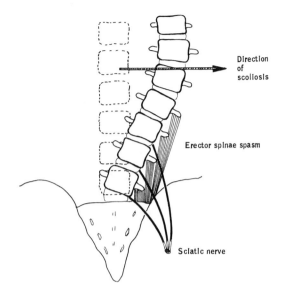

Figure 11–20. Mechanism of acute protective scoliosis. Irritation of the nerve root at its emergence through the intervertebral foramen causes reflex spasm, usually on the same side as the site of irritation. By its segmental distribution, only a small portion of the paraspinous muscles is involved, and thus a segmental lateral curve of the spine results.

to Fajersztain who explained the mechanism of the SLR test. He added dorsiflexion of the foot to the SLR and also neck flexion (Fig. 11–21). These two additions are now well-documented as being dural stretch, which causes the pain. The nerve is stretched in performing SLR but the inflamed dura is stretched by subsequently flexing the neck and dorsiflexing the foot. Without the positive dural component **the SLR test cannot be considered positive**.

Fajersztain, later in his paper, described and discussed the "crossed" (contralateral) sciatic nerve stretch. This will be subsequently discussed.

In the SLR test only one leg usually is painful, and as the sciatic nerve is primarily of L4-5 to S1, a positive SLR tests only these roots.

A similar test can be performed for higher root levels (L2-3), which go down the leg within the femoral nerve. To stretch the femoral nerve the patient is placed in the prone position and the foot is gently brought to the buttocks. This stretches the front of the thigh and thus the femoral nerve. Again, in performing this test, comparison of stretch in the normal leg to the suspected abnormal leg, care must be exerted to differentiate muscle stretch pain from nerve stretch pain (Fig. 11–22).

(d) Positive neurologic signs can be elicited implicating a specific nerve root and thus a specific disk level. These have been listed in previous illustrations (Tables 11–1, 11–2, and 11–3 and Figs. 11–1 to 11–18) as weakness and fatigue of the myotomes and sensory impairment of the dermatome.

The disk level, however, may be difficult to relate to a specific nerve

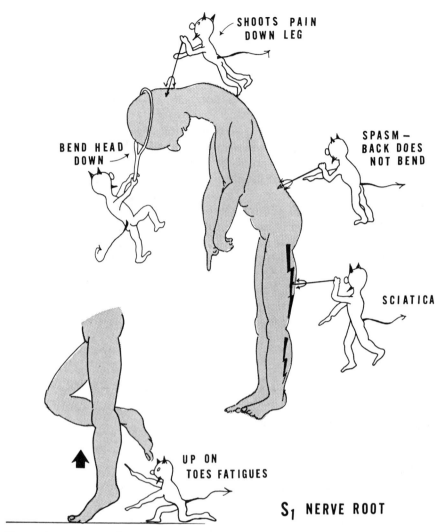

SHOOTS PAIN
DOWN LEG

BEND HEAD
DOWN

SPASM –
BACK DOES
NOT BEND

SCIATICA

UP ON
TOES FATIGUES

S₁ NERVE ROOT

Figure 11–21. Limited flexibility and pain pattern in a ruptured disk. The low back is "rigid," does not bend, and is straight. There is pain in leg in attempting to bend forward, aggravated by bending neck. If the S_1 root is involved, there may be difficulty getting up and down on the toes. (From Cailliet, R: Understand Your Backache. FA Davis, Philadelphia, 1984, p 88, with permission.)

root and vice versa. This is because the nerve root passes obliquely by the disk before it exits through the foramen (Fig. 11–23).

Crossed Sciatic Stretch Pain

This is an ominous sign indicating that the involved nerve root may be entrapped and frequently by an extruded fragment. This is a condition that

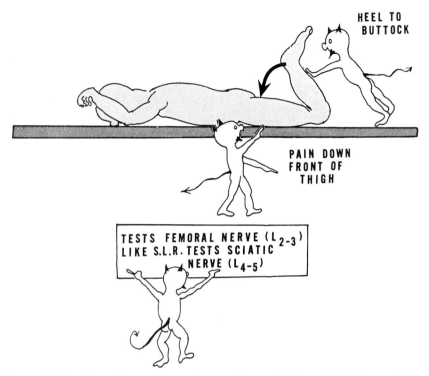

Figure 11–22. Femoral nerve stretch test. (From Cailliet, R: Understand Your Backache. FA Davis, Philadelphia, 1984, p 89, with permission.)

may mandate surgical intervention. This test is positive when SLR the **opposite** (normal or uninvolved) leg causes pain to radiate down the involved sciatic nerve distribution.

The mechanism for this reaction was described by Fajersztain. The test is consequently named as a positive Fajersztain test. In raising the opposite (uninvolved) leg the nerve roots within the spinal canal move medially a slight degree. If the involved nerve at this level is significantly entrapped **no** lateral movement will be permitted from SLR of the uninvolved leg.

A positive contralateral SLR test exists when pain occurs down the sciatic distribution of the involved leg by SLR of the contralateral uninvolved leg. This positive reaction indicates a significant entrapment of the involved nerve root at that specific level.

CONFIRMATORY TESTS

On suspecting or diagnosing a herniated disk as the cause of sciatic neuropathy, there are confirmatory tests that enjoy wide acceptance.

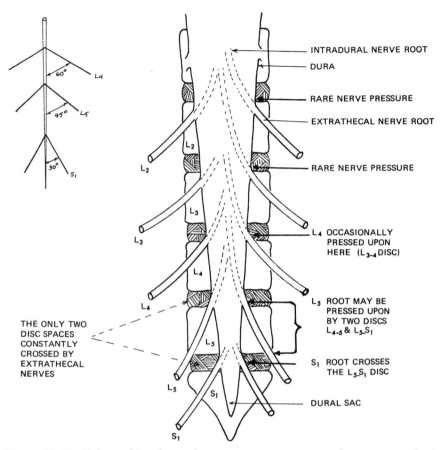

Figure 11–23. Relationship of specific nerve root to corresponding intervertebral disk.

The diagnosis of sciatic radiculopathy should never be made merely on the basis of an abnormal test, be it an x-ray or an EMG. These tests merely confirm the clinical impression gotten from a careful comprehensive history and a careful comprehensive physical examination. The "confirmatory" tests imply the site of pathology and may rule out unexpected pathology not indicated by the history. **It is the patient that is treated, not the x-ray, CT scan, MRI or the EMG. The symptom of pain can never be removed surgically unless the exact pathology causing the pain is confirmed as present and potentially causing the pain.**

X-rays considered "routine" reveal the bony alignment and functional unit integrity. These "routine" x-rays do not reveal the status of the intervertebral disk, the nerve roots, the fat pads, the ligamentum flavum, or the ligaments. Routine x-rays may reveal spondylolisthesis, spondylolysis, degenerative changes, malignancy, Paget's disease, osteoporosis, or fracture, and may even suggest the possibility of stenosis, but as a rule they are not specific. All too frequently a diagnosis is given to the patient based on the x-ray report that does not explain the cause of that patient's symptoms or findings.

Myelography is invasive diagnostic injection of a dye into the dural sac that outlines the contents of the dural sac within the spinal canal. A bulging disk and an entrapment of a nerve root sleeve may be revealed and its location depicted. Again, this test may be misleading as unfortunately many disk herniations are not revealed and there are many "false" positives.

Again, it must be emphasized that it is the clinical evaluation—a significant thorough history and a meaningful examination properly interpreted—that reveals the problem. The myelogram, if positive, confirms the presence and the site of the pathology.

CT scans have proven more precise in diagnosing the internal soft tissues within the spine. CT scanning adds views not available on anteroposterior, lateral, and oblique intradural routine x-rays. They reveal oblique, coronal, and sagittal views and indicate soft tissue views not seen on routine x-rays. CT scanning is also being done with the addition of injected intradural dye.

MRI scans are the latest diagnostic procedure. These examinations reveal, in a noninvasive method, the inner contents of the spinal canal and the foramina. They give less detailed bone configuration but reveal what may be encroaching on the nerve roots or the articular surfaces.

Within the limits of this text, other radiologic procedures and modifications of those mentioned will not be discussed. The state of the radiologic art and technique is progressing so rapidly that by the time this edition is printed, newer methods will have evolved and those mentioned may have been discarded, modified, or reinterpreted.

An EMG is also of confirmatory value. This test reveals the integrity of the nerve root, its site, and its status. Again, the interpretation of the EMG only confirms what the clinical picture has indicated and may help more specifically localize the precise root level. It must be remembered that some 14 to 21 days, after nerve injury from whatever cause, must elapse before demyelination of the nerve is noted on the EMG. Many "false" positives can occur. The time of occurrence of the nerve injury, be it recent or previous, is not always clear.

TREATMENT OF DISK HERNIATION

Treatment of low back pain has been discussed, but the difference of treating a disk herniation, be it nuclear or annular, merits discussion.

All the modalities used in mechanical low back pain—rest, heat, ice, oral anti-inflammatory medications, traction—have a role in treating disk herniation, but there are major differences that must be emphasized.

The major difference is that **disk herniation has potential nerve root injury with residual sequelae**. Pain is not the primary concern although it plays a major role as concerns the patient.

The question is also usually raised as to whether surgery is indicated—when, why, under what conditions, by whom and with which technique.

Which patient will benefit from surgery is also not completely accepted. This question relates to the symptom of pain and the resolution of the pathology causing nerve involvement. Pain is the basis of a complete chapter to follow. Resolution of objective neurologic involvement is also unpredictable with current diagnostic methods.

Recently, a provocative article (Kopp 1986) appeared that offered a simplistic clinical method to determine which patient, having classic acute disk herniation signs and symptoms, will need or benefit from surgery.

Inadvertently, this article also highlighted the controversy as to the value, if any, of exercise in the treatment of herniated disk and which type of exercise is of value in treating a patient with low back pain **and** sciatic radiculopathy.

The value of exercise in treatment of the average "mechanical" low back pain has been discussed. The controversy of abdominal exercises to create an "air bag" that supposedly unloads the lumbar spine has been evaluated. The controversy of the abdominal obliques affecting the width and strength of the erector spinae muscle fascia has also been developed as it relates to the fascia being the major tissue component that supports the low back during re-extension to the erect posture in the act of lifting.

The recent discrepancy between extension exercises versus flexion exercises in the treatment of low back pain has yet to be resolved, but the choice of either depends on the mechanism of low back pain as determined from a meaningful examination.

Traditionally the "Williams" flexion-type exercises have been routinely prescribed for low back pain in lumbar diskogenic disease with radiculopathy. This is the question that has been raised in the article mentioned (Kopp 1986).

Intradiskal pressures were measured by Nachemson and the pressure in the third lumbar disk compared in numerous positions and activities, including exercises. The pressure in mere standing with arms dangling at the side was considered the basis or norm (100). Laying supine (50) or on one's side (75) revealed the effect of gravity. Sitting erect (140), sitting bent forward (185), and sitting bent forward with weight in the dangling arms (275). These studies revealed that sitting and especially, sitting, leaning forward with weighted arms, markedly increases the interdiskal pressure in the lumbar disks. This is the position assumed by many people during their daily occupations and home activities.

If the nucleus, within an intervertebral disk, migrates posteriorly during the flexed trunk position, an increase in intradiskal pressure further migrates the nucleus posteriorly. If the posterior annulus is intact this nuclear migration is of no significance, but if the annulus has been impaired, weakened, or damaged then posterior movement of the nucleus may have adverse effects on the disk.

Exercises have also been studied as to their effect on intradiskal pressures. Related to the norm of 100 in the standing erect posture, sit-ups, even with hips and knees flexed, generate comparable pressures of 210. Raising the legs while in the supine position and with the hips and knees flexed, a pressure of 140 is generated. It becomes obvious that flexion exercises can intensify the posterior migration of the nucleus. The use of flexion exercises (William's type) theoretically can aggravate posterior migration of the nucleus with resultant posterior "bulging" of the annulus and even nuclear herniation through a weakened annulus.

The provocative test (Kopp 1986) for determining whether the disk nucleus is merely internal herniation with an intact annulus bulging or if there is a frank extruded nucleus fragment outside the annulus, is accomplished by having the patient assume the prone position and then raise the head and shoulders, which causes an increase in the lumbar lordosis.

In this extended lumbar position, the nucleus presumably (theoretically) is forced anteriorly back to its central normal position within the annulus (Fig. 11–24). This also forces the centrally extruded nucleus and the resultant annulus bulge to move away from the nerve roots and the posterior spinal canal.

From the prone position the patient is asked to rise up on the elbows (1) as in Figure 11–25, then (2) up on the extended arms (Fig. 11–25). This is an arm push up, **not** a low back extension exercise. An extension exercise increases the intradiskal pressure (Fig. 11–26) whereas "passive" maximum extension (push up) theoretically forces the nucleus further anteriorly.

If the nucleus has herniated from its central position but has not extruded through a tear in the posterior annulus, assuming this position becomes not only a test but a treatment. The posterior annulus can then "heal" and the nucleus remains centrally placed.

If the nucleus has migrated posteriorly and extruded out of the annulus into the foraminal or spinal canals (see Fig. 11–24B), assuming this extended position compresses the posterior nucleus and annulus further, forcing more extrusion. This compresses the contents of the foramen which are now nerve roots, its dura, and the nuclear fragment.

In the extended spine position, the foraminal exits are narrowed even though the nerve roots are more slack. A "positive" test, indicating an extrusion, causes radicular pain down the leg from this position and mandates **no further extension—either test or treatment exercises**.

The extruded fragment cannot return to the central disk position as it is no longer within the disk. Treatment now becomes more clear.

It must be reiterated that the position of lying prone and arising up on

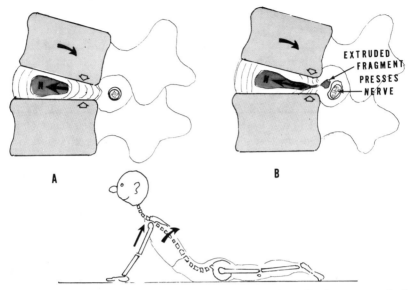

Figure 11–24. Provocative nuclear extrusion test. To clinically determine whether the nucleus merely has an intrinsic extrusion without annular disruption, or whether it has external extrusion through the posterior annulus, place the patient prone and extend the low back by extending the arms. The nucleus (theoretically) is forced anteriorly away from the nerve root (A). If there has been an external extrusion through a tear in the posterior annulus (B), there will be posterior pressure on the disk (*small arrows*), further extruding the nuclear fragment with resultant pressure upon the nerve root.

Using the results of the provocative test, if there is merely intrinsic extrusion (A), further conservative treatment is indicated. If there is extrusion (B), surgery may be required to prevent nerve damage.

the elbows then the extended arms must be done solely by the arms and not by extending the low back against gravity. This is true in the test and in prescribing subsequent exercises.

The standard exercises prescribed as Williams Protocol are essentially flexion exercises. In the average mechanical low back pain these may be warranted and beneficial, but in the presence of a herniated disk they may be contraindicated.

Flexion of the functional unit (theoretically) normally forces the nucleus posteriorly. If the nucleus has extruded from its central annular fibers, the resultant pressure is posterior migration of the nucleus. This forces the remaining annular fibers to "bulge" into the foramen or the spinal canal (see Fig. 11–6).

Based on the studies of Nachemson, the intradiskal pressure varies with numerus positions assumed daily. With a standard of 100 N in the

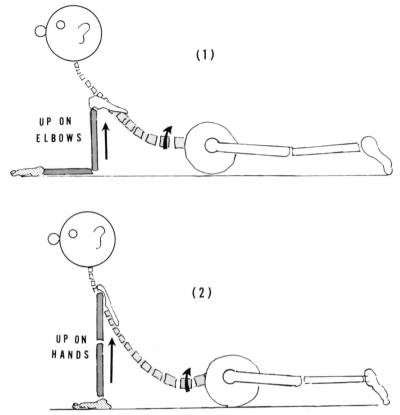

Figure 11–25. Provocative extension test for disk herniation. As stated in text, to determine if the disk "herniation with radiculitis" is an annulus bulge or a disk nucleus extrusion, the patient goes from lying prone to (1) getting up on elbows then (2) up on hands. This position is held for a few minutes then slowly return to prone. The low back is "passively arched." All the effort is with the arms. The effect upon the disk is shown in Figure 11–24.

erect posture, there are decreases in assuming the supine position, but there are also significant increases in forward bending and sitting postures (Fig. 11–27). These adversely affect the nucleus position within the disk, especially when there has been annular damage.

SCIATIC RADICULOPATHY WITHOUT DISK HERNIATION

There are numerous patients who present with low back pain and sciatic radiculopathy, yet upon radiologic examination and surgery show no

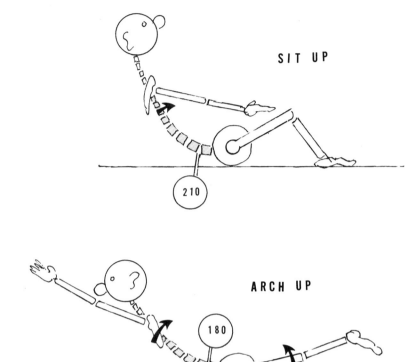

Figure 11–26. Comparative intradisk pressures in exercises. The "sit up," a flexion exercise, increases the intradisk pressure in the lumbar spine by more than twice (280) the normal pressure in standing. This is one of the William's exercises and (theoretically) should be avoided in an acute disk hernia.

The "arch up," done from the prone position, increases the intradisk pressure in the lower lumbar disks by almost twice (180) the pressure from erect standing. This exercise also (theoretically) should be avoided in an acute disk herniation. The exercise advised in provocative disk hernia position testing (Fig. 11–25) should, therefore, be an arm pushup and *not* an active low back arch up.

evidence of disk herniation. The pathomechanics of this aspect of sciatic radiculopathy remains unclear, but there is recent evidence that the causative factors may be a chemical derivation.

In his Presidential Address to the International Society for the Study of the Lumbar Spine, in 1986, Mooney posed the question "Where is the pain coming from?" All considered aspects were discussed and the possibility of the pain being chemical was raised.

In the same issue of *Spine*, a provocative article was published in which homogenized autogenous nucleus pulposus was injected into the intradural space of animals, causing the nerve roots to undergo inflammatory

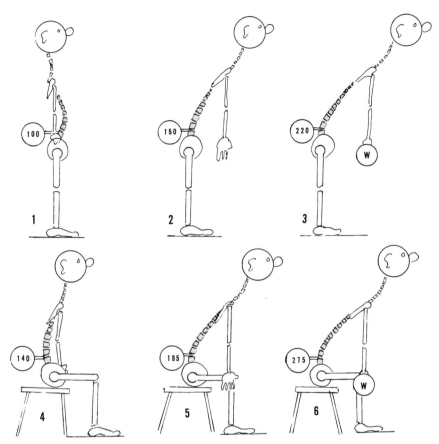

Figure 11–27. Relative intradisk pressures. As depicted by Nachemson, the intradisk pressures vary according to the position of the body. In the erect posture with arms at the side (*1*), the basic pressure is 100. Merely leaning forward with the arms dangling (*2*), the pressure increases by one fifth. Leaning forward with weights in the hands (*3*), the pressure more than doubles. The seated position with arms dangling (*4*) almost equals the intradisk pressure of the forward standing posture (*2*) and seated leaning forward with arms dangling posture (*5*); the pressure (185) is almost double that of standing erect. The highest intradisk pressure is the seated position with a weighted arm (*6*). This last pressure is what many people sustain in everyday occupational activities.

reaction. The inflamed nerve roots were considered very sensitive. Any pressure or traction upon these inflamed nerves could conceivably cause radicular sensations such as are experienced by patients with "sciatica."

Macnab had previously demonstrated that pressure upon an "inflamed" nerve caused pain whereas pressure upon an uninflamed nerve root, within the intervertebral foramen, did not. He reached this conclusion by inserting an inflatable catheter tip within the foramen against the nerve root in postoperative patients with known disk herniations.

The results of the homogenized nucleus pulposus studies postulated that when there is some annular tearing the nucleus tends to extrude outward and can "leak" into the epidural space inflaming the nerve root dura. A sciatic radiculopathy results with a positive straight leg raising (positive dural signs) due to traction or compression upon this inflamed nerve.

The possibility of the nuclear material leaking is implicated when there has been annular tearing resulting from a rotatory injury to the intradiskal space. The annulus tear may be central, near the nucleus, and ultimately progress outward (Fig. 11–28). With small tears the nuclear material, being liquid, leaks outward and ultimately leaks out of the outer annular fibers into the epidural space.

Further pressure upon the intervertebral disk from activities such as lifting, coughing, straining, and so forth force more nuclear material to extrude. Prolonged sitting in a forward flexed position is considered such a compressive force as is sustained emotional tension.

Further extrusion of nuclear material causes more irritation which is consistent with the average clinical picture of "aggravating factors" causing increased sciatica. CT scans, MRI scans, myelograms and surgical explora-

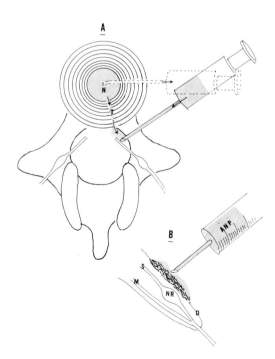

Figure 11–28. Extrusion of nucleus pulposus material into epidural space. *A* depicts removal of nucleus material (N) into syringe (*dotted line syringe*) and reinjected into epidural space (*solid line syringe*) near nerve root. The tear in the annulus (T) shows the pathways (*small arrows*) of the extruded material. *B* is the injection of homogenized autogenous nucleus pulposus material into the vicinity of the dura (D) which envelopes the nerve roots (NR) and their component branches: motor (M) and sensory (S). The dark material around the dural sheath is the nuclear material.

tions may be "negative." Fernstrum reported 35 cases of operations performed upon patients with diagnosis of herniated lumbar disks in which no herniation was found. All that was discovered was a tear in the annulus.

The normal dural sheath is a thin, translucent, fibrous membrane. The epidural fat normally enclosing the dura is firm, lobular, and slightly yellowish with a delicate vascularization. After exposure to the homogenized autogenous nucleus pulposus there was noted cellular involvement consistent with "inflammation." There was minimal polymorphonuclear inflammation. There were, however, granular tissue, fibrosis, large giant cells, and plasma cells. An immune reaction was postulated.

This postulated reaction may explain the benefit from chemonucleosus with the benefit occurring in spite of the persistence of abnormal CT scans, MRI, and myelograms. The clinical benefit apparently occurs from the nuclear material being "removed" with some residual annular bulging. The pressure upon the nerve may remain but the chemically irritating material is removed.

The extrusion of nuclear material as being a major factor in low back and sciatic pain may also explain why symptomatic disk herniation is more prevalent in physically active laborers who have greater exposure to annular tears and subsequent disk pressure activities. The "young" disk is well known to be more liquid and under greater pressure.

The older disk has greater annular fibrous reaction and the nucleus and annulus matrix is less hydrodynamic. Activities are also less stressful. All these factors add a new perspective to understanding low back pain and sciatic radiculopathy. If this chemical implication is sustained and clarified a more specific treatment may evolve in which a chemical intervention to the nucleus pulposus proteonucleosides will result.

It becomes apparent that a careful history will often depict which daily function or position aggravates the patient's symptoms. From an ergonomic viewpoint, modification of daily activities plays a vital role in the School curriculum for the low back.

TREATMENT OF DISK HERNIATION

The concept of four major types of low back pain can be reiterated as follows: (1) mechanical, (2) discogenic-sciatic, (3) fibromyositic, and (4) psychogenic.

An algorithm* regarding the treatment of low back pain and with disk herniation can now be summarized (Fig. 11–29).

---

*Algorithm: any special method of solving a certain kind of problem. (Webster Dictionary)

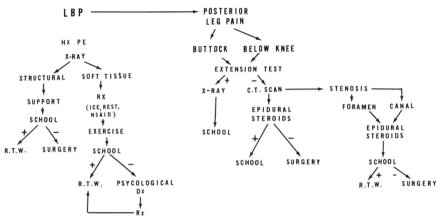

Figure 11–29. Algorithm of low back pain treatment.

With a suspected disk herniation, be it intrinsic nuclear herniation with an annular bulge or a frank extrusion, it has been postulated that a different approach to the mere mechanical low back injury is warranted.

As stated, after the "extension provocative test" has been performed, the question of external extrusion has been, to a degree, substantiated.

If there is no external extrusion suspected, then a period of extension position (not extension exercises) is initiated for several weeks. The period remains unconfirmed as the exact time it takes for any annular insult to heal is unknown. It is accepted that collagen fibers heal best with gentle compression and by gentle elongation. The disk hydrates best, as does cartilage, by gentle repetitive compression and relaxation; thus, within a reasonable time gentle exercises can be started.

Stressful flexion exercises are best deferred and isometric abdominal contractions suffice. Full flexion also needs to be curtailed. Walking is an excellent exercise, providing it is done with the entire body and gradually increased.

The School for **low back training** should be mandatory to teach the person the **proper** way of bending, lifting, pushing, and pulling, including all aspects of activities of daily living. Daily practice to ultimately make these functions **normal habit** will ensure proper function. Anxiety and stress should also be a School agenda and put into practice.

Exercises also play a vital role in which isometric low back extensor exercises gradually progressing to isometric strengthening exercises are advocated. Gentle hamstring stretch is also desirable **provided that the posterior leg stretch pain is muscular and not dural**. Stretching an inflamed dural sheath of a nerve root is counterproductive.

Strengthening of all the other muscles of the body is valuable as by so doing the general conditioning—both physical and psychological—is enhanced. Exercising the larger muscles of the extremities also has been reported to enhance the production of endorphins—a valuable asset in the person with low back pain.

As the dural sheath, as well as the posterior longitudinal ligament, may be inflamed resulting in pain and reflex muscular contraction, the use of anti-inflammatory medication is valuable. Even the use of epidural injection of steroids has its advocates as well as its opponents.

Pelvic traction has been advocated in the treatment of the bulging and/or herniated disk, but its physiologic basis and clinical value are far from totally accepted. The value of traction assumedly decreases the lordosis, elongates the spinal canal, and overcomes the erector spinae spasm. There have been reports that the intervertebral disk spaces also become elongated, but this effect on the dynamics of the disk are yet to be confirmed.

If there is a definite disk herniation with neurologic deficit that does not respond to conservative management within 3 months, surgical intervention has been recommended and justified (Weber).

The decision to intervene surgically mandates, however, that there is clear **objective** evidence of nerve root involvement consistent with the clinical findings and complaints, that the confirmatory tests are also precisely related, and **that the patient's psychological status is not a contraindication.** Waddell (1984) has clearly indicated that if pain persists for more than 3 months, the psychological make-up of the patient changes and complete "recovery" is impaired.

NEUROGENIC BLADDER
(CAUDA EQUINA SYNDROME)

There are cases where a massive extrusion of an intervertebral disk results in a neurogenic bladder with sudden partial or complete loss of voluntary bladder function. This bladder function loss is bladder extrusion tone, sphincter function, and loss of bladder capacity sensation.

In young adults this disk extrusion is usually found above the level of L4-5, but in older people the extrusion may be at that level or, occasionally, lower.

There is a general agreement among surgeons that **urgent decompression is mandatory to prevent irreparable damage to ultimate bladder function.** The time factor for decompression of the cauda has actually been stated to be **within hours,** with 12 hours being maximum before permanent impairment results. There are contradictory reports claiming that as much as 3 months can pass before irreparable damage is done to the bladder innervation. The decision must be the surgeon's based on his or her experience.

Bladder function impairment must always be suspected in a person with neurogenic deficit considered to be from a herniated disk or any other possible cauda equinal encroachment. The history must always elicit whether the patient:

1. Has full awareness of bladder fullness;
2. Has the ability to initiate and sustain bladder evacuation;
3. Completely empties the bladder after micturition.

The standard neurologic examination of patients with symptoms of possible nerve root compression from a herniated disk consists of dermatomal and myotomal examination of the specific nerve root levels, limited trunk movement, and a positive SLR dural sign.

The sacral segments should also be a significant part of the neurologic examination. This consists of perianal sensation being tested as well as rectal tone from a digital insertion test.

Cystometric testing should be performed more frequently than it currently is. By cystometric testing, a larger number of patients will be found to have bladder neurogenic dysfunction. This will confirm neurologic deficit others missed and will prevent the residual bladder impairment that may result.

Cystometric testing is relatively simple:

1. The patient is asked to void and completely evacuate the bladder.
2. A catheter is then inserted and the residual urine measured.
3. The catheter is connected to a cystometer, which is adjusted to the level of the symphysis pubis.
4. Sterile water is then dripped into the bladder at the rate of 50 mL per minute. This water may be at room temperature or be iced.
5. The patient is asked to report when the sensation of "fullness" is noted. This "sensation" may be the desire to urinate, a "cramping" sensation, or actually be painful fullness.
6. The amount of water in the bladder is now noted. An amount of 500 mL is considered "normal." If the amount exceeds 500 mL, the bladder is considered to be hypotonic (having loss of normal tone) and to have impaired sensation (both are signs of neurogenic impairment).
7. While in the supine position, the patient is asked to void. The pressure is measured by the cystometer and recorded on a graph. If there is inadequate force expended and inadequate urine expelled, the test is repeated in the sitting or standing position.

The mechanism by which abnormal urinary bladder function is produced is not clear. There is clinical evidence that blockage of the spinal canal—in this case a herniated disk—results in bladder dysfunction. This occurs probably from a reflex neural mechanism via the caudal nerves descending the lower spinal canal.

On discovering abnormal bladder function, initiated by a careful history, and confirmed by examining the perianal sensation and confirming the impaired bladder function by a cystometric examination, a CT scan, MRI, or myelogram must immediately follow.

Again it must be stated that the decision as to when to surgically intervene is left to the experience of the consulting surgeon and the significance (extent) of the neural impairment of the bladder. If conservative treatment is initiated, periodic testing of bladder function (by cystometry) must ensue to ascertain whether the condition is persisting, ameliorating, or deteriorating. It must be remembered that prolonged nerve encoachment on the sacral nerves to the bladder often, if not usually, results in permanent bladder dysfunction.

SURGERY FOR THE HERNIATED LUMBAR DISK

The indications for surgery have been alluded to throughout the text, and a text of this nature is not intended to delve into the specifics of surgical techniques. There are numerous texts that deal with this subject, and they are constantly being upgraded. Each surgeon also develops a specific technique and procedure.

It is the hope, in fact, the responsibility, of the primary physician to refer the patient considered to need surgery or need a surgical opinion. The patient should be referred to a surgeon with excellent training and experience in the field of spine surgery. Not every orthopedic surgeon or neurosurgeon has specialized in spine surgery and thus should not be given the opportunity to operate because he or she is labelled a "surgeon."

There are numerous terms that are bandied about varying from laminectomy, diskectomy, laminotomy, fusion, chymopapaine injection, to foraminotomy. The usual surgical procedure for a herniated disk is a **nuclectomy**. In essence it is the nucleus that has extruded from its central position to protrude the annulus or that has extruded through the annular tear. It is the nucleus therefore that usually requires removal.

Laminotomy, a removal of a small portion of the lamina, is the approach to the disk. Laminectomy is the removal of the lamina—a procedure of its own. Facetectomy is removal of a portion or all the facet. Foraminotomy is widening of the orifice (diameter) of the foramen. Fusion is the consolidation of two adjacent bones (vertebrae) into one mass to prevent further movement.

There is further breakdown in technique now as to whether the exposure of the offending disk material should be grossly achieved by removal of bone or should be accomplished via a scope. The scope is an instrument that requires a small incision, and the entire procedure is done through this instrument.

The terms "micro" or "macro" have evolved to depict the extent of the procedure and with the intent of minimizing the amount of normal tissue invaded to accomplish the procedural intent. The final acceptance of this procedure as being the most effective and least traumatic remains to be confirmed.

MICROLUMBAR DISKECTOMY (MLD)

This form of surgical intervention for the herniated lumbar disk was introduced in the medical literature in 1978. This technique was devised and recommended for patients with a "virgin" lumbar anatomy and a current soft herniated lumbar disk herniation. "Virgin" meant that there had not been previous surgery or significant structural abnormality such as spinal or foraminal stenosis. It meant initially surgery as a treatment for **one** specific lumbar condition—a single soft disk herniation.

The advantages for this procedure are

1. Minimal skin incision.
2. No muscular incision, therefore, no muscle suturing at the close.
3. No lamina or facet structural surgical encroachment.
4. Minimal removal of ligamentum flavum.
5. No excessive loss of extradural fat tissue.
6. Direct visualization of the nerve root during the entire surgical procedure.
7. Dilation of the annulus rather than direct incision.
8. No curettement of the disk nucleus or annulus.
9. No electrocautery extradurally.
10. No foreign bodies remaining within the surgical site after termination of the procedure.

The technique of the MLD procedure can be summarized as follows:

1. A 1 inch incision at the desired intervertebral level.
2. Lateral reflexion of the fascia and muscle at the site of the herniated disk down to the lamina.
3. Insertion of a Williams microscopic lumbar diskectomy instrument (a Zeiss Opmi #1 surgical microscope), which follows the piercing of the ligamentum flavum. The facet is lateral to the incision and no lamina is removed.
4. The nerve root is identified and is gently retracted.
5. No extradural fat is removed and only the necessary coagulation of extradural vessels is performed.
6. The annulus fibrosus of the herniated disk level is visualized and tear identified. The annulus is penetrated by the blunt probe instrument.
7. The disk material causing the herniation is removed by repeated small evacuations of nuclear tissue with a microscopic instrument. The disk

space is **not** curetted. The material dissected is aspirated by the suction retractor.

8. The instrument is removed and the incision sutured.

Postoperative care permits possible discharge on the third day with the SLR test performed daily, and ambulation and bathroom privileges allowed. For 3 weeks postoperatively no car riding is permitted and gentle exercises are instituted. Vocational evaluation follows to determine what the person can expect vocationally. This procedure has proven effective in recent years.

REFERENCES

American Health Consultant Publication, Atlanta, Georgia, 1968, p. 1.

Anderson, KS and Sneppen, O: Comparative study of myelographic filling defects in root sheaths and operative findings in cases of suspected lumbar intervertebral disk herniation. Acta Orthop Scand 39:312, 1968.

Breig, A: Effect of biomechanical phenomenon on function of central nervous system. Acta Neurochir 26:345, 1972.

Breig, A and Marions, O: Biomechanics of the lumbosacral nerve roots. Acta Radiol 1:1141, 1963.

Charnley, J: Orthopaedic signs in the diagnosis of disk protrusion. Lancet 1:186, 1951.

Crock, HV: Practice of Spinal Surgery. Springer-Verlag, New York, 1983.

Dilke, TFW, Burry, HC and Grahame, R: Extradural corticosteroid injection in management of lumbar nerve root compression. Br Med 2:635, 1973.

Edgar, MA and Park, WM: Induced pain patterns on positive straight-leg raising in lower lumbar disk protrusion. J Bone Joint Surg 56-B:658, 1974.

Falconer, MA, McGeorge, M, and Begg, AC: Observations on the cause and mechanism of symptom production in sciatica and low back pain. J Neurol Neurosurg Psychiatry 11:13, 1948.

Farfan, HF: Mechanical Disorders of the Low Back. Lea & Febiger, Philadelphia, 1973, pp 63–92.

Farfan, HF, et al.: The effects of torsion on the lumbar intervertebral joints: The role of torsion in the production of disk degeneration. J Bone Joint Surg 52-A:468, 1970.

Fernstrom, V: Discographical study of ruptured lumbar intervertebral discs. Acta Chir Scand (Suppl) 258, 1960.

Fernstrom, V: Disk rupture with surgical observations. Acta Chir Scand (Suppl) 258, 1960.

Forst, JJ: Contribution a l'étude dexique de la sciatique. Paris Thèse, no. 33, 1881.

Froning, EC and Frohman, B: Motion of the lumbosacral spine after laminectomy and spine fusion. J Bone Joint Surg 50-A:897, 1968.

Geiger, LE: Fusion of vertebrae following resection of intervertebral disc. J Neurosurg 18:79, 1961.

Goald, HJ: Microlumbar diskectomy: Follow-up of 147 patients. Spine 3:183, 1978.

Goddard, MD, and Reid, JD: Movements induced by straight leg raising in the lumbo-sacral roots, nerve and plexus, and in the intrapelvic section of the sciatic nerve. J Neurol Neurosurg Psychiatry 28:12, 1965.

Goodgold, J and Eberstein, A: Electrodiagnosis of Neuromuscular Diseases. Williams & Wilkins, Baltimore, 1972, pp. 6, 164.

Gunn, CC, and Milbrandt, WE: Tenderness at motor points: a diagnostic and prognostic aid for low back injury. J Bone Joint Surg 58-A:815, 1976.

Hakelius, A, and Hindmarsh, J: The significance of neurological signs and myelographic findings in the diagnosis of lumbar root compression. Acta Orthop Scand 43:239, 1972.

Hakelius, A, and Hindmarsh, J: The comparative reliability of preoperative diagnostic methods in lumbar disc surgery. Acta Orthop Scand 43:234, 1972.

Hause, FB and O'Connor, SJ: Specific management for lumbar and sacral radiculitis. JAMA 166:1285, 1958.

Herschensohn, HL: Disability of the back in industrial workers. Cal Med 92:31, 1960.

Hirsch, C: Efficiency of surgery in low back disorders. J Bone Joint Surg 47-A(5):991, 1965.

Inman, VT, et al.: Referred pain from experimental irritative lesions, in Studies Relating to Pain in the Amputee, Series II, Issue 23, June 1952, pp. 49–78.

Inman, VT and Saunders, JB: The clinico-anatomic aspect of the lumbosacral region. Radiology 38:669, 1942.

Kao, FF and Kao, JJ: Acupuncture Therapeutics. Eastern Press, New Haven, 1973.

Kirgis, HD, and Llewellyn, RC: Diagnosis and treatment of injuries to the lumbar intervertebral disc of industrial workers. J South Med Assoc 52:895, 1959.

Knuttson, B: Electromyographic studies in the diagnosis of lumbar disc herniation. Acta Orthop Scand 28:290, 1959.

Kopp, JR: The use of lumbar extension in the evaluation and treatment of patients with acute herniated nuclear pulposis. Clinical Orthopaedics 202:211, 1986.

Krusen, EM and Ford, DE: Compensation factor in low back injuries. JAMA 166:10, 1958.

Lindahl, O: Hyperalgesia of the lumbar nerve roots in sciatica. Acta Orthop Scand 37:367, 1966.

Lindahl, O and Rexed, B: Histologic changes in spinal nerve roots of operated cases of sciatica. Acta Orthop Scand 20:215, 1951.

Maigne, R: Orthopedic Medicine: A New Approach to Vertebral Manipulation. Charles C Thomas, Springfield, IL, 1972.

Maroon, J: Percutaneous diskectomy rated "safe" in clinical trials. Back Pain Monitor 4:33, 1987.

Mathews, JA: Dynamic discography: A study of lumbar traction. Ann Phys Med 9:275, 1968.

McCarron, RF, Wimpee, MW, Hudkins, PG, and Laros, GS: The Inflammatory Effect of Nucleus Pulposus. A Possible Element in the Pathogenesis of Low Back Pain. Spine, Vol. 12, Number 8, 1987, 760–764.

McKenzie, RA: Manual correction of sciatic scoliosis. NZ Med J 76:194, 1972.

McKenzie, RA: The lumbar spine: Mechanical Diagnosis and Therapy. Waikanae, New Zealand Spinal Publications, 1981.

MacNab, I: The Mechanism of Spondylogenic Pain in Cervical Pain. Edited by C. Hirsch and Y Zoherman. Oxford, Pergamon Press, 1971, pp 89–95.

McNab, I: Chemonucleolysis. Clin. Neurosurg. 20:183, 1973.

McNab, I, Cuthbert, H, and Godfred, CM: The incidence of denervation of the sacrospinalis muscles following spinal surgery. Spine 2:294, 1977.

Melzack, R, Stillwell, DM, and Fox, EJ: Trigger points and acupuncture points for pain correlation and implication. Pain 3:3, 1977.

Mensor, MC: Non-operative treatment, including manipulation, for lumbar intervertebral disc syndrome. J Bone Joint Surg 37-A:925, 1955.

Nachemson, A: The influence of spinal movement on the lumbar intradiscal pressure and on the tensile stresses in the annulus fibrosis. Acta Orthop Scand 33:3, 1963.

Nachemson, AL: The lumber spine: An orthopedic challenge, Spine 1:59, 1976.

Nachemson, A, and Morris, JM: In vivo measurement of intradiskal pressure. J Bone Joint Surg 46-A:1077, 1964.

Nachemson, A and Elfstrom, G: Intradiskal dynamic pressure measurements in lumbar discs. Scand J Rehab Med Suppl. 1, 1970.

Newton, MJ and Lehmkul, D: Muscle spindle response to body heating and localized muscle cooling. J Am Phys Ther Assoc 45:91, 1965.

Oudenhoven, RC: Paraspinal electromyography following facet rhizotomy. Spine 2:299, 1977.

Rosomoff, HL, et al.: Ceptometry in the evaluation of nerve root compression in the lumbar spine. Surg Gynecol Obstet 117:263, 1963.

Rosomoff, HL, et al.: Cystometry as an adjunct in the evaluation of lumbar disk syndromes. J Neurosurg 33:67, 1970.

Scott, JC: Stress factor in the disc syndrome. J Bone Joint Surg 37-B:107, 1955.

See, DH and Kraft, GH: Electromyography in paraspinal muscles following surgery for root compression. Arch Phys Med Rehab 56:80, 1975.

Smith, L and Brown, JE: Treatment of lumbar intervertebral disc lesions by direct injection of chymopapain. J Bone Joint Surg 49-B(3):502, 1967.

Smyth, M and Wright, V: Sciatica and the intervertebral disc. J Bone Joint Surg 40-A:1401, 1955.

Snoek, W, Weber, H, and Jorgensen, B: Double-blind evaluation of extradural methyl prednisone for herniated lumbar disc. Acta Orthop Scand 48:635, 1977.

Spangfort, EV: The lumbar disc herniation: A computer-aided analysis of 2504 operations. Acta Orthop Scand (Suppl.) 142:1, 1972.

Taylor, TKF and Weiner, M: Great toe extension reflex in the diagnosis of lumbar disc disorder. Br Med J 2:487, 1969.

Travel, J and Rinzler, SH: The myofascial genesis of pain. Postgrad Med 11:425, 1952.

Waddell, G, et al.: Chronic low back pain, psychological distress and illness behavior. Spine 9:209, 1984.

Weber, H: Lumbar disc herniation: Part I. J Oslo City Hosp 28:33, 1978.

Weber, H: Lumbar disc herniation: Part II. J Oslo City Hosp 28:89, 1983.

Weber, H: Lumbar disc herniation: A controlled prospective study with ten years of observation. Spine 2:131, 1983.

Wiberg, G: Back pain in relation to the nerve supply of the intervertebral disc. Acta Orthop Scand 19:211, 1949.

Wiesel, SW, et al: Effectiveness of epidural steroids in the treatment of sciatica: A double blind clinical trial. The International Society for the Study of the Lumbar Spine, Toronto, 1985.

Williams, PC: The Lumbosacral Spine: Emphasizing Conservative Management. McGraw-Hill Book, New York, 1965.

Williams, RW: Microlumbar diskectomy: Conservative surgical approach to the virgin herniated lumbar disk. Spine 3:175, 1978.

Williams, RW: Microlumbar discectomy: A 12-year statistical review. Spine 11:851, 1986.

Wilson, JC: Low back pain and sciatica. JAMA 200:129, 1967.

Wiltse, LL, Widell, EH, and Yuan, HA: Chymopapain chemonucleolysis in lumbar disc disease. JAMA 231:474, 1975.

Woodhall, B and Hayes, GJ: The well leg-raising test of Fajersztain in the diagnosis of ruptured lumbar intervertebral disk. J Bone Joint Surg 32-A:786, 1950.

Yoshizawa, H, O'Brien, JP, Smith, WT, and Trumper, M: The neuropathology of intervertebral disks removed for low back pain. J Pathol, 132:95, 1980.

CHAPTER 12

Degenerative Disk Disease: Developmental and Acquired

The integrity of the functional unit depends on the adequacy of the intervertebral disk. In the anterior weight-bearing portion of the functional unit the hydrodynamic properties of the disk maintain the separation of the two adjacent vertebrae. The portion of the disk that accomplishes this function is primarily the nucleus, but it also demands integrity of the annular fibers.

With full function of the hydrodynamics of the disk and thus separation of the vertebrae, the spine is elongated, the longitudinal ligaments are kept taut, and the posterior zygapophyseal joints are kept separated. The intervertebral foraminal openings are maintained, the ligamentum flavum is elongated, and the annular fibers are kept under tension. The functional unit is in a state of balance.

Flexibility of the functional unit requires competence of all these component elements: the ligaments, the facet capsules, and the erector spinae muscles. The disk annular fibers also maintain flexibility before failure occurs and this failure exists primarily with excessive rotation.

Degeneration of the disk is expected of all humans as a matter of "normal" attrition. Püschel (1930) claimed that by the age of 20, the disk has reached maximum development and degeneration begins to be noted.

The mucopolysaccharides undergo attritional chemical changes. A change occurs in the water-binding capability of the matrix. Naylor (1979) has expounded a degradation of protein polysaccharides with resynthesis of these polysaccharides to a lower level with an increase in the imbibition capability. This increased imbibition capability allows the disk to "swell" as well as to deteriorate.

252

The annular fibers comprised of collagen fibers enmeshed within a matrix undergo fibrillation. These altered fibers lose their integrity and decrease flexibility, which enhances the possibility of failure. External physical forces enhance these changes and increase the rate and extent of "failure." Annular tears that occur allow a loss of dynamic balance controlling the nuclear forces.

Tears in the collagen container appear early in the border between the nucleus and the cartilaginous vertebral plates. These tears gradually extend toward the center of the nucleus. These tears are enhanced by the trauma of everyday activities.

Initially the "tears" are concentric and resemble a separation of parallel collagen fibers (Fig. 12–1A).

Gradually the intradiskal pressure causes radial tears within the annulus (Fig. 12–1B).

As the tears progress and the mucopolysaccharides degrade, the fluid balance is impaired. With less hydrodynamic support, there is abnormal movement. The vertebral endplates approximate Figure 12–2. More shear is permitted of adjacent vertebrae. From prolonged trunk flexion, "creep" occurs between vertebrae and further degeneration results.

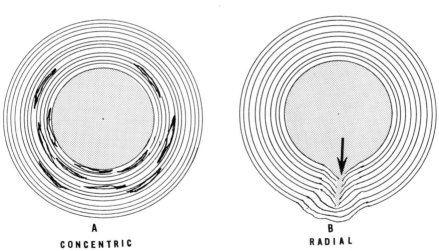

A
CONCENTRIC

B
RADIAL

Figure 12–1. Annular changes in the degenerating disk. A reveals concentric tears in the annulus that are first noted at age 15. They originate near the nucleus and are at first discrete. As the patient ages, they are found in greater number in the outer margin and tend to merge into larger tears. B depicts radial tears. These too begin centrally and proceed outward. They are more numerous in the posterior portion of the disk. The pressure of the disk matrix pushes the torn fiber margins outward. When they reach the outer margin they "bulge" and deform the disk.

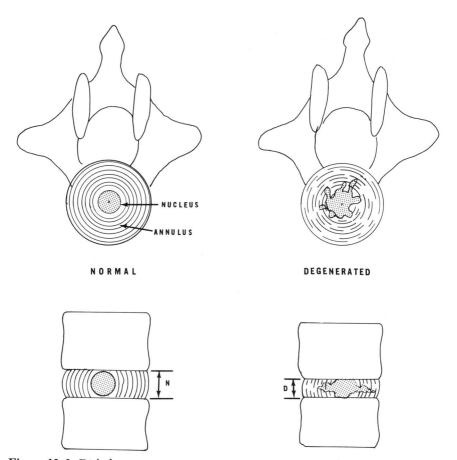

Figure 12–2. Disk degeneration. *Left*, Normal disk with intact nucleus and annular fibers. The space is normal (N). *Right*, Degenerated disk with the nucleus outside its boundary and fragmented annular fibers and narrowed space (D).

The normal growing spine allows the intervertebral disks to develop into their contours to form the lordosis of the lumbar spine. Once fully developed, maintenance occurs from as yet unknown sources: chemical, nutritional, hormonal, and mechanical. Which of these factors contributes to which aspect of degeneration remains unknown. Heredity also probably contributes to degenerative changes as some degeneration has been noted in the disks of 20-year-old individuals. There does not seem to be any sex variation and varying occupational forces are being studied.

The greatest degree (75 percent) of disk degeneration is noted at lumbar 4-5 and L5-S1. This may be because it is at this level that there is the greatest degree of angulation and the greatest degree of normal movement.

As the anterior weight-bearing portion of the functional unit narrows (i.e., there is approximation of the adjacent vertebral endplates) due to disk dehydration, the posterior joints (the zygapophyseal or facet) also approximate. These posterior joints are now exposed to attritional changes by abnormal weight-bearing and shear forces.

These attritional changes are capsular thickening, cartilage degeneration from fibrillation and microscopic fissures, and invasion into the cartilage of fibrous repair tissue. There are numerous unmyelinated nerve fibers of the thickened capsule and within the invading fibrous tissue that can transmit pain. The denuded bone, normally covered by cartilage but now exposed, also is supplied by sensory nerve fibers. The posterior facet joints now restrict movements and are capable of transmitting painful nociceptive impulses.

All these changes—in the disk, the ligaments, of the foramina, of the facet capsules and facet cartilage—are gradual and lead to a condition that has been termed **spondylosis** (Fig. 12–3).

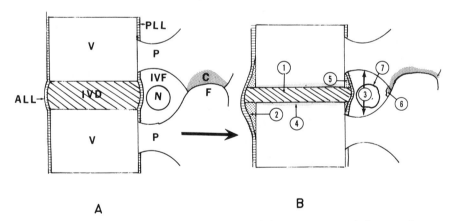

Figure 12–3. Sequence of degeneration: spondylosis. *A*, Normal functional unit: V = vertebral body; IVD = intervertebral disk; ALL = anterior longitudinal ligament; PLL = posterior longitudinal ligament; P = pedicle; N = nerve; IVF = intervertebral foramen; F = facet; and C = cartilage. *B*, Disk (1) degenerates; longitudinal ligament (2) slackens and pulls away from vertebral body; foramen (3) narrows; cartilaginous endplates (4) show sclerotic changes; posterior spurs or osteophytes (5) begin to form; degenerating cartilaginous changes (6) occur in facets; foraminal stenosis appears (7), leading to nerve root compression.

SPONDYLOSIS

This term is synonymous with the accepted term degenerative osteoarthritis. In the spine it is a sequela of disk degeneration. The ultimate degenerative changes within the posterior facet joints are more consistent with the concept of degenerative arthritis, but there are concurrent changes that occur within the adjacent vertebrae of the anterior portion of the functional unit.

In the intact functional unit, the intrinsic pressure within the disk—both nucleus and annulus—keeps the adjacent vertebral bodies separated. The longitudinal ligaments and the intervertebral annular fibers are kept taut. A pressure gradient is maintained.

As the intrinsic pressure within the disk is upset by the impaired imbibitory quality of the mucopolysaccharide of the disk, the tension on the longitudinal ligaments is diminished. The intrinsic pressure, within the disk, persists and causes the now slacker ligaments to avulse from their periosteal attachments to the vertebral bodies (Fig. 12–4).

The nuclear matrix now can extrude from between the vertebral endplates into the space between the detached longitudinal ligaments and the periosteum. The "raw" area of the vertebral periosteum now can undergo inflammatory changes. Invasion of this region is by hemorrhage and fibrous tissue. There is also extruded nuclear material.

At first this extruded material that has dissected the longitudinal ligament from its periosteal vertebral attachment forms a "soft" spurlike tumor. As calcification of this tumor occurs, the tumor, now calcified, becomes an osteoarthritis "spur."

At first during the evolution of this "spur" formation the long ligaments is kept taut and allows no "instability" of the unit. As changes occur within the disk and within the long ligaments, this stability is jeopardized and excessive abnormal movement is permitted.

These "spurs" encroach within the foramina and lead to **foraminal stenosis**. In conjunction with these posterior exostoses of the vertebral bodies (spurs), the cartilaginous degenerative changes of the zygapophyseal joints also create degenerative osteoarthritic changes. They also encroach upon the foramina (Fig. 12–5).

Before a meaningful discussion can be had regarding the pathology that is caused by encroachment into the intervertebral foramen, a simplification of the contents of the foramen is indicated.

The foramen (lumbosacral lateral foramen) is an oblique irregularly ovoid-shaped canal approximately 3 to 5 cm in length. It traverses between two adjacent vertebrae forming a functional unit. It is formed by two adjacent laminae and bounded by the vertebrae anteriorly and the facet joints posteriorly.

The canal (foramen) has three distinct zones with varying neural con-

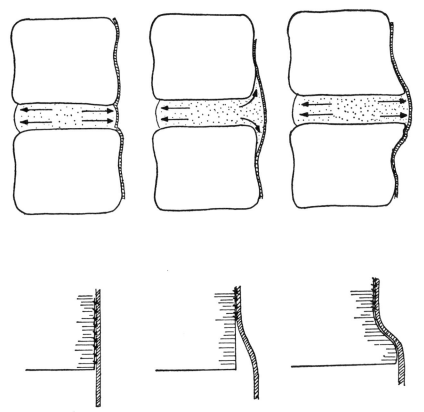

Figure 12–4. Mechanism of spondylosis. *Left,* The normal anterior portion of the functional unit with an intact disk, normal interspace, and a taut posterior longitudinal ligament that is totally adherent to the vertebral body periosteum. *Center,* Disk degeneration permits approximation of the two vertebrae, causing a slack in the posterior longitudinal ligament, and intradiskal pressure permits dissection between periosteum and ligament. *Right,* The extruded disk material becomes fibrous, then ultimately calcifies into what becomes a "spur."

tents that have clinical significance. The entrance zone (1) is under the inferior facet of the superior vertebra (L5, for instance, in the functional unit L5-S1). In this foramen the nerve roots are ensheathed in the dural (arachnoid). It has been ascertained that it is the dura that is sensitive and not the nerve roots. The dura is supplied by the recurrent nerve of Luschka (Fig. 12–6).

The middle region of the canal is bounded by the pars interarticularis (of the lamina). In this zone, the nerve roots are not enclosed within a dura and thus not suspended in cerebrospinal fluid. Any enlargement of the pars from degenerative "arthritic" changes can entrap the nerve roots. The re-

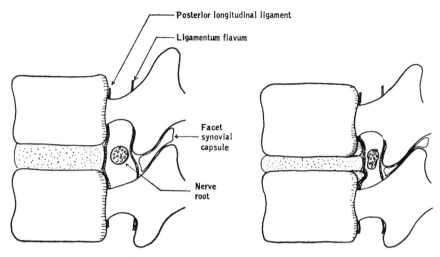

Figure 12–5. Intervertebral foraminal impingement in disk degeneration and spondylosis. The drawing at left shows the normal relationship of two vertebrae adequately separated by a normal disk. The foramen is open and the merging nerve root free. The drawing at right depicts the foraminal narrowing due to osteophyte impingement and posterior articular closure with synovial irritation. Movement is obviously restricted, and further nerve root pinch can be pictured by extension of this functional unit.

current meningeal nerve is contained therein, as are sympathetic nerve fibers. Encroachment on these nerves can cause paresthesias in their dermatomal distribution.

The outer zone of the funnel contains the division of the nerve root into the posterior and anterior primary divisions. The sinuvertebral recurrent nerve (R) is also contained within this zone. The superior facet of the inferior vertebra (S1 of the L5-S1 functional unit as an example) can encroach on the nerve fibers when there is hypertrophy or subluxation. The latter (subluxation) occurs when the anterior intervertebral space narrows from disk degeneration.

These pathologic changes are evolutionary and potentially progressive. They can be symptomatic or be merely radiologically perceived and yet not symptom producing.

Clinically there are symptoms that are attributed to these spondylitis changes. Which tissues are involved signifies which symptoms will be evoked. If the tissue of the functional units involves the facets or the posterior longitudinal ligaments, they are precise. If they involve the contents of the foramen they are also unique.

The symptoms of spondylosis, per se, can be enumerated as follows:

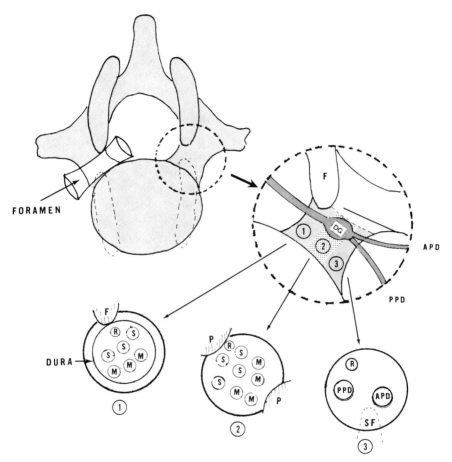

Figure 12–6. Contents of intervertebral foramen. The foramen is depicted in the upper figure as a funnel-shaped opening. The length of the canal is 3 to 5 centimeters. In the enlarged foramen on the circled area the canal is divided into three portions: the inner area (*1*), the middle (*2*), and the outer (*3*). The sensory (*S*) and motor (*M*) nerve root fibers with the dorsal ganglion (*DG*) are shown.

The inferior facet of the superior vertebra (*F*) encroaches into area (*1*) and when there are degenerative changes the facet may encroach upon the nerve roots and the dura (arachnoid). In the middle segment (*2*) there is no dural sheath but the pars (*P*) of the lamina line the canal. Degenerative changes of the pars can narrow the foramen in which is located the dorsal ganglion (*DG*). The outer segment (*3*) contains the posterior (*PPD*) and anterior (*APD*) primary divisions of the nerve root. The superior facet of the inferior vertebra (*SF*) can encroach upon these divisions when subluxed or enlarged.

1. Early morning stiffness. This is a feeling of lack of flexibility that gradually improves with local application of heat and gradual flexibility exercises.

2. Generalized low back "aching" with a sensation that, from prolonged inactivity, such as sitting too long, the low back loses flexibility. This is termed by patients as "freezing" or "jelling."

3. A limitation of movement either in bending over, twisting, or turning is noted.

4. A certain degree of relief is noted from local heat and from the ingestion of a salicylate.

Disk degeneration with root radicular pain or symptoms is a chronic, slightly progressive condition in which physical findings are sparse. The symptoms are related to the position and to specific movements and depend on which zone of the foramen is involved.

Generally, in patients suffering from spondylosis, there is noted poor general conditioning, poor muscle tone, excessive "flabbiness," poor posture, and limited flexibility.

There are many, however, who, between acute attacks, do not exhibit these findings and, in fact, are very active, flexible, and pain free. An "attack" may occur which transiently restricts their activities. What precipitates these "attacks" remains unanswered with statements such as cold damp weather, excessive physical stress, and acute emotional stress being causative.

Of greater importance, however, is **what movement** and **what position** causes which symptoms, which in turn indicates the nerve tissue involved and the site of the involvement. The movement and the position of the patient that had been determined to initiate the symptom, indicates the cause.

A condition termed "tropism" evolved to explain the spinal condition of a segmental asymmetrical scoliosis from assymmetrical disk degeneration. This scoliosis is usually found in the lower lumbar segments L5-S1 or L4-5.

By this segmental scoliosis, normal functional mechanics are impaired. The facets are "off center" and weight-bearing is not equally borne on the anterior intervertebral disk and the two posterior facets. The "tripod" weight bearing is impaired.

As flexion and extension occur, the concave element of this asymmetrical tripod (usually the facet on the concave side) becomes the point of rotation and torque forces evolve (Fig. 12–7). The approximated facet on the concave side may "lock." The separated facet on the convex side may excessively "sublux," and the annular fibers are subjected to excessive rotatory torques and can undergo some failure.

Clinically, the patient describes the movement that precipitated this situation. The spine assumes an acute scoliosis and limited motion. Flexion

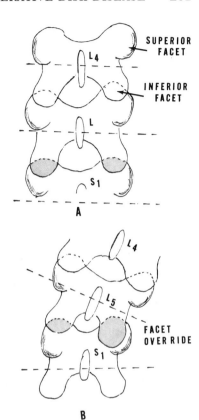

Figure 12–7. Tropism of lumbosacral spine. The term tropism has been applied to asymmetry of weight bearing and alignment of the lumbosacral articulation. With this asymmetry the vertebral bodies may be malaligned and the facet relationship also asymmetrical. Figure A depicts the normal alignment. In B, L_4 is off to one side with the disk having unequal thickness and the lower L_5 facet overriding the ipsilateral superior S_1 facet. It becomes apparent that static weight bearing poses unequal stress and that movement along facet alignment is unbalanced.

is limited and extension is painful. Pain is especially produced by extension with **simultaneous lateral flexion toward the concave side**. This motion obviously approximates the inflamed facets on that concave side. There is tenderness on deep digital pressure over the lower facet joint.

X-rays reveal this tropism. The segmental disk is narrowed irregularly. The segmental scoliosis is seen on A-P views, and on oblique views there is noted asymmetrical facet degeneration.

Treatment is to relieve the acute pain and to prevent or minimize recurrences. Local ice for 24 hours followed by deep heat is beneficial. Oral anti-inflammatory nonsteroidal medication for a few days affords relief. This is a condition that may be benefitted by gentle flexion rotatory manipulation **in the opposite direction of the concavity**. Deep local injections of an anesthetic agent and soluble steroid also may help.

Prevention of recurrence is difficult because the problem is anatomically mechanical. Here "Back School" principles offer the best remedy. Informing the susceptible person of "how" the spine normally functions and how this segmental scoliosis prevents normal motion is instructional. Explanation of the mechanical encroachment on pain-sensitive tissue of the functional unit helps the patient understand the reason for the necessary position and movement. Proper bending but, more important, proper re-extension to the erect posture, is mandatory. Instituting this proper body function in everyday activities is obviously important. Lateral flexibility exercises **away** from the concavity are beneficial.

DISK DEGENERATION (TROPISM) WITH ROOT IRRITATION

Many patients with disk degeneration experience radicular symptoms. This "sciatica" is veritably root entrapment, but from foraminal stenosis rather than from the protrusion or extrusion of nuclear material.

The foraminal narrowing has been described above. The nerve root, therefore, emerges through a narrowed foramen. Any further closure of the foramen, be it acute, recurrent, or chronic closure, further entraps the nerve root.

This closure is a body function such as acute extension of the low back from lifting an object over the head. Bending over in a twisting manner and returning improperly can cause an acute closure of the concave side and an entrapment of the nerve root. Any maneuver that initiates the occurrence of sciatica can be elicited from a precise history.

The findings are the history of radicular pain after an activity. The pain is a paresthesia into the lower leg, into the calf, or at least below the knee if S1 is involved. Often the radicular pain is only into the buttocks area. Neurologic findings are usually not present, with the sensory root symptoms predominant.

The radicular symptoms are reproducible by extension and lateral flexion of the low back and relief from flexion and simultaneous lateral flexion in the contralateral direction. The x-rays are as described above, but with lateralization of the foraminal closure on the clinically ascertained side.

Treatment is that of brief general rest in a comfortable position. This position is determined by the position assumed that relieves the severe symptoms—usually flexion and lateral flexion **away** from the involved side. Oral anti-inflammatory medication, local ice followed by deep heat, and gentle manipulation in the **opposite** direction may minimize the duration of the condition. Local deep injections into the facet region are beneficial. Prevention of recurrence is as the same condition of spondylosis without radicular symptoms.

In this condition, the proper exercise is that of flexion and avoidance of lumbar extension. In the flexed position the foramina are opened and the nerve roots given more space. Strong abdominal muscles benefit this lumbar kyphotic posture. Instruction in activities of daily living ("Back School") to avoid or minimize lumbar lordosis and proper re-extension from the flexed position in bending over and lifting are essential.

In the presence of severe and persistent symptoms and with continued neurologic deficit, surgical intervention (foraminotomy), once the condition has been confirmed by CT scan, MRI, or myelography, may be needed. As noted in the **contents of the intervertebral foramen,** any surgical invasion must be cognizant of the contents at each zone. The middle zone, wherein the dorsal ganglion is contained, requires careful observation, when opening the foramen is considered, that the dorsal root is not injured.

SPINAL STENOSIS

The condition of **spinal stenosis** was initially described by Verbiest (1954) as an anatomic variation that leads to specific neurologic symptoms. The diagnosis of spinal stenosis is being made with increasing frequency and variants of this condition are also evolving. There is now frequent diagnosis of foraminal stenosis and hypertrophic superior facet syndrome and others—all examples of stenosis of one of the canals, be it spinal canal or intervertebral foramen.

Initially the depth of the canal that constituted "narrowing" was an anterior-posterior measurement. Various figures were considered as evidence of stenosis: 12 mm (Verbiest, 1954), 14 mm (van der Heiden and Vinken, 1952) and 15 mm (Epstein, 1962). More recently, the lateral width of the spinal canal has been studied and related to symptomatology, especially with encroachment of the mouth of the intervertebral foramen.

There are numerous causes proclaimed as leading to and causing stenosis varying into two major categories: congenital (developmental) and acquired. The congenital is subdivided into idiopathic or achondroplastic. The acquired varies from spondylolisthetic (with pars interarticularis defect to secondary from degenerative disk disease) and iatrogenic such as postdiskectomy; surgical or chymopapase; post-fusion; or metabolic bone disease, such as Paget's.

The clinical picture that alerts the physician to the possibility of stenosis is the presence of paresthesias of one or both legs occurring after a period or distance of walking or after a period of standing. This picture is further suggested by the statement that the symptoms subside or disappear after sitting or bending forward, not merely by stopping walking such as occurs in arterial claudication. This factor is responsible for the diagnostic term "pseudoclaudication" or neurogenic claudication.

The factors that lead to "neurologic claudication" as a result of ischemia to the emergent nerve root are postulated on the following:

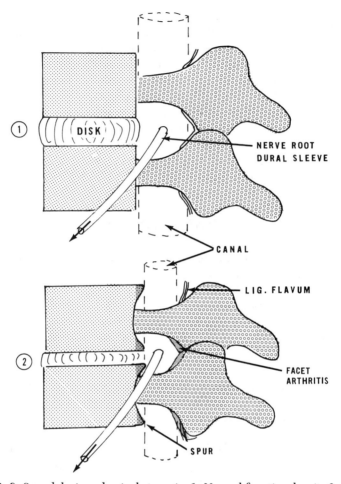

Figure 12–8. Spondylosis and spinal stenosis. *1*, Normal functional unit. *2*, Narrowing of intervertebral disk, approximation of adjacent pedicles, spur formation, facet arthritis with resultant narrowing of spinal canal (*broken lines*) and the intervertebral foramen.

1. Exercise of the legs normally causes an increase in venous capacity (dilation) of the veins that accompany the nerve roots as they emerge into the foraminal gutters.

2. If there is compression of the nerves within the foramina, the arterial supply is limited by compression of the venous return.

3. The compression of the content of the foraminae is from several factors:

      (a) In lumbar lordosis the length of the canal is shorter than in lumbar kyphosis.

(b) The canal also shortened by disk degeneration at several levels causes the cauda equina to "bunch up" causing constriction.

(c) The foramen is already narrowed by anterior osteophytes, posterior exostosis of the foramen (Fig. 12–8), and a bunching up of the ligamentum flavum or from a hypertrophic superior facet of the inferior vertebra (Fig. 12–9).

(d) In extension of the lumbar spine the foramen are mechanically normally narrowed.

The claudication therefore caused by walking or by standing with a lordotic curve understandably results in nerve root ischemia and symptomatic claudication. Sitting flexed forward or standing flexed forward causes a lumbar kyphosis and the following results:

1. The canal lengthens.
2. The caudal equinal fibers elongate.
3. The facets separate and the foraminae open.
4. Venous capacity returns and blood flow to the nerve returns.

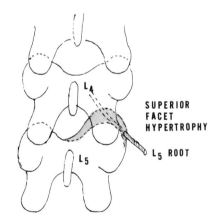

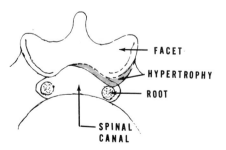

Figure 12–9. Foraminal stenosis: hypertrophy superior facet. *Top,* Posterior view of the L₄–L₅ functional units with hypertrophy of the right superior facet and widening of the lateral portion of the lamina that encroaches upon the foramen. The L₅ nerve root is extended, making it more vulnerable to compression and traction injury. *Bottom,* View from above showing how the enlarged facet forces the nerve root to be extended and actually compressed. The spinal canal opening is also evidently more shallow and may compress the thecal sac.

Other factors play a role in causing stenotic symptoms of the foramen-contained nerve roots. It is accepted that standing on one leg causes unequal pressure on the lower disks with compression on the side toward which a person leans. In essence, leaning to the left causes the disks to compress on the left side.

A normal disk increases its radius by 8 percent from merely standing on one leg with the lateral "bulge" to that side. If a disk is degenerated, the increase in radius may reach 30 to 35 percent with a greater bulge into the foramen. As we stand or walk, these bulges occur rhythmically with our gait. It also is apparent that normal walk causes alternate lordosis and kyphosis as we go through swing phase and alternately bear our weight in the stance phase. This alternate lateral bulging during walking contributes to foraminal compression by the disk on the nerve roots that already are within a constricted gutter.

If there is a disk bulge, be it an annular bulge from a nuclear extrusion or an extrusion of nuclear material out of the annulus, this protrusion into the foraminal gutter further causes ischemia of the nerve roots.

DIAGNOSIS

The diagnosis of neurogenic claudication from spinal stenosis thus is made when a patient complains of paresthesias of either one or both legs after a period of walking or a period of standing. Relief of these leg symptoms comes from leaning forward or sitting in a flexed position. The symptoms again recur from a period of walking or standing in a lordotic posture.

Neurogenic bladder symptoms frequently occur in spinal stenosis but are subtle and need to be considered so that the proper questions are asked and evaluated. These symptoms may not have concerned the patient. They include difficulty in maintaining the stream in the standing position (man) and greater ease of evacuation in sitting. External abdominal pressure may be used to completely empty the bladder (Credé maneuver). The symptoms of "frequent," urgent, and incomplete urination are pathognomonic. Dribbling and soiling may exist. Retention of residual urine leads to possible infection with enhancement of the symptoms of frequency and urgency.

Suspicion and ultimate confirmation of a neurogenic bladder require the consistent history, the possibility of rectal atonus on digital examination, possible perianal hypalgesia, and a confirmatory abnormal cystometrogram. This latter test has been previously discussed.

The specific diagnostic confirmation of spinal stenosis, whether it is the cause of the neurogenic bladder or the cause of neurogenic claudication symptoms, is confirmed by CT scan, MRI, or myelography. These diagnostic tests also assist in determining the type, the extent, and the tissue type involved, be it an enlarged lamina, herniated disk with a congenital predisposing narrow canal, or spondylolisthesis (Fig. 12–10).

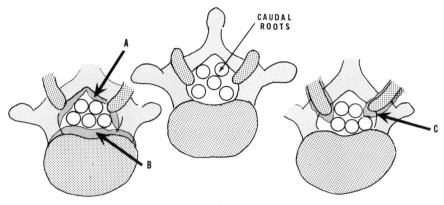

Figure 12–10. Spinal stenosis. The central drawing depicts a normal canal with adequate space for the cauda equina. The drawing at *left* reveals encroachment from changes in the neural arch (A) and vertebral body osteophytes. The drawing at *right* reveals degenerative arthritic changes of facets. Usually all factors have involvement in canal stenosis.

It may seem redundant to state that vascular (arterial) claudication rather than neurogenic claudication must be ruled out, but, in consideration of completeness of differential diagnosis, these differences are enumerated in Table 12–1.

TREATMENT

Nonoperative treatment should be undertaken before resorting to surgical intervention. This obviously applies when the symptoms are not too severe or are not causing progressive organic neurogenic impairment.

As the vast majority of patients increase the stenosis of the spinal canal with lumbar extension, this exercise, position, and posture must be prevented in activities of daily living. Pelvic tilting exercises of the William's protocol are, in this case, indicated and the extension protocol of MacKenzie avoided. Lying prone must be avoided. Strong abdominal muscles, especially the obliques, are to be fostered. Prolonged excessive flexion should also be avoided as it can cause tension on the caudal roots.

When there are urinary symptoms, the Credé method of evacuation must be taught and used. Occasional catheterization is diagnostic and therapeutic if a significant residual is encountered.

Oral steroids and then epidural steroids have their advocates and may help. Pelvic and gravity traction has value, albeit transient. Curtailment of walking distances is self-evident and will be decided by the symptoms felt by the patient. This test, however, recorded by the patient, details and re-

Table 12–1. DIFFERENTIAL DIAGNOSIS

	Aortoiliac Occlusive Vascular Disease	Pseudoclaudication/Spinal Stenosis
Pain site:	Hips, thighs, and buttocks-progress to calf (or in reverse direction)	Lumbar spine and buttocks Pain may occur from prolonged standing or lying with back "arched."
Onset:	After walking a long distance	After walking up inclines
Pain description:	Aching, squeezing, cramping quality increases with walking. Rarely paresthesias or "weakness"	Onset may be tingling, weakness, or clumsiness. "Pain" may be minimal, often numbness or burning, not "cramping."
Relief:	Fast relief by ceasing to walk. Slowing walk decreases onset or severity.	Must sit down and assume flexed trunk posture.
Impotence:	Frequent	May take 20 to 30 minutes for relief
Peripheral pulses:	May disappear after walking Loud bruits, frequently pale legs after walking, no neurologic findings	Saddle distribution of numbness frequent. SLR may not be present, and cough may not increase radicular pain. After prolonged walking, pain may occur from SLR. Ankle jerk may be absent after exercise.

cords the duration before claudication and aids in determining progression and ultimate surgical intervention.

Surgical decompression requires the surgeon know exactly the extent and type of canal encroachment. The facets must be examined as well as the disks and the laminae. The gutters (foramen) must be shown to be patent and, if not, need to be enlarged. Often the exploratory aspect of surgery is more revealing than the presurgical diagnostic studies. It behooves the referring physician to refer to an experienced, competent surgeon with wide experience in this field.

The patient must be apprised of the fact that all claudication symptoms may not improve. The neurogenic bladder may have residual effects, and the nerve roots, myotome, and dermatome also may have residual deficits. Pain, also, may not necessarily be "removed" by the surgery.

ARACHNOIDITIS

In 1974, 2614 surgical procedures for herniated disks were performed by neurosurgeons in the United States. How many more were performed by orthopedists was not recorded. What these figures were in 1986–1987 has not yet been computed, but they are numerous. Of all surgical procedures performed for this condition, some 10 to 40 percent are "failed back procedures." This diagnosis implies "failure" to properly interpret the subjective and objective factors leading to surgical intervention.

Although many failures are the result of poor or inadequate evaluation and standardized protocols leading to surgical intervention, many failures are ultimately attributed to the presence of arachnoiditis. In second and even third surgical interventions, this condition is more prevalent than in initial procedures. There is evidence that arachnoiditis may result from hemorrhage into the dura or chemical irritation by the contrast dyes of myelography.

Arachnoiditis is essentially inflammation of the pia-arachnoid of the spine and caudal equina. The arachnoid is a nonvascular membrane composed of fibrous and elastin tissue that envelops the cord and the dural sheaths of the caudal nerves.

There have been several progressive stages designated in the evolution of arachnoiditis (Fig. 12–11).

1. Pia-arachnoid inflammation with edema about the nerve roots. At this stage, there may be noted strands of collagen beginning to be deposited between the nerve roots. A fibrinous exudate (probably the main constituent of the ultimate arachnoiditis) forms around the nerve roots that have no cellular component.

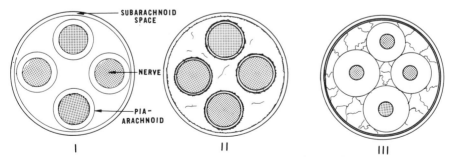

Figure 12–11. Arachnoiditis: natural evolution. *I*, The nerve roots with their enveloping pia-arachnoid in the normal state. *II*, The roots swell and the pia-arachnoid becomes inflamed and thickened. There are small adhesions between the roots and the arachnoid. *III*, The roots are atrophic and the pia-arachnoid is adherent with fibrous and collagen strands. The subarachnoid space is thickened as well.

2. There is an increase in fibroblastic activity and further collagen deposit. The swelling (edema) about the nerve roots decreases or disappears. The nerve root pia-arachnoid tissues begin to adhere to each other.

3. The adhesive phase marks the end of the "inflammatory" phase. The pia-arachnoid now is markedly thickened and the nerve roots become atrophic. No blood vessels, either arteriolar or venous, are visible.

Numerous theories have been postulated for the formation of arachnoiditis. These include infection, trauma, chemical irritation, allergic tissue reaction, autoimmune reaction, and even vascular abnormalities. No doubt previous surgery and preceding myelography constitute some of these causes in susceptible patients.

The presenting signs and symptoms are sparse and subtle. The symptoms may be continuous low back pain unrelated to specific activities or postures. Leg pains of a radicular distribution may be present with or without low back symptoms. Pseudoclaudication of spinal stenosis may be the presenting symptom.

Patients may exhibit a positive SLR test with dural confirmation. Crossed leg sciatica may be present. Pain is often aggravated by trunk flexion and relieved by trunk extension.

Treatment of arachnoiditis remains unsatisfactory, with limited benefit of any great duration. Surgical lysis of adhesions has been undertaken with limited success. Intrathecal steroids also have been advocated. Prevention remains the most desirable, but obviously this is stated after the fact.

REFERENCES

Armstrong, JR: Lumbar Disc Lesions: Pathogenesis and Treatment of Low Back Pain and Sciatica. E & S Livingstone, Edinburgh/London, 1952.

Barr, JS: Low back and sciatic pain: results of treatment. J Bone Joint Surg 33A:633, 1951.

Blau, JN and Logue, V: Intermittent claudication of the cauda equina: An unusual syndrome resulting from central protrusion of a lumbar intervertebral disc. Lancet 1:1081, 1961.

Blau, JN and Rushworth, G: Observations on the blood vessels of the spinal cord with their responses to motor activity. Brain 81:354, 1958.

Bradford, KK and Sperling, RG: The Intervertebral Disc, ed 2. Charles C Thomas, Springfield, IL, 1945.

Breig, A: Biomechanics of the Central Nervous System: Some Basic Normal and Pathological Phenomena. Year Book Medical Publishers, Chicago, 1960.

Brodsky, AE: Cauda equina arachnoiditis. Spine 3:51, 1978.

Burton, CV: Lumbosacral arachnoiditis. Spine 3:24, 1978.

Charnley, J: Orthopedic signs in the diagnosis of disc protrusions. Lancet 1:186, 1951.

Colonna, PC and Friedenberg, ZB: The Disc Syndrome: Results of the Conservative Care of Patients with Positive Myelograms. J Bone Joint Surg 31A:614, 1949.

Crisp, EJ: Massage, Manipulation and Traction. In Licht, S (ed): Orthotics Etc. Elizabeth Licht, New Haven, CT, 1969.

Cyriax, JH: Lumbago: Mechanism of dural pain. Lancet 2:427, 1955.

Davis, PR: Posture of the trunk during lifting of weights. Br Med J 1:87, 1959.

Edgar, MA and Nundy, S: Innervation of the spinal dura mater. J Neurol Neurosurg Psychiatry 29:530, 1966.

Ehie, N and Wehn, P: Measurements of the intra-abdominal pressure in relation to weight bearing on the lumbosacral spine. J Oslo City Hosp 12:205, 1962.

Ehni, G: Spondylatic cauda equina radiculopathy. Texas State J Med 61:746, 1965.

Epstein, JA, Epstein, BS, and Lavine, L: Nerve root compression associated with narrowing of the lumbar spinal canal. J Neurol Neurosurg Psychiatry 25:165, 1962.

Epstein, JA, et al.: Sciatica caused by nerve root entrapment in the lateral recess: The superior facet syndrome. J Neurosurg 36:584, 1972.

Evans, JG: Neurogenic intermittent claudication. Br Med J 2:985, 1964.

Falconer, MA, McGeorge, M, and Begg, AC: Observations on the cause and mechanism of symptom-production in sciatica and low back pain. J Neurol Neurosurg and Psychiatry 2:13, 1948.

Farfan, HF: Mechanical Disorders of the Low Back. Lea & Febiger, Philadelphia, 1973, pp. 63–92.

Feldman, S: Effect of intrathecal hydrocortisone on adhesive arachnoiditis and cerebrospinal fluid pleocytosis: an experimental study. Neurology 25:256, 1960.

Foerster, O: The dermatome in man. Brain 5:1, 1933.

Friberg, S, and Hirsch, C: On late results of operative treatment for intervertebral disc prolapse in the lumbar region. Acta Chir Scand 93:161, 1946.

Friberg, S, and Hirsch, C: Anatomical and clinical studies on lumbar disc degeneration. Acta Orthop Scand 19:222, 1949.

Friberg, S, and Hult, L: Comparative study of abrodil myelogram and operative findings in low back pain and sciatica. Acta Orthop Scand 20:303, 1951.

Goddard, MD and Reid, JD: Movements inducted by straight leg raising in the lumbosacral roots, nerves and plexus, and in the intrapelvic section of the sciatic nerve. J Neurol Neurosurg Psychiatry 28:12, 1965.

Grabias, S: The treatment of spinal stenosis: Current Concepts Review. J Bone Joint Surg 62-A:308, 1980.

Hadley, LA: Apophyseal subluxation: disturbances in and about the intervertebral foramen causing back pain. J Bone Joint Surg 18:428, 1936.

Hanraets, PRMJ: The Degenerative Back. Elsevier, Amsterdam/New York, 1959.

Harris, RI and MacNab, I: Structural changes on lumbar intervertebral discs: Their relationship to low back pain and sciatica. J Bone Joint Surg 36B:304, 1954.

Haymaker, W and Woodhall, B: Peripheral Nerve Injuries. ed 2. WB Saunders, Philadelphia, 1959.

Henderson, RS: The treatment of lumbar intervertebral disc protrusion: an assessment of conservative measures. Br Med J 2:597, 1952.

Hirsch, C: An attempt to diagnose the level of a disc lesion clinically by disc puncture. Acta Orthop Scand 18:132, 1948.

Hirsch, C: Studies on the mechanism of low back pain. Acta Orthop Scand 4:261, 1951.

Hirsch, C: Mechanical responses in normal and degenerated lumbar discs. J Bone Joint Surg 38-A:242, 1956.

Hirsch, C: Studies on the pathology of low back pain. J Bone Joint Surg 41-B:237, 1959.

Hirsch, C: Efficiency of surgery in low back disorders. J Bone Joint Surg 47-A:991, 1965.

Hirsch, C, Ingelmark, BE, and Miller, M: The anatomical bases for low back pain: studies on the presence of sensory nerve endings in ligamentous, capsular and intervertebral disc structures in the human lumbar spine. Acta Orthop Scand 33:1, 1963.

Hirsch, C, and Nachemson, A: New observations on the mechanical behavior of lumbar discs. Acta Orthop Scand 23:254, 1959.

Hirsch, C and Schajowicz, F: Studies on structural changes in the lumbar annulus fibrosus. Acta Orthop Scand 22:184, 1953.

Hovelaque, A: Le Nerf Sinu-Vertebral. Ann Anat Pathol 2:435, 1925.

Howland, WJ and Curry, JL: Pantopaque arachnoiditis: Experimental study of blood as an attenuating agent and corticosteroids as an ameliorating agent. Acta Radiol Diagn 5:1032, 1966.

Inman, VT and Saunders, JB: The clinico-anatomical aspects of the lumbosacral region. Radiology 38:669, 1942.

Inman, VT and Saunders, JB: Anatomical and physiological aspects of injuries of the intervertebral disk. J Bone Joint Surg 29-A:461, 1947.

Johnston, JDH, and Matheny, JB: Microscopic lysis of lumbar adhesive arachnoiditis. Spine 3:36, 1978.

Kaplan, EB: Recurrent meningeal branch of the spinal nerves. Bull Hosp Dis NY 8:108, 1947.

Kavanaugh, GJ, et al: "Pseudoclaudication" syndrome produced by compression of the cauda equina. JAMA 206:2477, 1968.

Keegan, J: Alterations of the lumbar curve related to posture and seating. J Bone Joint Surg 35-A:589, 1953.

Key, JA: Indications for operations in disc lesions on the lumbosacral spine. Ann Surg 135:886, 1952.

Knutsson, F: The instability associated with disc degeneration in the lumbar spine. Acta Radiol Scand 25:593, 1944.

Knutsson, B: Electromyographic studies in the diagnosis of lumbar disc herniations. Acta Orthop Scand 28:290, 1959.

Knutsson, B, Lindh, K, and Telhag, H: Sitting: An electromyographic and mechanical study. Acta Orthop Scand 37:415, 1966.

Kraft, GL and Leventhal, DH: Facet synovial impingement: a new concept in the etiology of lumbar vertebral derangement. Surg Gynec Obstet 93:439, 1951.

Lee, CK, Hanson, HT, and Weiss, AB: Developmental lumbar spine stenosis: Pathology and surgical treatment. Spine 3:246, 1978.

Lindahl, O: Hyperalgesia of the lumbar nerve roots in sciatica. Acta Orthop Scand 37:367, 1966.

Lucas, OB: Spinal Bracing. In Licht, S (ed): Orthotics Etc. Elizabeth Licht, New Haven, CT, 1969, pp 275–305.

Mennell, JM: Back Pain. Little Brown & Co, Boston, 1960.

Mensor, MC: Non-operative treatment, including manipulation for lumbar intervertebral disc syndrome. J Bone Joint Surg 37-A:925, 1955.

Mixter, WJ, and Barr, JS: Rupture of the intervertebral disc with involvement of the spinal canal. New Engl J Med 211:210, 1934.

Morris, JM, Lucas, DB, and Breslar, B: The role of the trunk in stability of the spine. J Bone Joint Surg 43-A:327, 1966.

Nachemson, A: In vivo discometry in lumbar disks with irregular nucleograms. Acta Orthop Scand 36:418, 1965.

Nachemson, A: The influence of spinal movements on the lumbar intradiscal pressure. Experimental studies on post-mortem material. Acta Orthop Scand Supp 43:1, 1960.

Nachemson, A: The effect of forward leaning on lumbar intradiskal pressure. Acta Orthop Scand 35:314, 1965.

Naylor, A: Factors in the development of the spinal stenosis syndrome. J Bone Joint Surg 61-B; 306, 1979.

O'Connell, JEA: The indication for and results of the excision of lumbar intervertebral disk protrusions: A review of 500 cases. Ann R Coll Surg Engl 6:403, 1950.

Püschel, J: Wassergehalt normalen und degeneraten zwischen Wirbelscheiben. Beitr Pathol 84:123, 1930.

Smyth, JJ, and Wright, V: Sciatica and the intervertebral disc: An experimental study. J Bone Surg 40-A:1401, 1958.

Spurling, RG, and Granthan, EG: Ruptured disks in lower lumbar region. Am J Surg 75:14, 1948.

Steindler, A: Lectures on the interpretation of pain in orthopedic practice, Charles C Thomas, Springfield, IL, 1959.

Steer, JC, and Horney, FD: Evidence for passage of cerebrospinal fluid along spinal nerves. Can Med Assoc J 98:71, 1968.

Taylor, TKF: Treatment of lumbar disk prolapse. Am Acad Gen Practice 23:141, 1965.

Verbiest, H: A radicular syndrome from developmental narrowing of the lumbar vertebral canal. J Bone Joint Surg 26-B:230, 1954.

Verbiest, H: Neurogenic intermittent claudication in cases with absolute and relative stenosis of the lumbar vertebral canal (ASLC and RSLC), in cases with narrow lumbar intervertebral foramina, and in cases with both entities. Clin Neurosurg 21:204, 1972.

Wiberg, G: Back pain in relation to the nerve supply of the intervertebral disc. Acta Orthop Scand 19:211, 1949.

Wilson, CB: Significance of the small lumbar spine canal: Cauda equina compression syndrome due to spondylosis. J Neurosurg 31:499, 1969.

Wilson, JC Jr: Degenerative arthritis of lumbar intervertebral joints: a clinical study. Am J Surg 100:313, 1960.

Wilson, JC Jr: Low back pain and sciatica. JAMA 200:705, 1967.

Wood, KM: New approaches to treatment of back pain. Western J Med 130:394, 1979.

Wright, J: Mechanics in relation to derangement of the facet joints of the spine. Arch Phys Ther 25:201, 1944.

Yamada, H, Ohya, M, Okada, T, and Shiozawa, Z: Intermittent cauda equina compression due to narrow spinal canal. J Neurosurg 37:83, 1972.

CHAPTER 13

Miscellaneous Low Back Conditions Relating to Pain and Disability

There are numerous "other" conditions of the lumbosacral spine, congenital or acquired, that do not fit the exclusive precise diagnosis of mechanical or diskogenic cause. They may be directly related to a mechanical factor and elicit diskogenic symptoms, but they are significantly unique to merit separate consideration.

SPONDYLOLYSIS AND SPONDYLOLISTHESIS

Frequently considered to be identical or specially interrelated, these conditions may exist alone and may be related. "Spondylo" relates to spine and "lysis" and "listhesis" to conditions of the functional unit of the spinal column.

Spondylolysis is an anatomic defect that exists as a defect in the continuity of the pars interarticularis. This portion of the vertebral body resides within the lamina. The defect may be unilateral or bilateral with separation or widening of neither, either, or both (Fig. 13–1). Normally this defect is considered a congenital failure of fusion during maturation of the bones of the growing body. There have been theories expounded that these are "fractures" that occur in the fetal or the neonatal development.

Often they are merely found during a routine x-ray and have no clinical significance. If bilateral, however, they pose a "weakness" in the arch of the neural canal and may predispose further separation leading to listhesis.

274

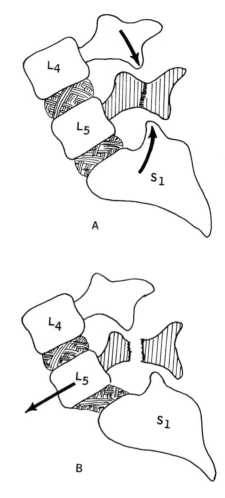

Figure 13–1. A mechanism of spondylolisthesis. *A*, The defect in the pars interarticularis but without listhesis. *B*, A fracture or separation of the pars occurs, causing forward sliding of L_5 upon S_1. A "pincer" effect of the opposing facets (*A*) is postulated as a cause of separation.

Spondylolisthesis is a forward or backward shearing subluxation of the body of a superior vertebra on its immediate caudal counterpart, for instance, L_4 on L_5 or L_5 on S_1. The term is derived from the Greek word **"olisthesis,"** which means slipping or falling. Although theoretically any vertebra may slide upon its adjacent vertebra within a functional unit, the common usage usually implies L_5 on S_1 with the next most frequent L_4 on L_5. Statistically, 70 percent of spondylolisthesis occurs at the fifth vertebra (on the sacrum), 25 percent at the fourth, and only 4 percent at higher levels.

In the lumbar spine, the superior vertebra reposes on its immediate inferior vertebra on an inclined plane. The superior surface of S_1 is at a sharp angle with the superior surface of L_5 at a lesser degree. The superior surface of L_3 is usually reasonably horizontal. The possibility of forward shear of L_5 on S_1 is obviously more marked than the more cephalic vertebrae (Fig. 13–2).

Forward sliding (shear) is normally prevented by the mechanical alignment and relationship of the posterior facet joints, their ligaments, their capsules, the integrity of the annulus of the intervertebral disk, and the longitudinal ligaments. The intact intervertebral disk nucleus expands the disk and places the annular fibers and longitudinal ligament under a tension that resists vertebral sliding. The contact of the facets and their planes also resists anterior subluxation of the vertebra.

Defects in any of these supporting structures may permit listhesis of the superior on the inferior vertebra of the involved functional unit. These have been classified into five categories according to the causative factors:

Type I (Isthmic): In isthmic spondylolisthesis, there is an anatomic defect in the pars interarticularis (see Fig. 13–1).

Type II (Congenital): In this type, the posterior elements are structurally inadequate due to developmental causes. This is a rare type.

Type III (Degenerative): In this type, the facets and their supporting ligamentous structure are deficient and listhesis results (Fig. 13–3). In this type, there is no defect in the pars interarticularis and the condition is related to trauma and aging and is potentially progressive.

Type IV (Elongated Pedicles): In this type, the neural arch is elongated, placing the facets more posteriorly. This may be considered an isthmic variant. Other traction forces occur that result in progression and symptomatology.

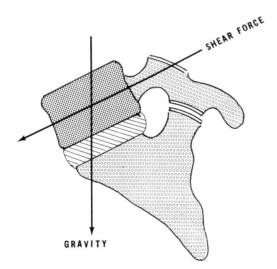

Figure 13–2. Gravitational forces acting upon the lumbosacral joint. The fifth lumbar residing upon the inclined sacral plane tends to glide due to shear force and gravity. Forward gliding is prevented by the facets, ligaments, and annular fibers.

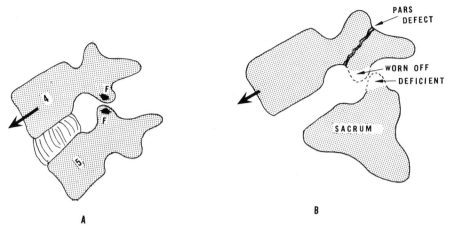

Figure 13–3. Type III spondylolisthesis. *A* depicts the facet factor that prevents listhesis (F–F). *B*, Facets are worn and permit listhesis. The pars defect is intact and does not cause listhesis.

Type V (Destructive Disease): This type is secondary to metabolic, malignant, or infectious diseases. Any "bone disease," be it primary or secondary, may result in listhesis.

The presence of listhesis noted on an x-ray does not imply that there are resultant symptoms. When present, however, in the presence of low back pain or radicular pain secondary to lumbar cause, listhesis is considered contributory if not causative.

Listhesis may exist throughout a person's life without symptoms. Traumas of various types are considered to occur when a listhesis becomes symptomatic.

Spondylolisthesis of isthmic type between L_5-S_1 usually does not progress after age 20 until age 70, but recent studies have concluded that listhesis above L5-S1:

1. has a higher incidence of neurologic signs;
2. has a higher incidence of causing or contributing to spinal stenosis by forming a large mass at the pseudoarthrosis of the pars defect;
3. has a higher incidence of further listhesis in later life, which is rare (as stated) at L5-S1.

SYMPTOMS

The major symptom of spondylolisthesis is that of a low back pain with referred pain laterally into the region of the sacroiliac joints. Pain, although vague in its characteristics, may radiate into the hips, thighs, and even in the feet but not precisely as a dermatomal pattern. Often the referred symptom is not pain but rather numbness or tingling paresthesias.

The low back is considered "stiff" with limited flexibility claimed by the patient and observed by the examiner. The patient frequently claims discomfort from lifting, excessive bending over, or from prolonged standing in a nonmoving manner.

The examination frequently reveals a palpable "ledge" on passing the fingers down the lumbosacral spine. A segmental lordosis may be evident, and pain can be reproduced or accentuated by holding the person in an excessive lordotic posture for an extended period of time.

During the performance of a rectal examination a hard mass may be palpated in the front of the sacrum. Percussion over the lumbosacral area may elicit tenderness or pain.

An interesting finding associated with spondylolisthesis but as yet unexplained is the presence of limited extensibility of the hamstring muscles. The hamstrings are "tight" on straight leg raising but with negative dural signs. A peculiar gait has been described due to a posterior tilting (rotation) of the pelvis, decreasing the lordosis and causing slight flexion of the hip joints. In an uncomplicated spondylolisthesis, the neurologic examination is normal.

The cause of the tight hamstring muscles is conjectural and has been attributed to caudal equinal traction with irritation to the nerve roots de-

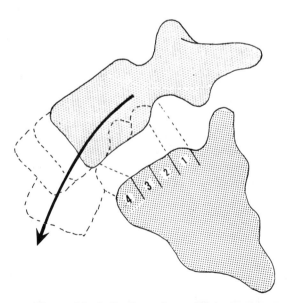

Figure 13–4. Grading of spondylolisthesis.

scending to the hamstring muscles. Electromyographic examination, however, fails to demonstrate nerve root involvement.

X-rays and now CT scans may reveal the pathognomonic factors: a defect in the pars interarticularis, an elongated arch, a fracture, severe lumbosacral angulation, and/or severe disk degeneration with measureable listhesis.

Lateral views of the lumbosacral spine x-rays afford measurement of the degree of subluxation (Fig. 13–4). Besides mechanical low back pain resulting from spondylolisthesis as a result of excessive facet weight bearing (and shear resisting), the foraminae are deformed and sciatic radiculopathy may result. The foraminae are normally narrowed during the process of extending the lumbar spine. In spondylolisthesis this narrowing is enhanced and nerve entrapment more probable.

As the superior vertebra slides forward on the lower vertebra, the spinal canal also narrows. This factor contributes to spinal stenosis and foraminal stenosis as was discussed in a previous chapter. Thickening of the pars interarticularis defect from fibrous closure also encroaches on the foramen and the canal, with encroachment on the nerve roots or the thecal sac. Neurologic symptoms and signs result.

TREATMENT

The treatment obviously depends on the severity of the symptoms and the objective extent of neurologic deficit. It is redundant to state that the symptoms **must be directly related to the spondylolisthesis**.

In a condition where there is low back pain that has a mechanical basis as determined from the history and physical examination, the objective of nonsurgical treatment is to decrease the forces of gravity as expended on the incline plane of the sacrum. The pelvis must be rotated to decrease the lumbosacral angle. This minimizes the extent of forward gliding of the superior on the inferior vertebrae and relieves the stress on the facet joints.

"Pelvic tilting" is a type of exercise in which the anterior aspect of the pelvis is elevated and the posterior lowered. Strong abdominal muscles, especially the obliques, must be gained and maintained. The school curriculum must emphasize the need for avoiding lordosis in all activities of daily living and occupational activities. The extensor muscles must also be strengthened, so that bending and lifting activities rely on muscles as well as ligaments.

A corset or a brace, as depicted in a previous chapter, may be of value in that the brace decreases the lordosis, reinforces the abdominal component, and minimizes excessive motion during bending and lifting. A brace must be an adjunct to exercise and must never be used without or to replace simultaneous exercises. Prolonged use of support tends to diminish the proprioceptive response of activities to the musculature of the lumbar spine, as it "does it for the spine" and does encourage atrophy and loss of flexibility of the trunk muscles and fascia.

Surgery becomes more pertinent when there is neurologic deficit— root entrapment with radicular symptoms, cord symptoms from canal stenosis, bladder symptoms from thecal sac encroachment, evidence of object listhesis from Grade I to Grade II, Grade II to Grade III, or a Grade IV with neurologic deficit (see Fig. 13–4), or intractable pain causing functional impairment that does not favorably respond to conservative treatment.

Surgical treatment varies from fusion of L4 to L5, L5 to sacrum, or an anterior interbody fusion. Laminectomy is performed when the arch is involved in nerve root entrapment.

Prophylactic fusion has had its advocates, but the results have been disappointing. It must be remembered that many, if not most, of listhesis does not progress between the ages of 20 and 70 if there is no intervening trauma or a definite physical deconditioning.

PIRIFORMIS SYNDROME

This is a controversial syndrome that implies that the extraspinal nerve of the lumbosacral plexus nerves forming the sciatic nerve becomes mechanically entrapped within or by the piriformis muscle (Fig. 13–5). The piriformis muscle is an external rotator of the hip by virtue of its origin and insertion.

This muscle arises within the pelvis in the region of the sacrum and inner aspect of the sacroiliac joint, then passes laterally out of the sciatic notch to attach posteriorly to the greater trochanter of the femur. The sciatic nerve passes between the two bellies of the muscle.

Pressure on the sciatic nerve at this pelvic level causes pain to radiate in the dermatomal regions of the nerve roots similar to that of disk entrapment previously described. Often the description of the pain is imprecise with no objective neurologic findings.

This condition is diagnosed most frequently in women who also have a symptom of dyspareunia. A history of stress on a hip joint position, such as faulty lifting, walking, running, or twisting may be elicited, but mostly no causative factors are elicited.

The physical examination that suggests that the "sciatica" is of piriformis rather than "diskogenic" causation is that the SLR done with foot in straight coronal position is mildly positive or actually negative, unless there is incorporated into the SLR a forceful internal rotation of the upper leg. This internal rotation of the hip places the piriformis muscle under tension and then the SLR stretches the inflamed nerve root against the tensed muscle.

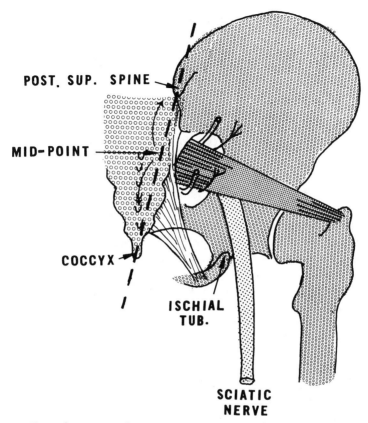

POST. SUP. SPINE

MID-POINT

COCCYX

ISCHIAL TUB.

SCIATIC NERVE

Figure 13–5. Piriformis muscle. Anatomical relationship of the sciatic nerve to the piriformis muscle is noted.

The test can be performed in the seated position by also simultaneously internally rotating the hip or by resisting abduction of the legs. Abduction of the legs is accomplished by active contraction of the piriformis as well as the gluteal muscles.

There is, in this syndrome, no causation of sciatic radiculopathy from trunk flexion or trunk hyperextension, which would implicate the lumbosacral diskogenic factors. Rectal examination or pelvic examination may reveal deep tenderness over the anterior pelvic wall lateral to the sacroiliac joint and lumbar spine. X-rays are essentially nonconfirmatory.

Treatment requires direct local injection of an anesthetic agent and a soluble steroid into the belly of the piriformis muscle. The anesthetic agent is diagnostic and may be therapeutic. This injection may be given in one of two routes: vaginally by direct insertion into the tender muscle that has been identified by manual palpation or via a 3-inch spinal needle through the gluteus muscle and the sacral notch aimed at the tender spot located by the gloved rectal examining finger. The latter is less direct and also more capable of failure.

Both of these injections must be done with the patient fully alert and responding to the sensation of the inserted needle and informing the treating physician as to when and if the sciatic nerve is touched before any agent is injected.

SACROILIAC PATHOLOGY CAUSING LOW BACK PAIN

The sacroiliac joint is the **bête noire** of low back pain with avid enthusiastic proponents and equally avid enthusiastic opponents of this clinical entity. Goldthwaite and Osgood (1905) introduced the concept of "sacroiliac strain" as a common cause of low back pain. There are currently still many that adhere to this concept and "adjust" or "reduce the joint with resultant alleviation of low back pain."

Bourdillon (1970), a recognized expert and proponent of manipulative therapy, noted: "The range of motion in the sacroiliac joint is small and demonstration by direct palpation is both difficult and unconvincing. . . . Indeed the existence and importance of sacroiliac mobility is still a subject of argument."

Unless there has occurred or there exists a definite subluxation of the sacroiliac joint following severe trauma, no motion can be noted on x-rays, which has been the strongest rejection of the concept of sacroiliac subluxation and pain.

The sacroiliac joint is an extremely stable joint by virtue of its multifaceted incongruous articular surface and powerful ligaments located anteriorly and posteriorly (Fig. 13–6). The mechanical analysis of the weight-bearing pelvis (Fig. 13–7) indicates further the structural aspects of stability of the S-I joint. After age 45 it has been demonstrated that 35 percent of the population has ossified sacroiliac joints.

The sacroiliac joints(s) can be indirectly damaged by a forceful injury that disrupts the pelvic "ring" (Figs. 13–8 and 13–9). The injury, as a rule, is severe and from external trauma. Other musculoskeletal or visceral injuries may distract the attention of the patient or the physician. Only later when the other, and possibly primary, injuries have subsided is the discomfort of the S-I joint noted.

Trauma to the ring structures with involvement of the sacroiliac joints (usually both joints, as it is difficult to envision a defect in the right that would spare one of the participating joints) is suspected by:

1. tenderness over the sacroiliac joint.
2. tenderness over the symphysis pubis (anterior aspect of the ring).
3. pain or discomfort on attempted mobilization of the joint. This test

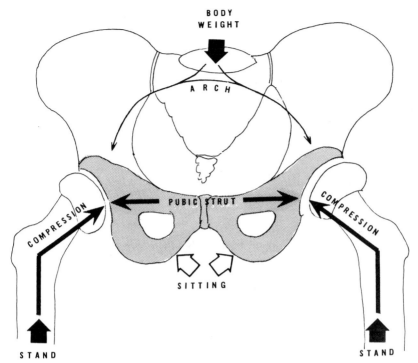

Figure 13–6. Forces acting on the pelvis. The body weight is imposed upon the fifth lumbar vertebra which lies on the sacrum. This weight is transmitted through the sacrum, across the sacroiliac joints, through the ilia, into the acetabula, and finally to the femora. The two compressive forces of the femoral heads are resisted by the superimposed pubic strut. When the body weight is borne in the sitting position, the forces tend to spread the ilia. This is resisted by the symphysis pubis and the sacroiliac ligaments.

is performed by placing the patient supine on a firm surface and pushing down hard on both anterior superior spines. In this same position, pressure can be exerted by placing both hands on the outer pelvic rims and compressing (bringing the hands together with force). The pelvis can be "rocked back and forth" by pressing downward on one anterior superior spine and raising the opposite ilium manually.

4. Pain noted in the S-I joint by hyperextending the hip on the affected side. This was termed the Gaenslen test, but its specificity has been refuted as the maneuver also hyperextends the low back and conceivably may cause referred radicular pain from this low back hyperextension.

5. Resisted abduction of the extended leg stressing the hip joint with the patient side lying may reproduce the S-I pain (Fig. 13–10).

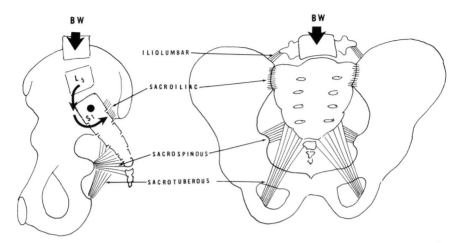

Figure 13–7. Ligamentous support of the pelvis. The side view of the pelvis indicates the stress of the superincumbent body upon the fifth lumbar vertebra. The downward pressure initiates a rotation about the axis at S_1 with depression of the upper sacral structure and posterior movement of the lower sacrum. This rotation is resisted by the sacrospinous and sacrotuberous ligaments. The front view shows these ligaments and the sacroiliac ligaments that firmly support the posterior border of the pelvic rim.

In pregnancy the iliac joint, as well as all the articulations of the ring, are more "unstable" due to hormonal laxity of the ligamentous structure to prepare for parturition.

X-rays are usually negative unless the trauma has been severe and the ring disrupted. A "heavy leg," anterior-posterior x-ray view with a weight suspended from the affected side (leg), may reveal minor subluxation of that joint as compared to the opposite "normal" joint. Oblique views of the pelvis are also worth evaluating.

Treatment

The S-I joint can be infiltrated with an anesthetic agent as a diagnostic test. If this affords relief, it can be repeated with the inclusion of a soluble steroid. Wearing a pelvic belt that essentially approximates the two ilia may afford relief. Oral anti-inflammatory nonsteroidal drugs are valuable, as is a series of ultrasound tests. To prolong **any** treatment for any length of time with no benefits is unacceptable and indicates that the S-I joint is **not** the source of pain.

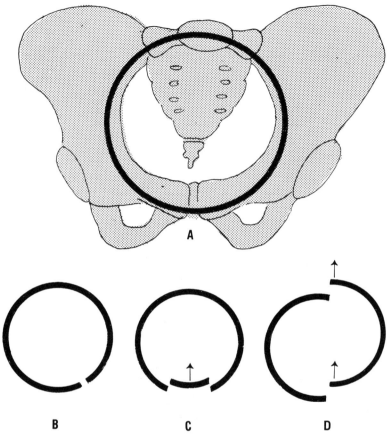

Figure 13–8. Pelvic ring. The pelvic ring is bounded laterally by the ilia, anteriorly by the pubic rami, and posteriorly by the sacrum and the sacroiliac joints. An intact ring of great strength is thus formed. The lower drawings depict the various types of fracture-dislocations that may occur and their effects upon the integrity of the ring.

RHEUMATOID SPONDYLITIS

In a young person, especially a young male who complains of persistent pain in the region of the S-I joints, the diagnosis of rheumatoid spondylitis (Marie-Strumpell arthritis) must be suspected. The x-rays are usually negative in the early stages of the disease, but a bone scan may reveal a greater uptake over the joints and may be diagnostic. HLA-W27 should be requested as well as a sedimentation blood test. If either, in the proper titer, is "positive," the result is significantly diagnostic to justify treatment. The diagnosis is ultimately evident by subtle then characteristic changes in

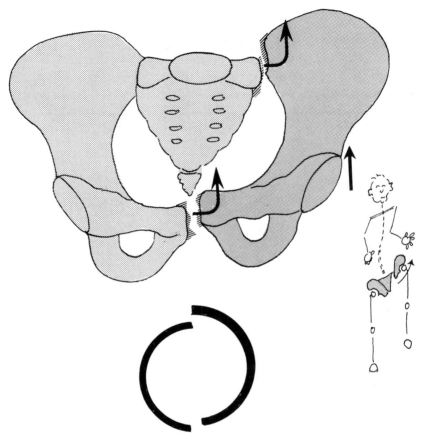

Figure 13–9. Combined sacroiliac and symphysis pubis separation. Injury resulting in combined separation of the symphysis pubis and the sacroiliac joints disrupts the pelvic ring. The fractured segment rotates posteriorly behind the sacrum and elevates. The involved leg is "shortened."

routine oblique x-ray views. Usually the diagnosis is entertained in males in their second or third decades who may have a family history of the disease.

In summary the diagnosis is suspected then confirmed by the following factors:

1. Usually found in men.
2. Age of onset: 20 to 30 years.
3. Aching of low back with nocturnal discomfort—unrelated to any specific motion.
4. Limited trunk flexibility.
5. Decreased chest expansion on "deep breath."
6. Ultimately a positive antigen HLA-W27 on blood testing. Possibly

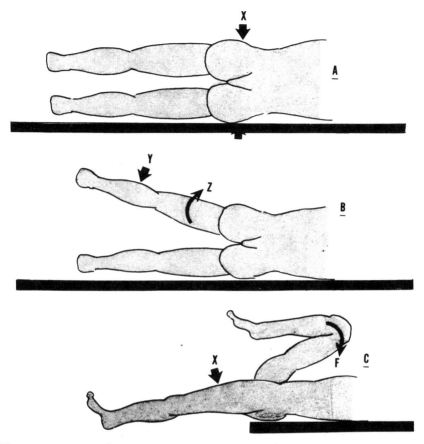

Figure 13–10. Sacroiliac tests. *A*, Direct pressure upon the iliac crest with patient side-lying on a firm surface. *B*, Resisted abduction of the involved side with hip extension. *C*, Hyperextension of the hip on the side of the painful sacroiliac joint.

also an elevated sedimentation rate, but other evidence of infection is missing.

    7. "Fuzziness" of the S-I joints on oblique view x-rays.

    8. Concavity of the manubrial-sternal joint.

    9. Increased uptake on bone scan.

Treatment

    The treatment is usually symptomatic with the expectation that in many patients the disease becomes quiescent with the spine "fused" in the final stage; treatment is to modify the expected abnormal posture.

The anticipated posture is dorsal kyphosis (round back) with compensatory cervical lordosis from the forward head posture. The head may not allow sufficient extension to permit direct vision. The neck usually also solidifies, and thus, the ultimate desired cervical head posture must be controlled throughout the activity of the disease.

Treatment may be summarized as follows:

1. Salicylates are of value for symptom relief.
2. Nonsteroidal anti-inflammatory drugs are also valuable.
3. Local heat decreases the discomfort.
4. More specific drug therapy such as gold, steroids, and x-ray therapy will rely on the state of rheumatology at the time of diagnosis.

To minimize the deformity anticipated the following guidelines are valuable:

1. Proper sleeping posture on a firm mattress without a pillow. The prone position is to be encouraged.
2. Daily exercises to increase erect posture, upper back extension without creating excessive lumbar lordosis.
3. Deep breathing exercises to maintain rib cage excursion as well as abdominothoracic breathing.
4. Range of motion exercises to the:
   (a) hips to maintain full extension;
   (b) knees to prevent flexion contracture;
   (c) neck-head to maintain cervical range of motion.
5. Periodic rest periods to minimize fatigue.
6. Bracing or corsetting, as indicated. This may include the consideration of a molded plastic cast to use at night during sleep.

Surgery may ultimately be needed to correct deformities that have not or could not be prevented or minimized. These surgical procedures include osteotomies or soft tissue releases.

SACRALIZATION OF TRANSVERSE PROCESS

There can be a congenital elongation of a transverse process of the lowest lumbar vertebra that forms a pseudoarthrosis with the sacrum or the ilium. The usual site is the fifth lumbar vertebra and the point of pseudoarthrosis is the medial aspect of the ipsilateral ilium.

Usually this condition is seen on x-rays and is asymptomatic. It can, however, cause a partial immobilization of the lumbosacral joint and result in a similar clinical condition as the tropism previously mentioned. By immobilizing the lumbosacral joint, excessive motion results in the functional units above.

Should there be a sciatic root radiculitis (Fig. 13–11) and a sacralization be noted, the condition must be differentiated from a disk herniation

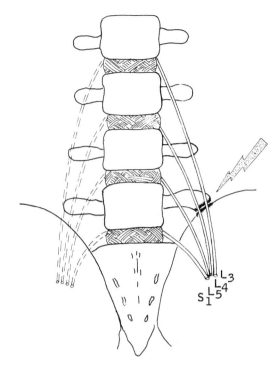

Figure 13–11. Sacralization of the transverse process. The elongated left transverse process of the fifth lumbar vertebra forms a pseudoarthrosis at its point of contact with the sacral wing. The passage over the area of pseudoarthrosis of the L_{3-4} nerve roots irritates the contiguous branches. The mechanism of pain due to mechanical irritation on left lateral flexion can be visualized.

or a hypertrophied superior facet. This is difficult and may be summarized as "being suggested with radiculitis being caused by lateral trunk flexion but not forward or backward flexion and a sacralization being noted on x-ray." A CT scan or MRI may not reveal disk herniation or superior facet hypertrophy.

Tenderness may be noted at the site of the pseudoarthrosis, and a local injection of an anesthetic agent often affords diagnostic and possibly therapeutic relief.

SPINAL INFECTIONS

Infections of the spine are rare but when they occur are potentially serious and recalcitrant to treatment. Infections are specified as to where in the spine they occur.

OSTEOMYELITIS

This is an infection of the vertebral body. It may result from hematogenous spread or local tissue spread from an adjacent abscess. Frequently it begins and is transmitted as a complication of a urinary tract infection.

Staphylococci are often the culprit. Diabetics are more prone to this type of infection. If two adjacent vertebrae are involved, there may be a transmission to the disk that is usually avascular. The infected vertebral body may gradually collapse from destruction, and a local abscess may augment the neurologic complications already initiated by collapse or compression.

Suspicion of an osteomyelitis of the lumbar vertebral bodies is a nonspecific backache, not specifically related to movement, with deep tenderness, nocturnal pain, and severe muscle spasm. Generalized toxicity is noted and a low-grade fever may be experienced.

X-rays are initially negative, but the blood count can reveal evidence of infection and a markedly elevated sedimentation rate. Blood cultures, at first, may be normal.

As the condition progresses, all these tests become positive, and x-rays become diagnostic. These findings are noted usually within 4 to 6 weeks.

Treatment is to isolate and identify the specific bacterial agent then specific antibiotics must be designated. To prevent deformation of the spine from an irregular degeneration and collapse of the vertebra, a molded body cast or fiber-glass spinal orthosis to maintain correct body alignment and immobilization for recovery from infection should be worn day and night, then gradually only at night as the infection responds to specific treatment. Usually within 3 to 6 months fusion occurs at the site in the alignment assured by the brace or cast.

DISKITIS: DISK SPACE INFECTION

Infection of the disk space is becoming more frequent or is being recognized more often. There are reasons postulated for this increase. More surgical procedures such as diskectomy, surgical and chemical, and diskograms are being performed. A hematogenous spread of infection into the disk is more frequent because of the high incidence of "drug addicted" people who use the venous or injection route for their addictive drugs. The narcotic addict is a strong candidate for a disk space infection for reasons not yet clearly delineated.

A disk space infection must be considered if the patient is some days or weeks post surgery, shows injection into a disk space, or is a drug addict. **Severe,** called "excruciating," local pain and tenderness is pathognomonic of a possible diskitis. Marked protective spasm occurs that "splints" the low back from any movement.

The sedimentation rate is markedly elevated. A positive "bone scan" may be localizing and diagnostic before the x-rays become diagnostic. The disk space becomes "hazy" and the endplates become disrupted and irregular in contour. Gradual progression occurs with destruction of the adjacent vertebral endplates and a narrowing of the disk space.

Needle biopsy results will often reveal the causative bacteria responsible. Treatment is as in osteomyelitis—specific antibiotics and proper casting or bracing.

BONE TUMORS

Bone tumors, either primary or secondary (metastatic), must always be suspected when there is nocturnal pain, pain without precise movement relationship, pain that fails to respond to reasonable treatment for a reasonable time factor, or when there are concurrent findings such as weight loss or evidence of debility.

INTRASPINOUS TUMORS

Intraspinous tumors, of which a disk herniation is a type, but not in the context of a potentially malignant growth, may cause any or all of the symptoms of a herniated disk.

As in bone tumors, the same criteria alert the physician: pain unrelated or poorly related to specific movement, failure to respond to appropriate treatment, progression of neurologic signs, and symptoms and "other" signs of systemic disease.

Suspicion is corroborated by myelography, CT scan, MRI, bone scan, and ultimately biopsy results. Treatment is the primary care of the tumor and all the ancillary aspects of treatment given in osteomyelitis and diskitis.

REFERENCES

Bailey, W: Observations on the etiology and frequency of spondylolisthesis and its precursors. Radiol. 48:107, 1947.

Barash, HL, Galante, JO, Lambert, CN and Ray, RD: Spondylolisthesis and tight hamstrings, J Bone Joint Surg 52-A:1319, 1970.

Bartelink, DL: The role of abdominal pressure in relieving the pressure on the lumbar intervertebral discs. J Bone Joint Surg 39-B:718, 1957.

Bourdillon, JF: Spinal Manipulation. Appleton-Century-Crofts, New York, 1970.

Brooke, R: The sacroiliac joint. J Anat 58:299, 1924.

Craig, W McK, Svien, HJ, Dodge, HW, and Camp, JD: Intraspinal lesions masquerading as protruded lumbar intervertebral discs. JAMA May: 250, 1952.

Freiburg, AH: Sciatica pain and its relief by operation on muscle and fascia. Arch Surg 34:337, 1937.

Freiburg, AH, and Vinke, TA: Sciatica and the sacroiliac joint. J Bone Joint Surg 16:126, 1934.

Friberg, S: Studies on spondylolisthesis. Acta Orthop Scand 82:Supp 25:1939.

Grabias, S: The treatment of spinal stenosis. J Bone Joint Surg 62-A:308, 1980.

Gramse, RR, Sinaki, M, and Ilstrup, DM: Lumbar spondylolisthesis: a rational approach to conservative treatment. Mayo Clinic Proc 55:681, 1980.

Grieve, GP: The sacroiliac joint. Physiotherapy 62:384, 1976.

Hanraets, PRMJ: The Degenerative Back. Elsevier, New York, 1959.

Hause, FB, and O'Connor, SJ: Specific management for lumbar and sacral radiculitis. JAMA 166:1285, 1958.

Hensinger, RN, Lang, JR, and MacEwen, GD; Surgical management of spondylolisthesis in children and adolescents. Spine 1:1207, 1976.

Herz, R: Subfascial fat herniation as a cause of low back pain. Ann Rheum Dis 11:30, 1952.

Hilel, N: Spondylolysis. J Bone Joint Surg 41-A:303, 1959.

Howarth, MB, and Petrie, JG: Injuries of the Spine. Williams & Wilkins, Baltimore, 1964.

Jackson, AM, Kirwan, EO, and Sullivan, MF: Lytic spondylolisthesis above the lumbosacral level. Spine 3:260, 1978.

Jonck, LM: The influence of weight bearing on the lumbar spine: a radiological study. S Africa J Radiol 2:25, 1964.

MacNab, I: Backache. Williams & Wilkins, Baltimore, 1977, pp. 64–79.

Meyerding, HW: Spondylolisthesis. Surg Gynecol Obstet 54:371, 1932.

Meyerding, HW: The low backache and sciatic pain associated with spondylolisthesis and protruded intervertebral disk; incidence, significance, and treatment. J Bone Joint Surg 23:461, 1941.

Moore, DC: Sciatic and femoral nerve block. JAMA, October 11:550, 1952.

Morris, JM: Low back bracing. Clin Orthop 103:120, 1974.

Morris, JM, and Lucas, DB: Biomechanics of spinal bracing. Ariz Med 17:176, 1964.

Newman, PH: A clinical syndrome associated with severe lumbosacral subluxation. J Bone Joint Surg 47-B:472, 1965.

Pace, JB, and Nagle, D: Piriform syndrome. Western J Med 124:435, 1976.

Phalen, GS, and Dickson, JA: Spondylolisthesis and tight hamstrings: Proceedings of the Association of Bone and Joint Surgeons. J Bone Joint Surg 38-A:946, 1956.

Rabinowitch, R: Diseases of Intervertebral Disk and its Surrounding Tissues. Charles C Thomas Publishing, Springfield, IL, 1961.

Silver, RA, et al: Intermittent claudication of neurospinal origin. Arch Surg 98:523, 1969.

Soren, A: Spondylolisthesis and allied conditions. Am J Orthop 8:8, 1966.

Steindler, A: Kinesiology of the Human Body. Charles C Thomas, Springfield, IL, 1955.

Stone, WK: The etiology of spondylolisthesis. J Bone Joint Surg 45:B:39, 1963.

Teng, P, and Papatheodorou, C: Lumbar spondylosis with compression of cauda equina. Arch Neurol 8:221, 1963.

Thieme, FP: Lumbar Breakdown Caused by Erect Posture on Man: With Emphasis on Spondylolisthesis and Herniated Intervertebral Disk. Anthropological Papers No. 4: Museum of Anthropology, 1950.

Williams, PC: Conservative Management of Lesions of Lumbosacral Spine. In: Instructional Course Lectures, American Academy of Orthop. Surgeons, Michigan, J.W. Edwards, 1953, pp. 90–121:

Williams, PC: Examination and conservative treatment for disk lesions of lower spine. Clin Orthop 5:28, 1955.

Woolsey, RD: Notes of painful spondylolisthesis. J Neurosurg 11:67, 1954.

Wynne-Davies, R: Inheritance and spondylolisthesis. J Bone Joint Surg 61-B:301, 1979.

Young, HH: Non-neurological lesions simulating protruded intervertebral disk. JAMA 148:1101, 1952.

CHAPTER 14

Chronic Low Back Pain

Persistent and disabling **low back pain,** appropriately termed **chronic pain,** is not, statistically, the most prevalent site of pain (Nuprin Report), but it is probably the most costly.

It is estimated that more than 15 percent of all industrial injuries and more than 20 percent of compensation payments are related to low back symptoms.

The economics of medicine find that low back pain, and especially **chronic low back pain,** is costing the country millions of dollars daily in its care, including diagnosis and therapy. The cost is multiplied in its incurred compensable disability borne by insurance carriers such as workman's compensation, private insurance, and governmental agencies. There can be no accurate estimate of the cost of the emotional impact on the patients with low back pain, their spouses, families, or associates.

Low back pain, in its initial stages, can usually be explained neurophysiologically as nociception generated by tissue insult or injury. The concept of inflammation caused by injury cannot be refuted. Progression from acute pain into chronic pain, however, can rarely be explained so simply. Persistence of pain, especially in a person in whom adequate organic objective abnormalities cannot be found to explain the pain, presents the problem of chronic pain.

P.D. Wall has recently postulated that intractable (this term implying that no therapy has been effective) pain falls into three classes:

1. Deep tissue pain, of which low back pain is an example.

2. Peripheral nerve damage, some examples of which are causalgia, reflex-sympathetic dystrophy, or phantom limb.

3. Dorsal root damage, under which, in the low back syndromes, fall spinal foraminal stenosis, arachnoiditis, etc.

Tissue injury becomes the site of nociception. This tissue injury is direct action on the nerve endings—either chemical, thermal, or mechanical. There is subsequent tissue breakdown creating products of inflammation such as bradykinins, histamine, prostaglandins, peptides, leukotrienes, or proteolytic enzymes. These created impulses causing invoked stimuli are transmitted via complex neurophysiological pathways (Fig. 14–1) to the

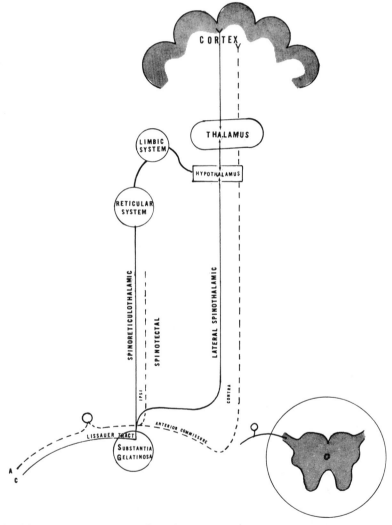

Figure 14–1. Two major neurophysiologic transmission systems: the spinothalamocortic system (A), which has spatiotemporal localization, and the spinoreticulothalamic system (C), which has no localization but is involved in emotional (limbic) and avoidance reaction.

brain, where they are conceived of as pain; this is considered the mechanism of pain transmission. Intervention of these pathways is the rationale for current treatment programs.

From the tissue site of nociception, sensation is transmitted via peripheral nerve fibers. The stimulated C fibers release chemicals such as substance P, neurokinins A and B, and other peptides. From the stimulated sympathetic fibers are released chemical substances such as adrenaline, adenosine, and acetylcholine.

Fibers A and C transmit pain sensation that enters the cord at the dorsal column of the grey cord matter. At this juncture of entry into the cord (gray matter), the released chemicals are probably amino acids that excite the dorsal horn ganglia.

Wall and Melzack postulated a neurophysiologic concept of a "gate" in this portion of the cord (Fig. 14–2). This concept postulates that fast-acting

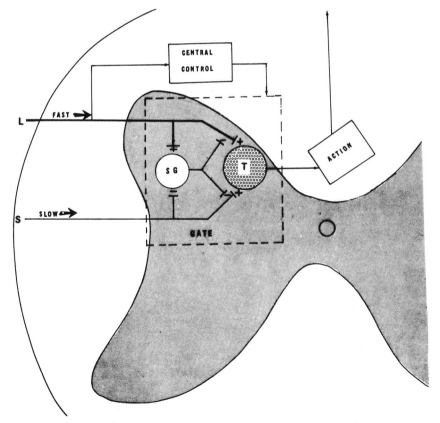

Figure 14–2. The Wall-Melzack gate theory of pain transmission. (SG = substantia gelatinosa; T = T cells.)

nerve fibers carry the sensation of touch and proprioception and can cause "blocking," at the substantia nigra (SG) into the "T" cells, of the oncoming slower C fiber impulses that carry the sensation of pain. These fast fibers actually are considered as "closing the gate" on the transmission of the slower C fiber impulses. The low-threshold impulses (afferents) excite **inhibitory** interneurones that decrease the excitability of the T cells. The chemicals so released are probably GABA (gamma aminobutyric acid) and endorphins (endogenous opiates).

The Wall-Melzack concept is used to explain and offer numerous methods of preventing pain sensation or, at least, "dampening" pain sensations that are transmitted from nociceptive tissue. Their concept also postulates impulses descending from the long tracts originating from the reticular foramation and the Raphe nuclei. These chemicals acting on the synaptic transmitters are serotonin, noradrenaline, dopamine, and peptides.

In chronic (albeit intractable) pain, there may still be nociceptive impulses emanating from injured tissues, yet, this concept applies. In chronic pain there may be a **pain pattern** (*pool* in Fig. 14–3) that has been engrammed into the central. A change in the nerve transmission pattern of the nervous system develops. Cells that normally would fire once now respond excessively to minor stimuli. Normally innocuous stimuli now may evoke pain response. It has been documented in animal studies that the dorsal ganglia actually undergo changes after prolonged painful stimuli.

According to the Gate concept, stimulation of more rapid transmitting fiber impulses is used to alter the **pool** and decrease the pain.

In the clinical situation, the tissue site of injury, the first stage of pain transmission mechanism, is repeatedly treated by various modalities such as rest, heat, ice, traction, and medication. These treatment modalities, in many patients, ultimately result in recovery from pain and disability. Although it has been claimed that 60 to 80 percent of most acute low back patients recover within 6 weeks to 3 months **regardless of any type of treatment,** treating the acute phase undoubtedly shortens the duration of acute pain. If appropriate, the initial treatment may prevent recurrence and possibly prevent progression into chronic pain.

Damage or impairment of tissues considered becoming a mechanical intrusion on nerve pathways that are capable of transmitting the sensation, that will become pain, is attacked surgically. Laminectomies, diskectomies, rhizotomies, fusions, and chemical nuclectomies, all aimed at eradicating or modifying this encroachment on nerve roots, are performed. The encroachment on the nerve may be relieved, but unfortunately pain may persist.

There are numerous concepts of pain and numerous classifications of pain evolving in medical literature. The symptom, the cause, and, therefore, the control of pain still remain in the domain of medical science. Admittedly, there are many ramifications into jurisprudence, legal, philo-

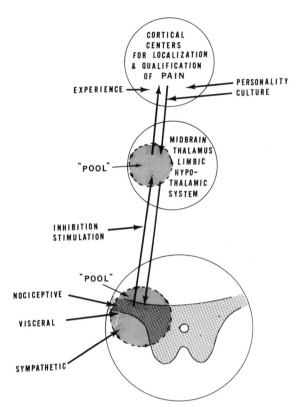

Figure 14–3. Neurone pool concept for generating pain patterns. The reverberating neurone pools that may become self-perpetuating are controlled or influenced by multiple inputs at various levels of the central nervous system. These inputs may sustain the pain behavior though no longer related to the initial nociceptive stimulus. Treatment is aimed at influencing any or all of these inputs. (Modified from Melzack, R., and Loeser, J.D.: Phantom body pain in paraplegics: evidence for a central "pattern generating mechanism" for pain. Pain 4:195–210, 1978.)

sophical, and even religious factors, and pain probably belongs to all those realms but, current thinking still isolates the concept into neurophysiologic and psychological domains (Fig. 14–4).

How one thinks of pain depends on the evaluator's learning and experience. In the medical realm, the neurologist considers pain a neurophysiologic abnormality. His or her counterpart, the neurosurgeon, also considers the basis for pain being a neurophysiologic condition that is amenable to surgical extrication or correction.

The psychiatrist considers pain to be an emotional response to internal emotional conflict that may respond to analysis, support, and, more recently, to psychiatric medication. The behavioral scientist considers chronic

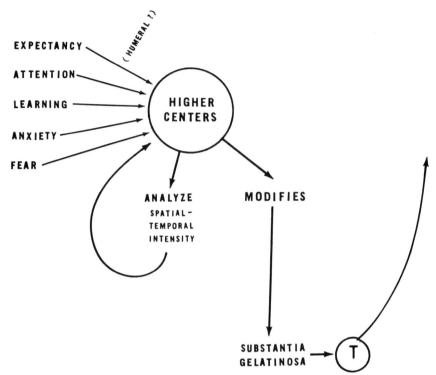

Figure 14–4. Higher center modification influencing gate in dorsal horns.

pain also an emotional response with psychosocial maladjustment. The pharmacologist considers chronic pain to be a biochemical aberration that can be therapeutically modified by medication.

The orthopedist evaluates the low back pain as a deviation of normal anatomical structure or an anatomical structural change caused by external forces that can be visualized by x-ray, CT scan, diskogram, or numerous other procedures. The "cause," once recognized, can be modified by physical therapeutic modalities or can be ameliorated or removed by surgical intervention.

The physiatrist views the pain to be the result of improperly conditioned and used tissues of the low back that can be improved, if not alleviated, by physical means such as heat, ice, exercise, electrical currents, etc.

Finneson did a three-year study and concluded that 50 percent of patients undergoing a conservative form of treatment found relief of their pain without surgery. He, therefore, concluded that any surgical procedure, to be considered effective, must have a success rate of greater than 50 percent. Medical records fail to reveal this percentage of successes from surgery to the low back.

Review of medical records shows that traditional surgical procedures fail to relieve pain in more than 30 percent of patients. Follow-up of surgery patients after 5 years revealed failure of the procedure to give relief of pain in more than 10 percent of the patients (Shealy and Beckner). Few, as well continuing to have pain, fail to resume gainful employment. It is also apparent that many patients who fail to receive benefit from surgical intervention seek to subject themselves again to surgical treatment.

Traditionally low back pain has been attributed to impaired neuromusculoskeletal function and treatment has been to correct or modify the abnormality. When appropriate treatment fails and the patients continue to have pain lasting approximately 6 months, the condition is considered as **chronic pain**. Whereas 6 months was originally considered to be the estimated point in time when acute pain became chronic pain, currently there are many who consider a time factor of 6 weeks when signs and symptoms of persistent pain can be considered to fall into the category of **chronic**.

Brena (1978) has enumerated five sequelae seen in chronic pain, termed the Five-D-Syndrome, which are the sequelae of low back pain that progress regardless of the considered causation or contemplated treatment. These are:

1. Drugs—abuse or misuse.
2. Dysfunction—a decrease in function, performance, and the achievement of good quality of life.
3. Disuse—loss of tissue flexibility, strength, endurance, and, ultimately, tissue degeneration.
4. Depression—significant loss, real or fantasized.
5. Disability—inability to perform activities of daily living or the pursuit of gainful employment.

These are sequelae and do not clarify the "cause" of why low back pain becomes **chronic**. Nor do these sequelae indicate the remedy.

Steinbach (1973) classified pain as an abstract concept that the patient describes as a personal sensation of "hurt." This sensation is conceived as a signal from damaged tissues aimed at protecting the individual from harm. Hurt implies harm with all its dire circumstances.

Bonica (1953) classified chronic pain into three groups:

1. Persistent peripheral noxious stimulants (from injured tissues);
2. neuropraxic pain;
3. learned pain behavior.

Bonica's first group pertains to the many persistent diseases such as rheumatoid arthritis, cancer, chronic infection, and metabolic diseases but not to too many conditions of the low back—especially those attributable to mechanical causes.

Unfortunately many practitioners treating patients with low back pain never entertain a departure from the presence and persistence of peripheral noxious stimulants. A "damaged, inflamed, irritated, malaligned tissue remains after injury" that is responsible for persistence of pain. **That** abnormality must be corrected or removed. Treatment modalities, including surgical "removal of the pain," continue ad infinitum and ad nauseum.

The patient has entered phase three of Bonica's classification—learned pained behavior. Now there is chronic pain that can be considered **central**. This implies that the concept of pain is in the psyche and no longer dependent on peripheral nociceptive stimuli. This also implies that interruption of these peripheral pathways can no longer be effective.

How this **central** engram is induced remains conjectural. The acute nociceptive impulses occur in many people, but few become chronically impaired. If this transition **from acute to chronic** were fully understood, there would be no chronic pain problem. It can be accepted that severe chronic diseases such as malignancy, osteomyelitis, and rheumatoid arthritis become "chronic" because the site of nociception remains active and pain-transmitting. Here the appreciation of pain may be attenuated but not necessarily completely eradicated.

It is the pain that begins as an acute nociceptive response that persists after the nociceptive irritant is no longer present that becomes chronic.

Acute pain is often, if not always, accompanied by anxiety. Anxiety may be a manifestation of fear, concern of the ominous, anger because of inconvenience, a feeling of helplessness, and many other numerous postulates. The anxiety over acute pain is what usually causes the patient to seek a remedy for the discomfort. Anxiety worsens pain.

It is the pain that begins as an acute nociceptive sensation and persists long after the irritant and tissue inflammation are no longer present that constitutes **benign chronic pain**.

Acute pain often is not always accompanied by the reaction of anxiety. This anxiety has various forms. It may be a manifestation of fear, fear of the possible ominous nature of the pain. Anxiety may occur as a resentment of the inconvenience of the disabling pain. Anxiety may be a feeling of helplessness at controlling the symptom and of decreasing the intensity and duration of the annoyance. Anxiety may be the conjuring of similarly previously experienced pain and its sequelae in one's self or in an acquaintance.

This anxiety has been experimentally shown to maximize the intensity of the pain and its resultant impairment. Anxiety has, as well as psychologically enhancing pain appreciation, been considered to have a hormonal and a chemical relationship. Anxiety also increases the muscular reaction by inciting exaggerated muscular contraction and tonus which, in itself, becomes a source of pain. This muscular excessive tonus has an adverse effect on the tissues that are involved at the nociceptive site (Fig. 14–5).

The cycle of stress, anxiety, tension, and pain is well established. The initial stress in the low back pain may be mechanical and hormonal-chemi-

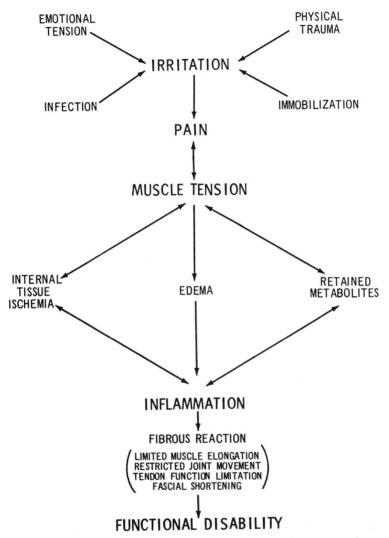

Figure 14–5. Schematic functional disability related to soft tissue involvement.

cal from an external insult. This can be considered as **somatic** in that it originates as a nociceptive tissue locus. If, at the onset or shortly after onset, there is added **anxiety** the cycle is initiated. **Tension** enters the picture as a muscular component of the cycle.

This tension may be protective at first in keeping the "injured part" immobilized to allow healing and avoid further injury to inflamed parts. This tension is at first reflexive, but with the onset of anxiety becomes a psychological component and can, per se, become the site of tissue pain.

On the cycle progressing, the aspects of pain expounded by Brena (1978) emerge: **Disability, drugs, dependence, disuse, and depression**. The true cycle is **SAD: Somatic going to Anxiety to Dependency and Disability**.

The somatic aspect has been thoroughly covered in the preceding chapters. The anxiety now must be addressed.

A question was posed by Cailliet (1974) of "Chronic Pain: Is It Necessary?" His point was that if acute pain were adequately addressed, fewer, if any, **benign chronic pain syndromes** would result.

Many cases of acute low back pain fail to address the presence of acute anxiety. Modalities of questionable value are used for excessive duration, allegedly to relieve or remove the "cause" of the pain. The duration of this treatment reinforces, to the patient, that the "condition is severe and serious . . . **and completely organic.**"

Heat, ultrasound, massage, and electrical stimulation are used indefinitely without concern to the normal needs for injured tissue to avoid becoming immobilized, contracted, and atrophied.

Terms are given patients by physicians: the meaning of these words is obscure yet conjure an ominous "medical condition." "You have arthritis of the spine" is blandly extolled yet although limited in meaning, implies an ominous, serious, disabling, incurable condition.

Dislocations, malalignments, and subluxations are implied and "corrected" when they do not, in fact, exist. The patient is led to believe these allegations and succumbs to their expected sequelae. The treatments given for these "conditions" fail, thus reinforcing the impression that the patient veritably has a serious "organic" condition.

If there is a personality correlate in the patient, the cycle progresses. The patient who may be low in self-esteem, mildly depressed, anxious, angry, prone to helplessness, susceptible to hysteria, or not assertive succumbs to these labels ("diagnosis") and treatment failures. Chronic pain results.

Recognition of the patient who is prone to become a chronic pain patient is difficult and often impossible. Numerous tests, examinations, and treatments ensue, and the organic pain causation factor becomes deeply engrained. An astute observer, early in the management of the acute pain patient, should recognize obvious symptoms and signs in the history and examination that indicate dormant, if not subtle, psychological signs. These signs and symptoms are numerous and have been well-documented in the voluminous psychological literature; to make their full expression here is not necessary nor possible.

Examples of chronic pain proneness are excessive manifestations of the severity of symptoms with a paucity of objective findings. Terms such as "killing, unbearable, excruciating, devastating" are a few that have been given chronic pain authorities. Symptoms that have no possible correlation to any organic physical cause should alert the examiner. Grimacing is a form of play acting that must be judged carefully as to its significance.

There are certain observations that lead to ascertaining the proneness for development of chronic pain:

1. Chronic anxiety that the patient manifests by being irritable, anxious, and overreactive to essential minor incidences. Neck and shoulder tension, chronic headaches, temporomandibular joint (TMJ) symptoms are just a few examples.

2. Misuse of medicines that may be relaxants "needed" for sleep, for relaxation, to get through a trying experience or that may be "pain pills that are used in large doses, yet do not give any relief." Numerous medicines of similar nature and efficacy that continue to be used in larger doses "even though they are useless."

3. Unrecognized depression expressed by the patient such as "waking up tired every day even after a good night's sleep" or no desire to pursue normal activities. Disinterest in environment, spouse, children and social activities also indicates depression.

4. Presence of litigation in which "something or someone caused this and will pay for my torment." This is often compounded by a supporting attorney who is not brought into the medical problem by the physician.

5. Unresolved anger at "something or someone having caused or aggravated the low back problem."

6. Family influence in which the spouse, child, or near relative is "accused" of "not helping or even of being a causative factor."

7. Cultural factors have been claimed to be contributing factors to overreaction to pain. Patients of Italian, Mexican, and Jewish origin are claimed to be more emotional and less stoic whereas Irish, English, and Germanic cultures are more stoic and less demonstrative.

8. People who lack assertiveness or are indecisive tend to be prone to developing chronic pain behavior.

TREATMENT OF CHRONIC LOW BACK PAIN

There is, today, no one accepted concept of treating the patient with chronic pain, but there are many accepted components of programs that are effective. These are listed alphabetically rather than numerically, so as to dispel the factor of importance or sequence. Any or all factors may be needed for that particular patient with benign chronic low back pain.

A. The patient must be amenable to entering into a program aimed at reducing the reactions to chronic pain. Acceptance of the program is mandatory. In essence, a "contract," entered into by the patient to participate, is considered vital by many pain treatment centers.

B. The objective of the program must be discussed, **in meaningful terms**, to the patient. This is the **school** aspect of the program that is part of the **back school** but also must be part of the **low back pain school**.

C. Drugs must be decreased and gradually eliminated. Drugs as needed for pain are no longer a valid prescription. If drugs have been a patient dependency, they are given at a regular time sequence and in decreasing strength dosage **with the patient's knowledge** and acceptance.

Self-medication is advocated by certain centers in which the patient is given instructions, education, and the responsibility of taking drugs when needed and gradually discontinuing them voluntarily.

D. Individual, group, and family psychotherapy sessions are held to help the patient develop stress management procedures, decrease anxiety situation reactions, acquire constructive self-control skills, and learn assertive behavior.

E. If depression is a contributing factor, and it very frequently is, antidepressant medications are desirable until formal psychotherapy intervenes for the benefit of the patient.

F. Relaxation therapy, which may be one or more of various techniques:

(1) biofeedback using EMG or galvanic skin resistance (GSR);

(2) self-hypnosis training for daily use;

(3) tapes for relaxation visual imagery;

(4) Jacobson Progressive Muscular Relaxation techniques.

G. General physical reconditioning. This implies the concepts of **back school** function and low back abdominal exercises but also gradually **total general body conditioning**. Today there is also greater emphasis on nutritional reconditioning of patients with chronic pain with weight reduction and control with a balanced diet of high percentage of complex carbohydrates (60 percent) and less protein (20 percent) and fat (20 percent). Calories, of course, must be contained.

A "working-hardening exercise program" has also been currently effective in making exercise more meaningful, less boring, and a trend toward return to gainful occupation.

H. Establishing meaningful objective goals of the program by which the patient can monitor his or her progress and the therapist can also modify the program. The program outlined at Casa Colina (Koler et al 1977) gives several good examples of an assessment evaluation program.

I. Periodic conference attended by the patient, the family, and the pertinent staff to document the progress. A rehabilitation counselor should be included if the person needs to return to a gainful occupation.

J. Admitted that further concentration on the tissue site of nociception may be redundant, the use of transcutaneous electrical nerve stimulation (TENS) (Figs. 14–6 to 14–9) and acupuncture may initiate and enhance pain reduction. These modalities are good in the armamentarium of modalities along with exercises, diet, assertion training, etc., but these modalities should not be considered as a sole modality to the exclusion of the remainder of the program.

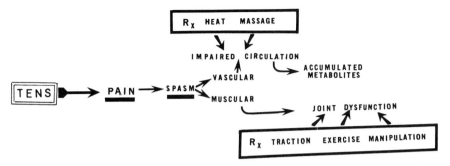

Figure 14–6. Concept of beneficial effect of transcutaneous electrical nerve stimulation (TENS).

The patient must be told that TENS can be expected only to:

1. Possibly give complete relief for a variable duration;
2. Give only partial or temporary relief;
3. May be of no value albeit not harmful.

The application of TENS requires varying the types of wave length, a form, and the site of application. TENS is not a muscle stimulator but merely mediates its efficacy via sensory nerve pathways according to the Gate concept of Wall and Melzack.

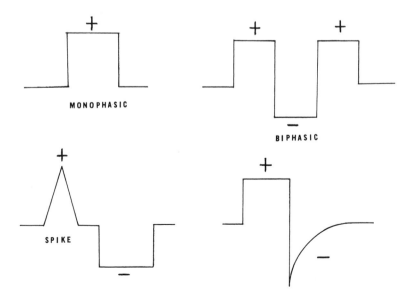

Figure 14–7. Wave forms of TENS.

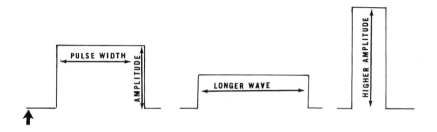

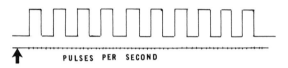

Figure 14–8. Characteristics of TENS application.

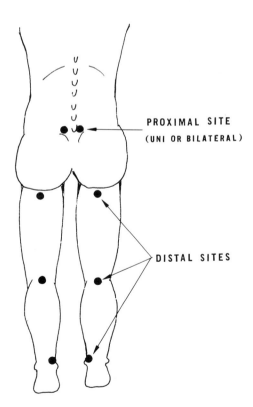

Figure 14–9. Sites of usual application of TENS.

MALINGERING

Insofar as low back pain is so frequent and is often related to compensation rewards and litigation judgments, there has been a tendency to claim that patients use the symptom of low back pain for ulterior gains. These gains are claimed to be psychological, environment manipulative, and financially remunerative. Pain is a way of life for some and "rewarding" for others, but the psychodynamics are far from clear and universal in their interpretation.

Malingering is a term not infrequently applied to patients with chronic low back pain who gain financial, social, and physical benefit. This term implies intentional falsification for fraudulent gains. It places the term as an accusation rather than a diagnosis.

True malingering is considered to be rare and by some as nonexistent. There are psychiatric concepts that consider the symptoms of malingering to be deep-seated psychiatric problems requiring therapy. As there are no objective tests that can be applied to patients with chronic low back pain that clearly unequivocally relate the symptoms to pure intentional volition, any psychological component of the pain resides within the framework of related, partially uncontrolled, and temporarily uncontrollable psychological factors.

CONCLUSION

Treating a patient complaining of benign chronic low back pain requires having a comprehensive evaluation by a meaningful comprehensive history and physical examination. Appropriate laboratory tests that clearly and objectively relate and confirm the findings with the symptoms and physical findings are needed. The personality of the person must be evaluated and the details of the pain progression cycle must be clearly ascertained.

Once the medical condition is considered as **benign**, which means without significant organic factors contributing to and persisting in the cause of the pain, the pain program must be initiated as outlined above:

1. drug control;
2. relaxation;
3. stress management;
4. control of depression;
5. development of assertive behavior;
6. physical reconditioning—as a hardening program, general fitness and low back school training;
7. psychological counseling;
8. vocational evaluation and counseling.

REFERENCES

Bonica, JJ: The Management of Pain. Lea & Febiger, Philadelphia, 1953.

Brena, SF: Chronic Pain: America's Hidden Epidemic. Atheneum/SMI, New York, 1978.

Cailliet, R: Presidential Address. American Congress of Rehabilitation Medicine. 1974.

Cailliet, R: Soft Tissue Pain and Disability. F.A. Davis, Philadelphia, 1977.

Crue, BL: Pain. Bull. Los Angeles Co Med Assoc Oct 4:10, 1973.

Davis, L, and Martin, J: Studies upon spinal cord injuries. II. The nature and treatment of pain. J Neurosurg 4:483, 1947.

Finer, B: Clinical use of hypnosis in pain management. In Bonica, JJ (ed.): Pain. (Advances in Neurology, Vol. 4) Raven Press, New York, 1974.

Fordyce, WE: Behavioral Methods for Chronic Pain and Illness. C.V. Mosby, St. Louis, 1976.

Fordyce, WE, et al.: Operant conditioning in the treatment of lumbar pain. Phys Med Rehab 54:399, 1973.

Forst, JJ: Contribution a l'etude clinique de la sciatique. Paris Thése, No. 33, 1881.

Gottlieb et al: Comprehensive rehabilitation of patients having chronic low back pain. Arch Phys Med Rehabil 58:101, 1977.

Hillman, P, and Wall, PD: Inhibitory and excitatory factors influencing the receptive fields of lamina 5 spinal cord cells. Exp Brain Res 9:284, 1969.

Holmes, TH, and Wolff, HG: Life situations, emotions and backache. Psychosomat Med 14:18, 1952.

Jacobson, E: Electrical measurements of neuromuscular states during mental activities. I. Imagination of movement involving skeletal muscles. Am J Physiol 91:567, 1930.

King, J, and Lagger, R: Sciatica viewed as a referred pain syndrome. Surg Neurol 5:46, 1976.

Kirgis, HD: Problems in the management of the "compensation" patient with lumbar disk syndrome. Southern Med J 57:1152, 1964.

Lampe, GN: Introduction to the use of transcutaneous electrical nerve stimulation device. Phys Therap 58:1450, 1978.

Laségue, C: Considerations sur la sciatique. Arch Gen Med 2 (Serie 6, Tome 4):558, 1864.

Malmo, RB, and Shagass, C: Physiologic studies of reaction to stress in anxiety and early schizophrenia. Psychosomat Med 11:9, 25, 1949.

Mannheimer, JS: Electrode placements for transcutaneous electrical nerve stimulation. Phys Therap 58:1455, 1978.

Melzack, R: The Puzzle of Pain. Basic Books, New York, 1973.

Melzack, R, and Loeser, JD: Phantom body pain in paraplegics: evidence for a central "pattern generating mechanism" for pain. Pain 4:195, 1978.

Melzack, R, and Perry, C: Self-regulation of pain: the use of alpha-feedback and hypnotic training for the control of chronic pain. Exp Neurol 46:452, 1975.

Minter, WJ, and Barr, JS: Rupture of the intervertebral disk with involvement of the spinal canal. N Engl J Med 211:215, 1934.

Nathan, PW: The gate control theory of pain: a critical review. Brain 99:123, 1976.

Newman, RI, Seres, JL, Yospe, LP, and Garlington, B: Multidisciplinary treatment of chronic pain: long-term follow-up of low back pain patients. Pain 4:283, 1978.

Papper, S: The undesirable patient (editorial). J Chron Dis 22:777, 1970.

Rees, WS: Multiple bilateral subcutaneous rhizolysis of segmental nerves in the treatment of the intervertebral disc syndrome. Ann Gen Pract 26:126, 1971.

Shaw, RS: Pathological malingering: the painful disabled extremity. N Engl J Med 271:22, 1964.

Shaw, RS: Pathological malingering. N Engl J Med 271:22, 1964.

Shealy, CN: Facets in back and sciatic pain: a new approach to a major pain syndrome. Minn Med 57:199, 1974.

Steinbach, R: Pain Patients: Traits and Treatment. Academic Press, New York, 1974.

Steinbach, RA: Pain and depression. In Kiev, A. (ed): Somatic Manifestations of Depressive Disorders. Excerpta Medica, Elsevier, New York, 1974.

Steinbach, RA, and Rush, TN: Alternatives to the pain career. Psychotherapy: Theory, Research and Practice 10:321, 1973.

Szasz, TS: The painful person. Lancet, January: 18, 1968.

Wall, PD: Future trends in pain research. Philos Trans R Soc Lond Biol 308:393, 1985.

Wall, PD: Introduction. In Wall PD and Melzack R (eds): The Textbook of Pain. Churchill Livingstone, Edinburgh, 1984, pp 1–16.

Wall, PD and Woolf, CJ: The brief and the prolonged fascilatory effects of myelinated afferent input on the rat spinal cord are independently influenced by peripheral nerve injury. Neuroscience 17:1199, 1986.

Wolkind, SN, and Forrest, AJ: Low back pain: a psychiatric investigation. Postgrad Med J 48:76, 1972.

Zborowski, M: People in Pain. Jossey-Bass, San Francisco, 1967.

Index

A "t" following a page number indicates a table. A page number in *italics* indicates a figure.